A SOCIOLOGY OF HEALTH

A SOCIOLOGY OF HEALTH

ANDREW C. TWADDLE and RICHARD M. HESSLER
Associate Professors of Sociology,
University of Missouri,
Columbia, Missouri

with 68 illustrations

with Foreword by **Talcott Parsons**

The C. V. Mosby Company
Saint Louis   1977

Copyright © 1977 by The C. V. Mosby Company

Printed in the United States of America

Distributed in Great Britain by Henry Kimpton, London

The C. V. Mosby Company
11830 Westline Industrial Drive, St. Louis, Missouri 63141

Library of Congress Cataloging in Publication Data

Twaddle, Andrew C   1938-
  A sociology of health.

  Bibliography: p.
  Includes index.
  1. Social medicine. I. Hessler, Richard M.,
1941-   joint author. II. Title. [DNLM: 1. Health
services. 2. Social medicine. WA30 T969s]
RA418.T92   362.1′04′2   76-41215
ISBN 0-8016-5153-0

VH/VH/VH 9 8 7 6 5 4 3 2 1

With affection and respect

to

our parents

Ruth and Paul Twaddle   *Doria and Hugh Hessler*

our families

Sarah, Lisa, and Kristin Twaddle   *Anne, Amy, Peter, and Angela Hessler*

and

our teachers

Kɛpe Ta Kišeləmuxsi

FOREWORD

I have long had the conviction that the study of health and illness and of the professional and other organizations devoted to health care is one of the most important fields in which sociologists and other social scientists, such as economists and psychologists, should work. After a rather promising start a good many years ago, medical sociology seemed to lag for a considerable period but recently has shown signs of revived interest and greater vitality. The appearance of this textbook is one of the signs of that renewal.

A textbook designed primarily for undergraduate courses seems to me to be one of the most important contributions to the development of the field, for the undergraduate years are probably for most students the most favorable time to awaken interest. Good courses open to undergraduates should therefore be a particularly important foundation of an expanding interest in the subject. And rather obviously the availability of good teaching literature is one of the most important resources needed by teachers of such courses.

It should be remembered that however deeply dependent medicine and the other health services are on the biological and physical sciences, health service organization, including the medical profession itself, is *social* organization and people trained in what are usually called the medical sciences have no special competence in the disciplines, on knowledge of which good organization rests. Since in such a highly complex society as ours health services, like other parts of the society, have been growing increasingly complex, there is a growing need for personnel with better knowledge of the relevant problems than that possessed by even the well-educated ordinary citizen.

Furthermore, though the main anchorage of medicine is in the biological sciences, there is an exceedingly important zone of interaction and interpenetration between the healthy and sick person as organism and as personality. I am indeed very far from sharing a still not uncommon view in medical circles that there is really "nothing to" these ideas of mental health and mental illness, which are not even finally reducible to organic terms. Insofar as this position is justified, there is another exceedingly important field in which many health service personnel need to be trained, not only in psychology, but especially in sociology, because of the importance of the social environment, both in the etiology of illness both organic and societal and in favoring or hindering the maintenance of good health and favoring recovery from illness.

Hence instruction in what has come to be called medical sociology can be important to a wide variety of different kinds of people. In one sense first come those planning for a career in social science, not only research and teaching in the field of health service and sociology of the professions, but definitely including them. Second, it can be highly important to future physicians and other health service personnel. By no means least it can be important to the intelligent ordinary citizen who has no specialized technical concern with these fields, but has a simple desire to understand better some of the features of the complex world in which he lives.

Health and the many forms of impairment to which it is subject are after all among the most fundamental of human concerns, completely transcending age and sex, social class, and cultural differences, as does the inevitable end of the "quest for health," the death of the individual, which is no fault of defective health services, but simply one of the fundamental "facts of life."

I repeat my hope that many a young person, especially, will initiate a lifelong interest in this fascinating field of knowledge, of human action, and of public policy by reading this book.

Talcott Parsons

PREFACE

This book has come about as a result of our experience in teaching courses in the sociology of health. We have been frustrated in searching for adequate teaching materials. Although several texts are currently available, most have addressed highly specialized audiences or they have adopted limited perspectives within the sociology of health. The two textbooks that have attempted an overview of the field are both seriously out of date, and there seem to be no plans for their updating.

Our first reason for writing this text is that there is need to take account of the rapid developments of the past decade. Our second reason is that all intellectual disciplines have been challenged in recent years by developments in the philosophy of science that have explored the limits of positivism and reintroduced humanistic concerns into the scientific enterprise. Although not addressing those issues directly, we believe there is a need for a text that reflects those changes.

In writing this book, we have collaborated in different ways. Chapters 1, 3, 11, 13, and 15 have been prepared jointly by drafting a detailed outline and dividing the preparation of specific sections. Most have been separately authored by one of us and critiqued by the other.

It is trite but true that any book is more than simply the product of the authors. The assistance of many people was vital to this book's successful completion. The staff of the Reference Center of the Section of Behavioral Sciences, University of Missouri Medical Center, Columbia, Missouri, performed heroic services in generating bibliographies, tracking down difficult-to-find references, and calling our attention to critical references. To Trudy Gardner, Mary Steiner, and Rhonda Anson, we give our deep appreciation and undying gratitude.

Several of our undergraduate and graduate students helped by summarizing articles and books and by sharing with us their insights into the organization of medical services. Karen Pecault, Sue Mahan, Karen Wind, Karen Kelly, Stu Plotnick, Bob Menamin, Emily Bonwich, Sue Beavert, Terry Bernhardt, Judith Maurin, and Jim Campbell provided these services, in addition to reading some portions of the manuscript and sharing with us their critical comments. Also, students in our introductory course in the sociology of health have suffered trial runs of the first drafts of about two thirds of the chapters and provided us with their reactions, which have been taken into account in subsequent revisions. To all these individuals, our thanks.

Vivian Smith, Mary Emerson, and Beverly McGee supervised the typing of the manuscript at various stages. Mrs. McGee typed the final copy. For consistently competent and occasionally heroic effort, we commend their efforts with deep appreciation.

To the several people who reviewed the entire manuscript, we are grateful for both criticism and encouragement. These include Dr. Michael L. Rainey, Director, Medical Education Preparatory Program,

Southern Illinois University, Carbondale, Illinois; Dr. Peter Kong-Ming New, Professor, Department of Behavioral Science, University of Toronto, Toronto, Ontario, Canada; Dr. Eugene S. Schneller, Chairman, Department of Sociology, Union College, Schenectady, New York; Dr. H. Hugh Floyd, Jr., Association Professor, Department of Sociology, University of New Orleans, New Orleans, Louisiana; and Dr. Minako K. Maykovich, Associate Professor, Department of Sociology, California State University, Sacramento, California.

Thanks are due our teachers, James Barnett, Alexander Burgess, Robert Burnight, Sidney Goldstein, Martin U. Martel, Kurt Mayer, Harold Organic, Bufford Rhea, James Sakoda, Ralph Spielman, Edward Stockwell, Robert von der Lippe, Helmut Wagner, Walter Wardwell, Jack Wheatcroft, Philip Withim, Basil Zimmer, Robert M. Avery, Morris Berkowitz, William Delaney, Ray Elling, David L. Ellison, Hugh Fox, John Hitchcock, Burkart Holzner, Alexander J. Humphreys, S.J., Floyd Jenkins, S.J., Bernard M. Kramer, F. Donald Laws, Jiri Nehnevasja, Peter Kong-Ming New, and Edward A. Suchman.

Finally, to Sarah Wolcott Twaddle and Anne Dietz Hessler; Lisa and Kristin Twaddle; and Amy, Peter, and Angela Hessler, we are indebted not only for providing the supporting environment essential to the completion of an extended project and our health but also, and more important, for being what makes life and health worth having.

Andrew C. Twaddle
Richard M. Hessler

CONTENTS

PART THREE

THE HEALING OCCUPATIONS

PART FIVE

SOME URGENT ISSUES

A SOCIOLOGY OF HEALTH

INTRODUCTION

The intent of this book is to consider critically societies and the models of health care organization that have evolved. As behavioral scientists and citizens, we have found it increasingly difficult to teach about medical sociology and do the kind of research that treats health care as if it existed in a social vacuum, somehow divorced from the larger society. There is a coherent and powerful set of relationships between the political economy of a society and its health care institutions. The student who takes into account the structure and contradictions of the total social system has the best chance of understanding what health care systems are all about. Ultimately this understanding can be applied to create a more humane and equitable health care system for patients and practitioners alike.

In this book, we have tried to maintain the focus on the larger society as we work toward understanding medicine and its fascinating forms of organization. Research careers tend to become narrowly focused on a specialized range of problems, and it is easy to lose sight of the broad issues, even in a subspecialty of sociology such as the sociology of health. Writing this text has forced us to take a broad perspective, to immerse ourselves in literatures that we had never before explored in depth, and, most of all, to organize and make sense of the total enterprise. In terms of our intellectual growth and renewal, the act of writing the book has been its own reward.

For the student, there are some tangible reasons why the subject matter of this text is important. For sociology students, the text offers an application of sociological theory to the particular social institution of health care. Because the health care system reflects the political and economic organization of the larger society, evanescent health programs, high technology, creative waste, mass production centralized development planning, and monopolistic capital forces are features of technologically advanced societies that are mirrored clearly in the health care system. For the student of sociology interested in the nemesis of corporate bigness, impersonality, insensitivity, and the worldwide trend toward concentrated power, the health care system provides one with an excellent laboratory for research. Medicine like other corporate monopolistic forces strives to gain control of as much of human behavior as possible. Wants and needs are created by health care organization as medicine moves its proprietary interest from control over disease to health care and, finally, to general well being. Behaviors that in past years would have been defined as "crime" and controlled by the legal system are more and more defined as "sickness" and controlled by medicine. Thus an analysis of the institution of health care should help one to understand the central control mechanisms of the society.

Today medicine is one of the largest industries worldwide. More than ever, it is

1

permeating all aspects of life. If we can understand the health care system, we may be taking steps toward understanding ourselves and where we are going in society. Billions of dollars, increasing annually, are spent on medicines, health professionals, and complex organizations that promise improved quality of living or greater length of life. The sociology of health is important for another reason. Health care is concerned with fundamental human issues involving life, death, and the quality of life.

For students in the health professions, there are important practical reasons for gaining an understanding of the sociology of health. After phenomenal growth and development in the late nineteenth and early twentieth centuries medicine has arrived at a theoretical crisis. The germ theory of disease, responsible for the successful control of acute infectious disease, has not proved useful in the control of the now dominant chronic and degenerative diseases. In this century, the expansion of epidemiology has led to the insight that most chronic diseases are closely associated with social structures and behaviors. The avenues for the control of these diseases seem to be leading to appreciation of the need for alteration of life-styles and the organization of the society. At the same time, there are important prices to be paid. Vested interests are being challenged, and the possibility of maintaining a free society that is also a healthy society is in dispute.

Although the health occupations have dramatically improved their capacity to effectively intervene in disease processes, they have lost much of their control over the forces that shape medical work. Both consumers and health professionals have become increasingly alienated as a result of rapid and sweeping scientific, technological, and organizational changes.

To interact in a competent and humane fashion, the health professional and consumer will need to understand the larger political and economic forces that impinge on their lives, at times forcing them to compromise values and commitments. Understanding the disease process is no longer adequate if treating the whole patient is the goal. Humane medical care is predicated on understanding the sociopolitical context of patients and the broader impact of medical practice in that context. This text is designed to foster that kind of understanding.

Finally, for students of the humanities, which we urge should include both students of sociology and the health professions, study of the sociology of health is important in helping focus some philosophical questions of major import, questions that need urgent debate and resolution if we are to face the future with assurance that life will continue to be worth the effort. Because medicine is centrally concerned with life and death, because it is a focus of major technological change, and because health is such a core human value, an understanding of medicine throws into relief many core concerns of ethical conduct. The scientific revolution and its technological aftermath have raised fundamental questions regarding the quality of life, the nature of morality, and the implications of knowledge as power. Nowhere are these better studied than as they affect the processes of death and disease.

In writing this book, we have tried to keep all three of these audiences in mind and to interweave all these concerns. This has not been as difficult as might be imagined because the three audiences and the many concerns are not mutually exclusive. Since sociology is taking on increasing responsibilities in the training of health professionals, it is increasingly important for those students to understand not only the facts about health and medical care generated by sociologists but also the frame of reference within which such information is generated. The sociology student must understand not only the theoretical and methodological issues but also the practical concerns to which they are applied. The humanist, to be effective, needs concrete problems to address and an appreciation of the social context within which philosophical problems are manifest.

The differences between this text and others are not apparent in the outline of the book. The topical coverage as indicated by chapter titles is not distinctive. Rather it is in the content of the chapters, the way in which each topic is addressed, that differences will be found. We have tried to equal the *range* of previous texts while increasing the *depth* of coverage, particularly with reference to historical and cultural context. Whether we have succeeded, the student will have to judge.

The text is divided into five parts, with two to four chapters in each part. Part One is designed to set the stage for the text by reviewing some developments in both medicine and sociology that have led to the development of the sociology of health and by stating the theoretical and value posi-

tions taken in organizing the book. In Part Two we look at the problems that the health care institution addresses, disease and sick people. Part Three explores one aspect of the societal response to disease and sickness, the emergence of specialized occupations that promise cure and relief. Part Four looks at the settings in which the sick person and the health specialist come together, the medical practice, the hospital, the clinic, and the organization of these at the national level. Finally, Part Five explores some issues that emerge from the analysis in the previous sections, specifically medical ethics and the effectiveness of the health care delivery system. Each of these parts is provided with an introduction giving more detail on the organization of that section of the text. We suggest that the student look over those introductions as the first step in using this text.

PART ONE

TOWARD A SOCIOLOGY OF HEALTH

The first two chapters provide a general orientation to the book and outline its context with reference to both sociology and medicine.

Chapter 1 explores the emerging relationships between medicine and sociology that have resulted in the creation of an identifiable sociological specialty labeled the "sociology of health." Medicine has been in ferment over the past century, facing a changing environment that it has had some part in shaping. At the same time, sociology has come into its own as a significant discipline that, while having its own roots, has become important for health care. This chapter explores some of the major changes in medicine and sociology that have resulted in a convergence of interests. Medicine has become theoretically important to sociology at the same time that sociology has become practically important to medicine.

The perspectives of sociology are distinctive, nevertheless. Chapter 2 explores the nature of sociology as a discipline, identifies the major theoretical paradigms, and provides a mapping of where this text stands with reference to core issues in both sociology and medicine. This is a difficult chapter that tries to condense a great deal into a few pages. While we apologize to the student for the labor that the chapter requires, we believe that the task is important and worth the effort. For the student new to sociology, it provides an orientation to the discipline in skeleton form. For the more experienced student, it is intended to provide a cognitive map of the text as a whole. For both, it will make explicit the stances taken by us relative to the discipline and the subject matter. We have tried to make our values explicit and to identify the master concepts that have informed the writing of the text.

We emphasize that the intention of these two chapters is to orient the student. What is important is that the student gain some sense of the historical context of the subject matter, not that all the information be learned in detail. To gain in-depth knowledge the student will have to pursue the literature referred to in the chapters.

CHAPTER 1

Medicine and sociology

Medical sociology is one of the youngest substantive specialties in sociology, which is one of the youngest intellectual disciplines. Although young, both sociology and medical sociology are well-established, important, vigorous, and exciting fields of study.

In this text, we plan to present the field of medical sociology and to summarize what is known about health, illness, and medical care from sociological perspectives. We will begin this task by reviewing the historical roots of the discipline to show how a set of developments extending over several centuries led to the creation of a field of inquiry that treats health, illness, and their management as problems in the understanding of society and how this understanding helps address problems in the management of health and illness. After introducing some basic concepts, we will explore the nature of health and illness as sociological concerns, the role of the sick person, and various healing roles. After that, the organization of health services will be explored, starting with small organizational units and working up to the health care system as a totality. Finally, we will outline some major issues in health care delivery and discuss some alternatives for the future.

What we hope to communicate is some of the nature of medical sociology as a substantive interest in sociology, the range of problems being addressed by medical sociologists, and some of the more important findings of the field. We would regard it a bonus if we succeed in communicating some of our excitement and enthusiasm sufficiently to encourage a few to explore this field in greater depth.

The following concerns inform this text and will be discussed in greater detail later.

1. *Health, illness, and their treatment are historically bound.* Any system of delivering health services and indeed the definitions of health and illness are social solutions to problems that have a history. These solutions are the product of past solutions and emergent problems. No social system is static. Accordingly an understanding of how any given society is currently solving problems requires that the problems and solutions be located in time, and this text will be concerned to place modern health and health care problems in a historical context.

2. *Health, illness, and their treatment are culturally bound.* Different peoples have worked out different solutions to problems, even when the problems they face are similar. In part this is because different peoples have different histories and they have faced different problems in the past, or different solutions have been tried and have worked in different places. Also different peoples

7

have different values and different conceptions of the meaning of life and what constitutes a "good" life. For this reason, this text will be concerned to place modern health and health care problems in a cultural context.

3. *In every known society, the definition of health problems and the response to them have been organized.* In each society, certain people have been given the responsibility to decide who is sick, what kind of sickness they have, and what kinds of treatment are appropriate. In some societies these tasks have been merged into a single role, whereas in others they have been divided into several, but nowhere is the response to illness random. Each society has made some organized provision to confront health problems, and this text will be concerned to identify the roles and structures that have arisen at different times and places to deal with the social problem of illness and death. In fact, it is this organized response that makes health and illness of interest to sociologists.

Our task is to convey an understanding of medical sociology. One avenue toward this goal is to explore the emergence of this field of interest. This would help in understanding why medical sociology came into being at all and what issues led to its development.

We have already said that medical sociology is a new interest in a young discipline. The history of sociology as an identifiable intellectual interest dates back just a little over a hundred years, although the groundwork for the emergence of sociology dates back several centuries.[1] During this brief period, many questions have been raised in an attempt to gain an understanding of the nature of social organization and its implications for the ongoing process of living. These questions have resulted in several theories that address different problem areas such as the workings of societies taken as total entities, complex organizations, intergroup relationships, and interpersonal interaction. These theories constitute the unique sociological perspectives

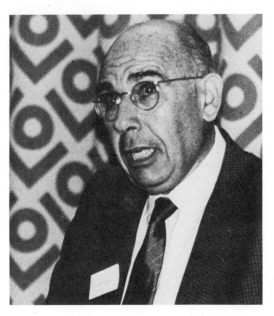

Fig. 1-1. *George Rosen.*

that are discussed in the next chapter. These perspectives have been employed to gain understanding of many substantive problems and events, including the family, industrial organizations, the economy, education, politics, work groups, religious organizations, leisure activity, interaction at social gatherings, prisons, and criminal behavior.

As an identifiable substantive specialty in sociology, medical sociology is generally thought to date back to the middle of the twentieth century, although as George Rosen (1944) (Fig. 1-1), a notable medical historian, correctly shows, "viewed as the study of the relationships between health phenomena and social factors and contexts, medical sociology is seen to have deep historical roots." These roots relate to concerns with developing health policies and in controlling disease. What Rosen refers to is a set of medical and social policy issues that preceded the development of a specifically sociological interest, wherein the study of medicine became relevant as a means of understanding the society. Understanding both the medical and sociological origins of medical sociology, however, is important to an understanding of the discipline, and our attention now turns to that problem.

MEDICAL ORIGINS OF MEDICAL SOCIOLOGY

A major force leading to the development of medical sociology can be found in the broad historical changes in the history of medicine, which have created a felt need on the part of the medical community for behavioral and social science knowledge. To provide an understanding of how this state of affairs came about, a brief review of some highlights of the social history of medicine is necessary. For convenience, medical history is divided into the following periods.

1. *Before germ theory (the Social Era).* In its early history, Western medicine was concerned with the social and environmental aspects of experience with illness. Early theories of disease emphasized a conception of the individual as organically related to his environment, and treatment often consisted of manipulation of the environment. Physicians were trained to be conscious of the conditions under which their patients lived, including their social relationships. With this perspective, effective public health measures were developed even in the absence of any knowledge about the causes of disease.

2. *The era of germ theory.* The discovery of microorganisms and their implication as causes of disease in the nineteenth century was a momentous event in the social history of medicine. Medicine became so preoccupied with disease and the development of a chemical armamentarium for combating disease that the patient receded to the background as a medical concern. At the same time, medicine became more technically competent as it became caught up in the movement of philosophical positivism. The public health movement and epidemiology flowered. Optimistic that disease was ultimately conquerable, public policy attempted to provide the means through national health insurance programs. In the United States and Canada the influential Flexner Report (1910) enthroned the germ theory of disease in medical school curricula.

3. *Post–germ theory (the Social Scientific Era).* The optimism of the germ theory has been short-lived. By the middle of the present century, it had become apparent that as acute infectious disease came under control, chronic diseases, in which microorganisms are not implicated, became more prevalent. This has led to the thought that disease may not be conquerable but is something that must be adjusted to as a permanent fact of life. This blow to germ theory was supported by the emergence of psychiatry, which held that nonbiological causes were to be found for at least some illnesses, if not most. Work in epidemology was demonstrating social patternings of illness, which demanded attention to factors in the social environment. Accordingly medicine adopted the survey technology of the social sciences for a number of health surveys, providing a major linkage between medical and sociological concerns.

Before germ theory

During the long period before the emergence of germ theory in the middle of the ninteenth century, Western medicine had a variety of theories that changed over time. These theories had one element in common: they focused attention on the environment, including the social dimensions of life. Hence relative to the germ theory era, these were broadly based and socially oriented.

The major impact of this period on modern times was to lay the groundwork for modern public health. It was a period when health became a matter of public policy, and many effective measures were developed for the control of disease in populations.

Early theories of disease. Early theories of disease emphasized the importance of the physical and social environment, a conception that was religious in origin long before it was medical or sociological. Leviticus in the Old Testament writes of a Roman senator, Epidaurus, who viewed the physical environment as a factor in controlling illness, which he considered to be spiritual in nature. The early Greek civilization embodied the Platonic value of sound mind and body and theorized that one could promote health by bringing the physical and social environment into harmony with Platonic values. Some of the measures taken by the Greeks included infanticide, control over diet, and the building of aqueducts. Hippocrates conceptualized health as a delicate equilibrium among the four humors within man (blood, phlegm, yellow bile, and black bile) and physical environmental factors such as seasonal changes, wind direction, and diet. Plutarch, in advising his contemporaries on keeping healthy, mentioned the role that the physical environment plays in determining mental well-being.

One of the most farsighted early efforts dealing with the relationship between environment and health was Galen's Hygiene, a six-volume work written soon after the death of Marcus Aurelius in AD 180. Galen was one of the most famous physicians of his time, and he gradually became the dominant authority in medicine through the Renaissance and up to the time of Paracelsus in the sixteenth century. Galen utilized Hippocrates' theory of health and illness, and he elaborated on the internal environmental factors that act on the equilibrium or balance called good health.

The influence of Galen's theory of disease declined during the Middle Ages for several reasons. The free citizens of the leisure class for whom *Hygiene* was written no longer existed in the manner of ancient Greece. Also Christianity was a powerful force teaching that concern with health and its maintenance was secondary to spiritual well-being and the salvation of one's soul.

A different kind of social order developed during the Renaissance period as compared with the world of medieval Europe. The old feudal order was beginning to crumble, and new trade centers began to spring up at old crossroads. A whole new economic order was evolving that demanded free initiative, free enterprise, and the individ-

uality of man. As a result of the discoveries of land overseas, the volume of trade increased and precious metals came into demand as a medium of exchange, with large increases in industrial production and mining. Thus it is no surprise that the first theories of occupational diseases emerged at this time, linking occupation, environment, and health status (Rosen, 1944).

Physical science was developing rapidly, with Copernicus presenting a new picture of the universe and Vesalius writing his book on anatomy. New vistas were opened, and the closed social and economic systems of the Middle Ages were openly rejected and revolted against. The concept of man as a pawn whose life was merely a short, nasty event preceding the glorious hereafter was replaced, and in its stead developed the value of freedom for the highest possible social and physical development of man. Man wanted to live longer because he was shown more to live for, and many theoretical works were written outlining various strategies for a long life. One work that stands out from the rest is *Liber de Longa Vita* written by Paracelsus in 1560. He was a firm believer in good mental health as the principal factor responsible for a long life. Luigi Cornaro, a contemporary of Paracelsus wrote *Trattoto della Vita Sobria* in which he developed a theory for the long life. He emphasized that man's control over the physical and social environment was critical, and he applied his theory by draining swamps around Venice, cleaning the Venetian harbor of pollutants, and leading an austere social life that included a rigid low-calorie diet. Indeed, he lived to be 98 years old, a remarkable feat for 1565!

The early public health movement. The early public health movement emerged more out of aesthetic and social welfare interests than from notions of technical efficacy in the control of disease. Effective public health measures, however, are found as far back as biblical times, as in the isolation of lepers in colonies.

Extensive sanitation systems have been

found in archeological diggings in the ruins of ancient Indian cities, and the Greek and Roman aqueducts are evidence of a measure to provide a sanitary water supply.

The medieval city was an unpleasant place. Sewage ran in the streets, water supplies were generally contaminated and often foul smelling, and housing was dense, allowing little light or circulation of air. During the late Middle Ages, efforts were mounted to clean up the environment. The motivation was to create a more pleasant environment, but the consequence was a healthier environment (Mumford, 1961).

Presumably people noticed their improved health and linked it to the environmental changes. Such would be consistent with the still-prevailing Greek doctrines in medicine that posited contamination as a cause of disease (although without any notion of the mechanism of contamination) and focused attention on the environment as the source of health changes.

After 1687, the date of Newton's *Principia,* major efforts were launched to establish quantitative reasoning, which spurred medical research. The emergence of mercantilism in England and cameralism in Europe emphasized rational productivity, wealth, and a viable industrial complex (Small, 1909). Accordingly the health of the population became the interest of the state, linked to the need for a productive labor force.

Hence health became both a matter for quantitative investigation and a concern of public policy. Nowhere was this more evident than in Germany where Johann Peter Frank proposed the establishment of a medical police force. Frank, writing between 1779 and 1817, was Director General of Public Health in Austria-Lombardy and Professor of Clinical Medicine at Pavia. On the basis of careful public health surveys, he concluded that illness was linked to poverty. The medical police concept was supported by Joseph II and Maria Theresa, but the idea dwindled with the shift to the individualistic philosophy of the Enlightenment (Rosen, 1953).

Even in the absence of any knowledge about infectious agents, many effective measures in the control of disease developed. In France, free medical services were established in Paris, health surveys were conducted, and theories of public health developed that saw the social and physical environment as a powerful instrument in the reduction of health problems. Many important associations were established between disease and housing, nutrition, life-styles, and physical geography.

Perhaps the most famous example of effective public health technique was John Snow's investigation of a London cholera epidemic in 1824. Snow noticed that the epidemic was centered in a single neighborhood and suspected contamination of the water supply from the Broad Street pump. On investigation he found that those with the disease had used the pump and those who did not get cholera used alternative water sources. On his recommendation, the handle was removed from the pump, and the epidemic subsided (Clendening, 1942).

The era of germ theory

The conception that disease is caused by germs came to fruition in the nineteenth century. It was the most powerful single idea in the history of medicine, being responsible for (1) a massive and effective assault on acute disease through immunization and treatment, (2) a refocusing of attention onto the disease process with an attendant loss of interest on the part of the medical profession in the nonbiological aspects of illness, (3) a period of optimism in which it seemed possible to eradicate all illness from human populations, and (4) a fundamental reorganization of medical training resulting in the modern medical school.

The rise of germs and the fall of people. The concept of microorganisms arose from an older theory of contagion that dates to the fifteenth century. The first bacteria were discovered in the seventeenth century by Anton van Leeuwenhoek, a Dutch microscope maker. It was not until the middle of the nineteenth century, however, that Louis Pasteur linked bacteria with the theory of contagion and demonstrated that germs caused anthrax, chicken pox, and cholera (Clendening, 1942). The work of Pasteur and several others gave force to a powerful germ theory of disease that was to dominate medical thinking for a century.

The medical importance of the germ theory can hardly be underestimated. It was probably the single greatest weapon in the so-called conquest of disease, a victory that had been declared prematurely. Nonetheless, the germ theory led to the development of pharmacology, and medications were developed that enabled cures of a wide range of human ills. It would not be an exaggeration to say that the germ theory is *the* success of modern medicine as viewed by the profession and the public at large.

Of major social importance is the fact that the discovery of germs marked a dramatic shift in medicine from a people-oriented to a disease-oriented profession. Physicians became absorbed in the study of disease, and their mission and training shifted from the care of sick people to the diagnosis and cure of disease. Skill at performing appropriate diagnostic tests and in selecting appropriate drugs became the hallmark of the good physician. The earlier focus on the social context of illness and on the public policy questions regarding health receded to the background as medicine experienced one triumph after another and received an exclusive public mandate to set health policy.

The flowering of the public health movement and epidemiology. Epidemiology, the study of diseases in populations, had its roots in Hippocratic theory. Its emergence as a special discipline and its application to problems of public health, however, resulted from the development of germ theory.

Whereas germ theory focused solely on the relationship between an individual (the host) and microorganisms (the agent), epidemiological theory retained from the Hippocratic tradition a focus on the environment. Hence epidemiological theory conceptualized the disease process as one that linked these three interacting elements, all of which are necessary to produce disease (McMahon and others, 1960) (Fig. 1-2).

This model became the basis for public health practice in the nineteenth century. With the identification of microorganisms, it became possible to specify the nature of the agent, thus making sense of earlier successes such as Snow's with the Broad Street pump, described previously. Manipulation of features of the environment became a way of preventing illness, along with immunization and isolation of infectious cases.

For example, one did not have to wait for a case of malaria and then initiate treatment. It was possible to recognize that certain mosquitos are vectors which carry the infectious agent to the host, that mosquitos need stagnant water to breed, and that clearing swamps is a way to reduce the mosquito population and thus the incidence of malaria. Hence preventive medicine and

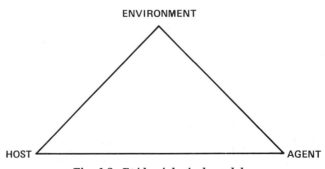

Fig. 1-2. *Epidemiological model.*

epidemiology became a powerful tool in the control of disease.

In the late nineteenth century, most large cities established departments of public health with responsibility for epidemic control and maintaining a sanitary water supply. Although the scope of responsibility varied from one jurisdiction to another, public health and epidemiology became established tools of public policy.

The Flexner Report. Although germ theory provided a firm base for medical practice in objective and observable data, medical training lagged behind the scientific developments. At the turn of the century in the United States, a segment of the medical profession was concerned that relative to available knowledge, the training of physicians was inadequate. To document this case the American Medical Association (AMA) contracted with the Carnegie Foundation to undertake a comprehensive study of medical education. Abraham Flexner, Dean of Johns Hopkins University, was given the task of doing a survey in which he visited all schools of medicine in the United States and Canada. The Flexner Report, which resulted from this study, caused a major reorganization of medical training.

Flexner (1910) found that the vast majority of medical schools provided little or no training in the basic sciences, most were not linked to universities or hospitals, many provided only apprenticeship training, and some were diploma mills. In short, medical training was inadequate and in many cases fraudulent.

Flexner made several proposals that were widely adopted and that set basic standards for medical education. The curriculum and organization of the present-day medical school largely resulted from the following demands pressed in state legislatures by the AMA:

1. Basic training must include two years of biological and physical sciences.
2. Clinical training must include two years of closely supervised experience in a hospital.
3. Medical schools should be affiliated with universities to take advantage of faculties in the sciences.
4. Graduates of medical schools must pass a rigorous examination before being allowed to practice medicine.

As a result of the Flexner Report, two thirds of the medical schools in the United States and Canada were closed. With few exceptions, the remainder affiliated with universities, and courses in basic sciences were uniformly adopted in all medical colleges. The result has been a marked improvement in the technical competence of the medical school graduate, so that Lawrence Henderson could say that between 1910 and 1912 "for the first time in human history, a random patient with a random disease consulting a doctor chosen at random stood better than a 50-50 chance of benefiting from the encounter" (Somers and Somers, 1961).

Two points must be made. First, high-quality, technically competent medicine is a recent historical innovation that resulted as much from the solution to a problem in organization as from technical advances. Second and more important to the principal argument, the reorganization of medical training on the Flexner model constituted the academic enthronement of the germ theory of disease in which disease became the sole point of focus in medical education.

Post–germ theory

For several reasons, the narrow focus on disease and the optimism attendant on the germ theory proved unsatisfactory in the long run. The decline in deaths due to acute illness was accompanied by an increase in chronic disease, leading to doubts as to the ultimate conquest of disease in general. As medical practices became further removed from common sense, patients became alienated from physicians. The result has been a renewal of social concerns in medicine but this time based on the social sciences rather than social philosophy.

Health as a mirage: the limits of germ theory. In 1959 a noted microbiologist, Rene Dubos, published a book entitled *Mirage of Health,* in which he presented the germ theory as an ideology[2] and rejected the "utopian assumption" that disease is ultimately conquerable.

Dubos' major point was that "complete freedom from disease and from struggle is almost incompatable with the process of living. . . . The very mastery of nature may release dangers that cannot be controlled." For him, health consists in the adaptation of man to his environment, and man's environment is constantly changing, resulting in some irreducable degree of maladaptation.

The mirage of health, the belief that health is attainable, was fostered by the myth that germs cause disease. Dubos was careful to point out that germs are a necessary but not sufficient cause of *some* diseases. The presence of germs does not lead to disease unless some other factors (genetic, nutritional, or environmental) are present. When Koch isolated the tuberculosis microbe, "most of the persons present in the very room where he read his epoch-making paper in 1882 had been at some time infected with tubercle bacilli and probably still carried virulent infection in their bodies," yet they did not have tuberculosis. As Dubos said, "the presense of pathogens in the body can bring about disease, but usually does not. . . . Disease, when it occurs, is due to a change in the conditions under which the ecological equilibrium had evolved." In short, the doctrine of specific etiology that was central to the germ theory of disease proved to be over simplistic and led to false promises.

Ultimately the self-proclaimed mission of the medical profession to cure all disease would have to be seen as a hopeless case, and physicians would have to learn to accept disease and shift attention to the care of sick people. To do this would require a much broader focus than that of the germ theory, one in which all aspects of man's adaptation to his environment are taken into account. Environment must be taken to include psychological and social states, as well as physical and biological ones.

The emergence of psychiatry. Another major impetus to the recognition of the limits of germ theory was the development of psychiatry, most importantly the work of Sigmund Freud. Working with hysterical patients, Freud demonstrated that some physical disorders were psychologically caused. Hence not only were germs insufficient to cause disease even when they were present and necessary to explain the presence of disease, but also some diseases were not physically caused at all.

This discovery led to the development of a classification of diseases into those that were physically caused and those that were psychosomatic. As investigation proceeded, a number of diseases were discovered to have a large psychological component in their etiology. In addition to hysterical paralysis and anesthesia, such diseases as asthma, gastric ulcers, hypertension, and ulcerative colitis are of this type. From several different theoretical perspectives, there seems to be an emerging consensus that social stress is an important cause of several physical diseases (Selye, 1950; Grinker, 1953; Wolff, 1953; Graham and Stevenson, 1963).

It was not a large step from the concept of psychosomatic illness to the position that all illness has significant psychological dimensions, and the personality system is implicated in the creation of disease, the response to symptoms, and the likelihood of recovery (Engel, 1962). Coupled with recognition of the importance of social environment for the development of the personality system (Erikson, 1959; Parsons, 1964) and the development in recent years of community psychiatry (Susser, 1968), it has become difficult to treat any illness as simply a physical problem.

The flowering of social epidemiology. In a sense, social epidemiology is an old discipline. Studies linking the incidence and prevalence of disease to occupation can be found in ancient times. However, during the biological era of medicine in which the germ theory of disease dominated, the major emphasis in epidemiology was on the

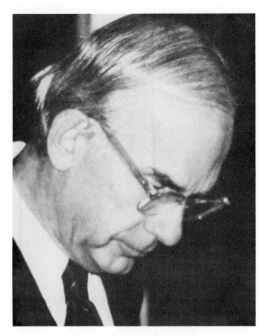

Fig. 1-3. *Saxon Graham.*

search for physical causes of illness in populations.

The conceptualization of population characteristics and behavior patterns as causes of disease was a logical development from observations that diseases were found to distribute differently by age, sex, social class, ethnicity, marital status, occupation, and migration patterns.

The major pressure toward social epidemiology, however, came from the success of the germ theory. Mortality and morbidity from acute illness dropped in part as a result of immunization and treatment based on the germ theory. At the same time, there was a marked increase, both relatively and absolutely, in the incidence and prevalence of chronic diseases (Twaddle, 1968; Graham and Reeder, 1972).

Unlike the case of acute illness, medicine has made little progress in the treatment of chronic disease, which seems not to be susceptible to a single-cause approach. In fact, many have no known physical cause at all. Accordingly, the rise of chronic illness has led to the development of multi-

causal theories of disease, and social patterning has been a major consideration, along with socioenvironmental stress.

With social epidemiology, attention has turned from disease vector analysis to the use of social surveys of health problems. The growth of survey research on social factors related to disease has had a profound impact on epidemiology. Recent investigations have explored the role of perceived stress and social disorganization in the cause of mental illness and investigated the relationships among life-styles, social values, and attitudes and heart disease, arthritis, and cancer (Langner, 1963; Syme and Reeder, 1967; King, 1972).

One recent development is the rejection of the concept of disease by some epidemiologists. Since many if not all diseases are associated with the same social events and diseases correlate highly with each other and disease is one of many alternative responses to social stresses, epidemiologists such as Leonard Syme (1966) have abandoned the concept of disease in favor of a concept of "brokenness." It is thought that humans subject to sufficient social stress are likely to "break," with the particular style of breaking being to some extent a matter of chance.

This, however, is an avant gard movement. As exciting as it is theoretically, the greatest current impact of sociological thinking is in the use of the social survey for investigating health problems.

Health surveys. The renewal of interest in the social aspects of disease was manifest in the development of the health survey. Sampling and survey procedures were developed in sociology relative to other problem areas and were later applied to the field of health.

The first modern statistical report of a population's health was carried out in Hagerstown, Maryland, from 1921 to 1924. Data relating to the prevalence of disease were collected, and on the basis of a twenty-year follow-up, the first reliable five-year incident rates were computed along with disease-specific death rates (Sydenstricker, 1930; Commission on Chronic Illness, 1957).

The first national survey was conducted by the Committee on the Costs of Medical Care between 1928 and 1931. The sample consisted of 9,000 households in 130 localities in eighteen states. Interviews covered many aspects of disease and medical care. For each illness, information was gathered on "the diagnosis . . . date of onset, duration of the illness, and many facts about the nature and extent of medical care provided by various kinds of practitioners and institutions. Costs were also obtained" (Commission on Chronic Illness, 1957). According to Suchman (1963), "These various studies raised serious questions concerning the adequacy of medical organization in the United States and pointed the way toward the growth of governmental interest in the provision of medical care." Thus health and illness once again became public issues, as well as technical medical problems.

In part because of renewed public interest and the success of the reports of the Committee on the Costs of Medical Care, the United States Public Health Service undertook a National Health Survey during the winter of 1935 and 1936. This survey covered over 737,000 households, including urban areas in eighteen states and rural areas in three states, and gathered detailed information on disease patterns and the use of medical services. Extensive checks on the validity of data were introduced, vastly improving the quality of health survey data (Perrott et al., 1939).

Similar developments occurred in other countries. In England and Wales, for example, a continuous survey of sickness was conducted from 1944 to 1951 in which 4,000 households were interviewed each month. In that country, hospital record forms were standardized in 1949, allowing for a summary of hospital data to be made from 1953 onward. In conjunction with other studies of reportable diseases, samples of general practitioners' records, and

the other information sources, much reliable data are being generated (Logan, 1959).

In Denmark a national morbidity survey was conducted in 1950, which sampled 100,000 people in their homes and 33,000 people in hospitals and allowed calculation of sickness rates and their relationship to social characteristics. Self-reporting of illness was checked against medical records, and a high degree of reliability was established (Lindhardt, 1959).

The National Health Survey Act of 1956 established a continuous program of data collection for the population of the United States to provide general background data on health, illness, and the use of medical services. Beginning in 1957 a program of health interviews was initiated with a national sample of households in which illness, disability, and the use of health facilities are reported. In 1959 a program of health examinations was begun with a subsample of the health interview survey, and in 1962, a survey of records in health care facilities was started. These three components, the health interview survey, the health examination survey, and the health records survey, constitute the ongoing National Health Survey, which is a major source of data on trends and differentials in the health and use of medical service in the United States (National Center for Health Statistics, 1963). The data generated constitute the most sophisticated and reliable information available on the health of any national population.

With the development of a continuous base of solid information based on publicly mandated health surveys, a technique developed in the social sciences and in conjunction with the growing recognition of deficiencies in a narrow, disease-oriented approach to health and illness, medicine became ripe for increased collaboration with behavioral scientists. At the same time, sociology was undergoing changes that led to sociologists becoming interested in studying medicine.

SOCIOLOGICAL ORIGINS OF MEDICAL SOCIOLOGY

Whereas the medical origins of medical sociology were rooted in a series of practical concerns relative to the understanding of illness and treatment, the sociological origins were related to developments in theory and methods. Some of sociological theory has roots similar to those informing much of biology, providing some common assumptions with medicine as a base on which to build collaboration. Other theory is based on different assumptions but makes medicine a naturally emerging interest of sociologists. At least one sociological tradition, that of demography and human ecology, has a long history in which it is not sharply differentiated from public health and epidemiology.

Demographic traditions: mortality and morbidity

Demography, the study of population, has long been concerned with the dynamics of population growth. A major component of this analysis has been mortality, the volume and distribution of death in societies. The study of mortality has led to concern with disease, first relative to the cause of death and later in its own right (morbidity analysis).

Records of births and deaths have been kept from the fourteenth century in Italy, but it was not until 1662 that John Graunt published the first systematic analysis of death rates. His study was based on weekly "bills of mortality," which listed deaths by cause for the city of London, England. From this study, not only the general rate of death for a population but also some major differentials by age and sex first became apparent. William Petty did a similar analysis for the city of Dublin, Ireland, in 1690.

The first national study of mortality was published by Per Wargentin for Sweden in the late 1750s based on a national system of population registers established by law in 1748. In 1837 England and Wales adopted a system of vital registration in which births, marriages, and deaths were recorded, and in 1839 William Farr became the Compiler of Abstracts in the General Register Office. Farr devoted a career to the compilation of statistical information and their application to questions of public policy. According to Dorn (1959), "He related causes of death to seasons of the year, residence, density of population, age, sex, and occupation," which initiated the base for most of what is known about differential mortality.

In the United States, the Massachusetts Bay Colony began keeping records of births, marriages, and deaths in 1639. From 1850 to 1900 information was collected with each census on deaths during the previous year. In 1880 a death registration area was established, consisting of states that provided accurate information in the form of vital records. This area expanded until all states were included in 1933 (Dorn, 1959).

The study of mortality has been recognized as one way in which the quality of life can be measured. Such indices as the death rate and life expectancy reflect levels of nutrition, public sanitation, and the toll of disease. Death is an important social cost not only to the individuals involved but also to the society at large. The study of mortality was hence an important aspect of sociological study from its earliest inception.

One way in which mortality figures have been used is as an indicator of the health of populations. Accordingly, one of the earliest demographic concerns was to measure the death toll from specific causes, or disease-specific mortality. However, there are several reasons why mortality figures are not good indicators of health, most importantly because not all diseases are equally likely to result in death. Some produce considerable disability while seldom causing fatalities.

Accordingly, many demographers have turned their attention in recent years to the analysis of morbidity. Special attention has been given to the incidence (number of new cases reported during a specified time period) and prevalence (total number of cases present during a specified time period) of diseases. In this interest the sociological field of demography parallels closely the medical field of social epidemiology discussed previously.

Theoretical developments

Relative to demography, other fields of sociology developed an interest in health and medical care late. In part, this is because demography is the most empirical of the sociological specialties and other fields had to await theoretical developments that created the feeling that health and health care issues were relevent to their concerns. Two aspects of sociology, which have a long historical standing, provide a base for medical sociology arising: the organic tradition, in which early sociological theory arose from developments in biology; and the debunking tradition, in which sociological findings often upset the ways in which people are used to conceptualizing the social order. The timing of the emergence of medical sociology partly depended on the emergence of specific landmark studies, most notably Durkheim's famous study of suicide; the concern with social change, cultural lag, and interaction of the Chicago school of sociology; the Lynds' study of Middletown and their discussion of keeping healthy; and the attention given to illness and medical care in Parsons' influential theory of social organization.

The organic tradition. Early sociological theory was closely linked with biological theory. Herbert Spencer, one of the first sociologists, presented a model of the organization of society based on an organic analogy. He suggested that societies were like biological organisms and were subject to change by a process of natural evolution. The work of Charles Darwin on the theory of evolution was influential, and a school of "social darwinism" dominated British and American sociology at the turn

of the twentieth century. Social stratification was explained as a natural result of natural selection and "survival of the fittest," and numerous theories were developed that explained social structure and process as determined by physical and biological factors such as climate and race (Sorokin, 1928).

In 1906 Ward presented an argument in which he called attention to the limitations of the organic analogy by listing significant ways in which societies are not like biological organisms. This document effectively brought to an end the idea that societies are organisms and that sociology can be seen as a biological specialty. From that point, sociology moved to develop its own distinctive theories.

Several concepts were retained from the biological era of sociological theory. One field in fact still operates on the basis of biological models. The conceptual apparatus of human ecology consists of adaptations of concepts borrowed from plant and animal ecology. Most important, however, is the retention of the concept of "system," in which wholes are seen as more than the sum of their parts and changes in one part of a system are seen as affecting each of the other parts. This concept is still central to several sociological theories, which are usually taken together as the "functionalist school."[3]

The debunking tradition. Inherent in the nature of sociological work has been a tradition of debunking common beliefs about the nature of the social order (Berger, 1963). When any discovery is made about social organization, cherished beliefs of many people are challenged, and over time a large number of popular beliefs have been disproved by empirical data. Moreover, many sociologists have selected research problems on the basis of the existence of common beliefs in an effort to assess their validity.

As stated by Berger (1963:38), "The sociological frame of reference, with its built-in procedure of looking for levels of reality other than those given in the official interpretations of society, carries with it a logical imperative to unmask the pretensions and the propaganda by which men cloak their actions with each other."

In addition, the debunking tradition is often deliberate. The recognition of this tradition and the development of the school of "critical sociology" has led to the puncturing of myths as a goal of many sociologists. It is the ideological posture of the most powerful and prestigious groups that is most often singled out for investigation. Hence groups like physicians and politicians are prime subjects.

Durkheim on suicide. In 1897 the French sociologist Emile Durkheim published *Le Suicide,* a work that has become a sociological classic. This was among the first empirical studies done in sociology, and it was to have enormous influence on the development of the discipline. It also represents the earliest empirical study to form a benchmark in the development of medical sociology.

At the time when *Le Suicide* was published, most sociologists were entangled in philosophical debates regarding the nature of social reality and the epistomology behind the operations of societies. Durkheim was active in this debate, although during his lifetime little attention was paid to his work. He asserted that social facts existed *sui generis* and were not reducible to psychological or biological facts. He had also presented a model of social change in which the social bonds in simple societies were characterized by common values and roles (mechanical solidarity), whereas those in more complex societies were characterized by mutual interdependence based on dissimilar roles (organic solidarity).[4] This assertion was important to the development of the social realism of Western European sociology, particularly in England.

Durkheim's impact on American sociology came later when attention turned from broad philosophical issues and demand developed for "careful description, exact comparison of concrete behavior, and inductive empirical study rather than a

priori deductive speculation. . . . With the emergence and ascendance of statistics, *Le Suicide* assumed a new relevancy" (Hinkle, 1960). It served as a model for the use of official statistics for the generation of sociological knowledge.

In *Le Suicide,* Durkheim tabulated official data regarding suicide in several countries. His careful analysis differentiated populations at different levels of risk of committing suicide according to age, sex, marital status, economic conditions, and other categories. From this analysis, he identified several types of suicide and related these to major aspects of social organization. The study showed not only how much knowledge could be gained from poor data but also how the analysis of official state data could contribute to the development of sociological insight.

In a sense Durkheim was the first medical sociologist, although at the time there was no conception of medical sociology and suicide was not then thought of as a medical problem. Its relevance developed with changes in both sociology and medicine.

The Chicago school on social change and cultural lag. Cultural lag occurs whenever one aspect of a culture develops more slowly than another, resulting in conflict within the culture as a whole. For example, in the medical institution, technological advances have moved well ahead of the political, economic, and family sectors of Western culture. Medical technology has cracked genetic codes and controlled human reproduction to the extent that it is now possible to determine the types of people produced by a society vis-à-vis sex, intelligence, personality, size, and so forth. However, the political, social, and economic technology is lacking to adequately control this development; in other words, there is cultural lag.

This concept was the brainchild of William Ogburn, a member of the Chicago school of sociology. Ogburn (1922) used a medical care example as his first case study of cultural lag, and the concept has been applied successfully to medical sociology research during the 1920s and 1930s. Syden-stricker (1933), in a study of the lag between available health care services and those received by the poor, demonstrated higher incidences of illness among the poor. Moore (1927) produced one of the finest examples of the application of cultural lag to medical sociological research. He analyzed all available data on medical care in the United States from the perspective of cultural lag, and his interest in adjusting medical services to meet the demands of rapid social and economic change set the tone of much of the research on medical care organization in the United States through World War II (Roemer and Elling, 1963).

Health in Middletown. In 1924 and 1925 and again in 1935 Robert and Helen Lynd studied the community of Middletown. This study constituted one of the major early works in American sociology and one of the first to focus on social stratification (Lynd and Lynd, 1929, 1937). It too has become a sociological classic.

In their study, the Lynds examined a wide range of behavior, including ways of earning money, life-styles at home and during leisure time, training the young, and religion. They demonstrated the pervasive influence of social class on behavior at a time when it was thought that social class was unimportant in the United States.

The Middletown studies were also important contributions to medical sociology, being among the first to explore health and illness behavior from a community perspective. Both books contained a chapter discussing the organization of medical practice, the use of medical services by members of the community, and the major alternatives to medicine along with patterns of their utilization.

As was the case with Durkheim's work, however, this study appeared before there was any conception of medical sociology as a field. Although many other aspects of *Middletown* soon were followed up in subsequent sociological literature, it was many years before the materials on health and illness were recognized as having major sociological importance.

Parsons on professions and clients. The major sociological breakthrough, which more than anything else made health, illness, and medical care sociologically relevant, came with the publication of Talcott Parsons' *The Social System* in 1951. In one chapter of this major work in sociological theory, Parsons focused his attention on medical practice and the role of the sick person. In part because health, illness, and medical practice were singled out for attention by the most prominent contemporary theorist, the study of such phenomena became legitimated, and many sociologists began to investigate the institution of health and illness care as a major concern in the study of societies.

Perhaps equally important is the fact that Parsons carefully linked the study of medical sociology to long-standing sociological concerns involving the process of social change and social control, thus bringing the study of medical phenomena into the mainstream of sociological thought.

Parsons has a long-standing concern with one of the most central issues in sociology, the modernization of societies. He entered the field when the dominant way of looking at social change was in terms of single dimensions, such as Tonnies' distinction between *Gemeinschaft,* or community based on face-to-face interaction and moral consensus, and *Gesellschaft,* or society based on contract and mutual interdependence. Durkheim's distinction between mechanical and organic solidarity, as well as several other formulations, reflected the same unidimensional thinking.

Early in his career, Parsons became dissatisfied with this approach and argued that change occurs in several dimensions and cannot be adequately discussed as a one-dimensional phenomenon. He was especially concerned that the dominance of the businessman in the occupational sphere was identified with the *Gesellschaft* side of the continuum and that the emergence of self-interest was seen as a hallmark of modern capitalist societies. What was troublesome was that the professions were emerging to a dominant position in the occupational structure at the same time and these occupations were characterized by a collectivity interest rather than self-interest. That is, the professional relates to his client in a cooperative venture, whereas the businessman relates to his customer in a competitive venture.

The merits of Parsons' case are not at issue here, and some aspects will be discussed in subsequent chapters. What is important is that the argument made it theoretically necessary to study the professional as an occupational type in comparison with the businessman and the client in comparison with the customer. It was therefore natural to study the physician as a prototype professional and the patient, or sick person, as a prototype client and sickness as the main situational variable controlling the interaction between the two. This step made the study of medicine as an institution sociologically revelant.

There is another important dimension of sociological relevance. As will be discussed in some detail in Chapter 4, Parsons has conceptualized illness as a form of deviant behavior. Abnormal behavior can be treated by the society as either crime, in which case it is punished, or illness, in which case it is treated. Hence from a sociological perspective, illness is linked to another major traditional interest of sociology, that of deviance and social control.

Drawing on the deviance perspective, several sociologists have developed the following theme, which is implicit in Parsons' work: in the control of deviant behavior, societies are shifting from a criminal-punishment model to a sickness-therapy model. In a sense, social control is becoming, in Pitts' (1968) term, "medicalized," and the study of sickness, therapy, and physician-patient interaction also provides a proto-type for the predictive study of deviance and social control.

Methodological influences

Both sociology and medicine share a common interest in and pursuit of quantitative, experimental, and predictive methodology, although the units of analysis are different for the two fields. Medicine is concerned primarily with the individual person and sociology with human group processes and institutions. Nevertheless, both disciplines share a methodological core consisting of a concern with large numbers. There is a mutual interest in statistical techniques for the analysis of multiple variables and in research designs that control for intervening or confounding variables.

Recent developments and innovations in survey research techniques and design have had great influence on the growth of sociology. There exists an extensive history of excellent survey research on issues germane to medicine (Cornaro, 1558; Villerme, 1830; Buret, 1845-1846; Sydenstricker, 1930; Shattuck, 1948), and the rapid growth of medical sociology during the last three decades can be linked with new methodologies developed in the area of survey research.

The major methodological landmarks in survey research that have had an impact on the growth of sociology occurred during the period since 1940. Survey research in sociology developed rapidly once the public opinion polls appeared on the scene. The 1940 presidential election found the Fortune Survey (Roper), the Crossley Poll, and the Gallup Poll fully operational. This advance allowed the researcher for the first time to gauge the strength of attitudes, as well as reasons behind the voters' decisions.

Gallup began to expand his research interests to include public opinion on social and economic issues of the time. The central public issue was the war in Europe, and Cantril devoted much of his survey research efforts to studies of shifts in war opinions and attitudes of families with potential soldiers for the war. Problems of the bandwagon effect, reliability, sampling, classification of socioeconomic status, and the validity of indicators were raised.

Lazarsfeld (1939) developed the panel design in 1938, and between 1940 and 1945 panel studies were applied to questions of international relations, communications, and propaganda research. A major breakthrough in panel design occurred as a direct result of Lazarsfeld's Erie County survey, in which an elaborate study design consisting of matched control groups, repeated measurements, and multivariate analysis was used for the first time in a sociological investigation.

The stage was set for the American Soldier Studies, perhaps the single greatest contribution to sociological methodology. During this period, the Research Branch of the War Department's Information and Education Division completed 300 surveys of the American soldier. These studies were directed by Samuel Stouffer and Associates. By the end of the war, 600,000 interviews were handed over for reanalysis to a research committee appointed by the Social Science Council. Published in four volumes, this study was without parallel in the history of social sciences in terms of theoretical and methodological advances. Louis Guttman developed a scaling technique that was a vast improvement over the earlier Thurstone and Likert scales in as much as a logical basis was provided for item selection and the acceptance of the scalability of a set of items. Furthermore, elaboration analysis, both marginal and partial, was developed and applied effectively, moving survey research away from the unsophisticated single cause–simple percentage analysis that characterized most survey research prior to this time, especially the epidemiological surveys.

Throughout this development of survey research, one finds rather profound efforts of sociologists to integrate theoretical sociology with empirical research on problems applicable to real human needs. It is not surprising then that the marriage of these two foci would occur in applied substantive areas such as education, crime, or the medical institution. Health needs and medical care organization provided quantifiable, real world data of significant national importance, and survey research sociologists, armed with remarkable innovations in technique and design, moved almost automatically into the medical arena to do research that would come to be called "medical sociology."

In the medical sphere, social epidemiological studies emerged that advanced multicausal theoretical models, multivariate analysis, and adequate sampling models. Hollingshead and Redlich's study (1968), *Social Class and Mental Illness;* a study by Srole et al. (1962), *Mental Health in the Metropolis;* and especially a study by Syme et al. (1964) on cultural mobility and the occurrence of coronary heart disease are examples of social epidemiological surveys that rank among the best of sociological surveys in methods and concepts.

On other fronts in medical sociology, research has occurred on rural and urban health needs of the population, the hospital as a complex organization, patterns of medical practice alternatives to the hospital, health personnel, and the patient. Survey research in these areas has advanced the substantive development of medical sociology to the point at which medical sociology can begin to consider research of great national and international scope and of tremendous potential benefit for communities and nations.

Comparative national studies on health care organizations, patterns of consumer and provider decision making, health manpower, issues germane to centralization-decentralization of facilities, power and control, and consumer participation in health care decision making are only a few of the fronts that medical sociology can advance, given the present level of technology and theoretical accumen.

THE MERGER OF MEDICAL AND SOCIOLOGICAL INTERESTS

The broad outlines of the merger of medical and sociological interests have been suggested. By concentrating on disease processes, medicine lost sight of sick people, and when the germ theory of disease proved to be limited, there was a need to recapture a human focus. In this task the behavioral sciences, including sociology, had potential utility. They had developed theoretically in ways that made medicine an interesting behavioral science subject and methodologically in ways that provided tools needed for medical and public policy problem solving.

Increasingly, medicine and sociology were finding common ground. Both were concerned with resolving the basic philosophical issues between the Western traditions of positivism and idealism, allowing for the simultaneous use of "hard" objective information and human meaning. In addition, external pressures on medical practice were changing in ways that not only made sociological expertise essential for understanding questions of medical policy but also understanding the pressures related to core sociological concerns. The emergence of medical sociology followed, with the specialty defined as both a basic and an applied field of study.

Philosophical tensions between idealism and positivism

The positive perspective asserts that natural events are real and not simply mental constructs. It further asserts that there are invariable laws of nature and that nature is subject to the control of man (Bury, 1955). This tradition laid the groundwork for modern science and technology by asserting that "we would be able to arrive at general laws and, thereby, be able to solve most of the problems that confront mankind" (Rose, 1965).

The idealist perspective in its extreme form asserts that there are no laws of human nature, and therefore there can be no science of human nature. The emphasis of the idealist tradition is placed on ideas about human nature, with concentration on detailed history or philosophy of history (Parsons, 1937; Rose, 1965). Whereas positivism focuses on causal relations, idealism focuses on systems of meaning.

Both the positivist and idealist traditions have made important contributions to Western thought. The logic of science, which arose as part of positivism, is responsible for the establishment of reliable, predictive knowledge that is objective and useful. The human meaning attached to the events of the world is validly approached through idealist assumptions on which history and subjective explanation are based.

In medicine the tension between idealism and positivism has manifested itself in alternative concerns with disease processes on the one hand and the patient on the other. Positivist, germ theory–oriented physicians take the position that technical competence relative to diagnosis and treatment is central. Idealist, care-oriented physicians see the cure functions as important but place emphasis on the care of sick people. One manifestation of the merger of these traditions is the changing definition of health and illness discussed in Chapter 4.

In sociology a like set of tensions has focused on the extent to which social behavior can be explained by objective events that exist independently of human will and that shape social relationships or the extent to which the ways in which humans define events is key to shaping those relationships. These tensions will be outlined in Chapter 2 in the discussion of theoretical domain.

Both sociology and medicine are moving toward a position that both objective and subjective phenomena are important. Sociology, however, is much further along in this regard, having dealt with the issues as far back as Max Weber's *verstehen* sociology at the turn of the century. Relatively speaking, medicine is still a positivist discipline, but it contains a movement of physicians and others who are interested in incorporating idealist elements. For those people, sociologists are important allies (as they are for the sociologists). One of the distinctive contributions of medical sociology may be to systematically bring to account the study of conceptions of health and illness in a discipline committed to the study and treatment of disease.

Changing pressures on medical practice

In addition to a variety of philosophical parallels between sociology and medicine, there are some concrete problems facing medicine that sociology and other behavioral sciences are uniquely qualified to address. Recently Twaddle and Stoeckle (1972) argued that attempts to solve the problem of technical competence raised in the Flexner Report have resulted in the emergence of several new problems, including the following.

1. *Changes in medical knowledge and the need and demand for medical services.* The merger of medical schools and universities produced a knowledge "explosion" that improved medical effectiveness in treating acute illness. A larger proportion of the population is in need of attention for chronic illness than was formerly the case, and there is greater demand for medical service as it becomes more effective.

2. *Increased work pressures on the medical system and technological change.* The increase in demand has increased the work load of the medical care system. Combined with changes in knowledge, this has resulted in a search for laborsaving machinery, and the technological sophistication of medicine has increased.

3. *Growth of the scale of organization and specialization and fragmentation of services.* Medical care has shifted out of the home and into the office, clinic, and hospital. Physicians have specialized in small subareas of medicine, and the patient is often faced with seeing several physicians to treat different problems. As a result,

medical care is less well coordinated and takes more time and sophistication on the part of the patient.

4. *Skyrocketing costs of medical care.* Medicine has become an area of high capital investment and overhead, requiring a large number of people to treat each patient. Because of the fragmentation of service, much medical care is inefficient and more expensive to the client. And provisions of some health insurance carriers have aggravated the cost problem by requiring that work be done in the most expensive settings for coverage to be provided.

As a result of these changes, many in medicine see a new set of problems that require the expertise of the social sciences for their solution. Among these are the need to make the system more efficient for its clients, the need for cost controls, the need for better organizational forms to improve coordination, and the need to deliver service in such a manner as to not alienate the patient, that is, in a more humane manner.

Problems of social organization, alienation, and interaction are central to the concerns of sociology. Their perception by the medical care system allows a true merger of interests in which the solution of theoretical problems in sociology can become an important input into the solution of practical problems in medicine. This merger of interests between a few sociologists and a few in medical care has contributed to the development of medical sociology.

The emergence of medical sociology

As suggested previously, medical sociology emerged as both a basic and an applied discipline. A *basic science* is one in which knowledge is pursued for its own sake. Problems are defined as a result of contradictions, inconsistencies, and gaps in the state of theory or in the outcomes of studies dealing with the same properties. An *applied science* is one in which knowledge is pursued for the solution of practical problems or in which the knowledge from basic science is used to solve practical problems.

Basic and applied sciences are often thought of as being antithetical to one another and as mutually exclusive pursuits. It seems more reasonable, however, to think of them as differing aspects of any research (Hudson, 1970). As described by Hudson, applied research is concerned with concrete events and objects, whereas basic research is concerned with the properties of events and objects. An applied researcher might be interested in understanding a particular organization; a basic researcher is interested in properties of organizations in general, such as size, stratification, and authority. Both may be interested in the same information, but they will differ in what they do with it. The applied researcher will be concerned to summarize all the properties of a given event or object, whereas a basic researcher will be concerned to summarize one or more properties as found in all events or objects. The goal of the applied researcher is a practical *model,* whereas that of the basic researcher

is a scientific *theory*. These relationships are diagramed in Fig. 1-4.

It is clear, where basic and applied interests intersect, that a given work may be either basic or applied. Also applied research may be used for basic ends and vice versa. The differences are more in how the information generated is used than in the kinds of information sought.

Relative to basic and applied concerns, a distinction is common among medical sociologists between sociology *in* medicine and sociology *of* medicine. This distinction was made first by Strauss (1957), one of the pioneers of behavioral science training in medical schools.

Sociology in medicine. The phrase "sociology in medicine" refers to the applied aspects of medical sociology. In extreme form, it designates a sociologist whose work consists of providing technical skills for the solution of medical problems or of problems in health care delivery without regard for contributions to sociological theory. For example, sociology in medicine may characterize the work of those who are mainly concerned with the prevention and

PROPERTIES	OBJECTS AND EVENTS							
	Hospitals	*Clinics*	*Physicians*	*Nurses*	*Diseases*	*Sick people*	*Other*	
Size								
Division of labor								Sum of rows = Basic theory
Social identity								
Roles								
Norms								
Sanctions								
Ideology								
Other								

Sum of columns = Applied model

Fig. 1-4. *Hudson's model of the relationship between basic and applied sociology. (Modified from Hudson, J. Social policy and theoretical sociology. Paper presented at the meeting of the Midwest Sociological Society, April 16, 1970.)*

treatment of illness, allocation of resources, and other similar problems (Freeman et al., 1972).

There has been much discussion in the literature about the value of sociology in medicine. Many believe that when sociologists allow physicians or other nonsociologists to define the problems they work on, they cease to function as sociologists. They are rather technicians. Others think that those who address applied problems contribute more to the parent discipline than others (Hall, 1951; Williams, 1953; Gouldner, 1957; Davis, 1964; Hyman, 1967).

The suspicion that they may have "sold out" to nonsociological interests has made many who work in the medical field defensive about their identities as sociologists (Suchman, 1963; Freeman et al., 1972).

Sociology of medicine. The term "sociology of medicine" refers to the basic research aspects of medical sociology. As with education, religion, the family, and the economy, medicine is a social institution worthy of sociological study in its own right. As with the study of other institutions, the study of medicine generates insights into the properties of social relationships and social organization. The goal of such study is to learn about societies rather than to understand disease processes or to otherwise contribute to medical ends.

Although their contributions to sociology are not suspect, sociologists of medicine have relatively more difficulty gaining access to meaningful research sites. Understandably the medical community is interested in results that serve its ends, and no group enjoys being subject to the debunking motif, which challenges treasured self-images. Relative to other types of settings, such as factories or governmental agencies, the tradition of privileged communication in medicine gives these settings more power and incentive to block access to meaningful data.

As Mechanic (1968b) suggests, medical sociologists are frequently caught in a dilemma. They can serve medical interests, thus gaining access to valuable information while running the risk of losing their unique perspective, or they can serve basic interests of the discipline, thus retaining their perspective while making access to information more difficult. Increasingly, workers in this field have learned to combine basic and applied goals in their research, thus attempting to serve both ends. To date, however, this has been a matter of personal style of research.

SOCIOLOGISTS AND HEALTH WORKERS

To the extent that medicine and sociology have become mutually useful to one another, it is possible to speak of a merger of interests between the fields. This merger is far from complete, however. The fields are distinct in their interests, sufficiently to suggest that they form separate subcultures. Medicine is not just indifferent to theoretical questions; it is intolerant of any investigation that does not serve immediate, practical goals.

From the perspective of medicine, sociology often seems to be a vague, impractical discipline, and the medical culture frequently seems profoundly anti-intellectual from the sociologist's point of view. Hence empirical work in the medical field by sociologists is frequently characterized by more tensions than may be the case in other substantive specialties. Even so, the payoffs are great enough on both sides to have established medical sociology in both its applied and basic aspects as a viable discipline.

Against the brief historical background outlined in this chapter, this text will provide an introductory survey of medical sociology. For the most part, it will concentrate on the sociology of medicine and only secondarily on sociology in medicine. However, since we do not see these aspects as radically distinct, the two will be intermixed.

In Chapter 2 the basic sociological framework for the text will be provided, with the introduction of core sociological concepts that orient the student to the language of the text and provide the basic assumptions that serve to order the remainder of the book. Thereafter the book is organized into four main sections.

NOTES

1. It is not the place of this text to review the history of sociology. The interested student is referred to any of several books in this area, including those by Barnes (1948), Bogardus (1960), Maus (1962), Nisbet (1966), or Mitchell (1968). References will be found by author and date at the end of this text.

2. Ideologies are defined by Tumin (1973) as "conceptions of how things should be." Ralph Spielman suggests that we all live by certain myths about the nature of the world around us, and "when we believe the lies ourselves, they are ideologies."

3. See Chapter 2.

4. This is not the place to describe Durkheim's contributions to sociology. The interested student is referred to Wolff (1960).

5. We do not imply that Durkheim's findings should be accepted in the light of more recent work (Douglas, 1969).

CHAPTER 2

Sociological viewpoints
THE STANCE OF THE DISCIPLINE
AND THIS TEXT

This chapter is intended to serve two purposes. First, it will provide a brief and broad orientation to the field of sociology for the benefit of students who have not had such an exposure. In so doing, it will help those students gain a frame of reference that will enable them to appreciate the relationship of the more substantive materials to the body of knowledge in the larger discipline. It should also provide a framework for understanding why some interesting topics (from the standpoint of other disciplines) may be left out. In short, it will show the broad guidelines that we have used to decide what is relevant and what is not when making judgments of inclusion and exclusion.

Second, we will try to be explicit about the stance we are taking relative to some key issues in the discipline. We reject the idea of a value-free sociology and agree with our colleague Derek Gill: "Sociology never was, never will be and never can be value free." Our only choice is to be as explicit as possible within the limit of self-understanding about the values we hold or to try and conceal those values while allowing them to color our subsequent analysis. We elect the former.

Some overview, necessarily brief and inadequate, of some issues in sociology will be necessary to make our position explicit.

THE SOCIOLOGICAL PERSPECTIVE

Relative to other intellectual disciplines, sociology lacks a single, integrated perspective. There is no one key historical figure who served as a "fountainhead" for the discipline, such as the case of Freud in psychology. Nor has a single body of theory been as influential and central as that of Darwin's in biology or Newton's in physics. Rather sociology is characterized by a relatively large number of theories that to varying degrees are in competition with one another. Marx and Weber in the nineteenth century and Parsons in the twentieth come the closest to being key figures in that much of the work of sociologists can be seen as a dialogue with one or more of these men. Even here, however, a large part of theoretical work in sociology treats these figures as benchmarks for staking out the differences in approaches. None has crystallized a majority of sociologists into a dominant school.

This is not to say that there is no common ground among sociologists. There are a number of metatheoretical positions that most sociologists would, we think, agree on at least broadly. These arise from the historical and political (ideological) roots of the discipline in the nineteenth century.

Historical roots

Sociology, as noted in Chapter 1, took shape in the middle and late nineteenth century. This was a time when the doctrines of positivism had been consolidated, and there were rapid and exciting developments in science. Objective and verifiable knowledge was being developed in physics and chemistry largely as a result of the breakthrough conceptually and symbolically in Newton's work. Biology was developing a new empirical base that would soon culminate in Darwin's theory of evolution. Positivism was working, and doctrines of the new sciences were coming to dominate all thought in Western Europe (Bury, 1955).

Science as an enterprise had captured the public imagination, and positivistic modes of thought permeated public thought, leading to the novels of Doyle as well as the theories of Einstein. In short, positivism was a widespread cultural phenomenon, not simply a development in philosophy as a discipline. One important development was an emerging attempt to apply scientific procedures to the study of human behavior, even to the extent of the application of physical science theories.

Freud, for example, developed a model of the human personality that was based on Newton's fluid mechanics (Yankelovitch and Barrett, 1970). The personality was divided into "compartments": the id, ego, and superego. The id exerted "pressures" on this closed hydraulic system that were resisted through the "counterpressures" of the superego, causing the danger of "blowouts" in the ego in the absence of appropriate "safety valves" provided through early childhood learning.

Adopting the view of the world from the physical sciences, early sociology also developed a number of deterministic and mechanical models of society (Sorokin, 1928; Ritzer, 1975).

Durkheim, for example, saw social facts as existing *sui generis* as a collective conscience, or body of norms, that determined the behavior of individuals in the society.

The social darwinists applied Darwin's theories of evolution to the social order and saw social arrangements as part of a natural evolutionary process (Hofstadter, 1955; Sumner, 1961).

The major counter to the rise of positivism was the German tradition of idealism, which dominated the intellectual style of historical work. Whereas positivists asserted that there were immutable laws of nature which awaited discovery and that events of the world were external to human definitions and objectively measurable, idealists asserted that there were no laws of human nature. All that existed of reality was human conceptions of reality (Parsons, 1937).

Not to put too fine a point on it, sociology can be seen as a field that has wrestled from its beginnings with the conflicts between these competing historical viewpoints. Marx in his early writings emphasized the humanistic traditions, focusing on the plight of men entrapped in the economic forces of the society. His attempt to resolve the conflicts was to take the idea of the dialectic from Hegel's humanistic philosophy and to "stand it on its head" by applying the model to materialistic (i.e., objective and observable) events. In so doing, he moved from a humanistic to a more positivist stance. Weber, although acknowledging the importance of economic forces, argued that ideas in and of themselves could cause changes in the social structure (Gerth and Mills, 1946; Weber, 1958; Marx, 1961). In this century, Parsons has tried to resolve the conflicts by focusing on the subject matter of the idealist tradition (ideas, norms, values) with the conceptual tools of positivism (the concept of structure, system).

It is important to note that the issues are not resolved. Radically positivist and radically idealist theories can still be found in sociology, as well as a variety of theories that have tried in various ways to resolve these tensions. For this reason, we will have to be explicit on our stance relative to this issue.

Political roots

The nineteenth century was also a time of political ferment. The emerging commercial middle class, committed to non-interference with profit making, developed an ideology of laissez-faire capitalism. From this perspective, government should be limited to certain essential services that could not be supplied by private enterprise. The public good demanded that business be unfettered by regulation.

At the same time, the situation of employees of the capitalist was one in which working conditions were grim at best. Hours were long, pay low, and factories dangerous. Under the new system, the product did not belong to the worker but to his employer. In short, the worker was alienated from his labor (Marx, 1961; Ludz, 1973). People in these circumstances tended to favor restrictions on the activity of the capitalists either through government regulation of business or through a reallocation of power in which the workers would become the owners of the means of production. Hence the ideology of socialism was born.

The political ideologies of the nineteenth century had a profound influence on the development of sociology and still have an influence on modern theory and research.

Classical liberalism: from Spencer to Parsons. Herbert Spencer, who must be regarded as one of the founders of sociology, proposed between 1842 and 1896 a view of society that was closely tied to laissez-faire capitalism. Spencer in fact was one of the major developers of the theory. There were two essential ideas that have had historical significance.

The first of these was that of evolution (developed independently of Darwin's but influenced in its later development by Darwin). Spencer held that societies naturally evolved from simple to compound forms of organization. Furthermore, this evolution was a natural phenomenon. Any attempts by the state to alter or accelerate progress would lead to disaster. The job of the state then was limited to protecting citizens in their individual rights and to

protect property. It should not attempt to interfere with social arrangements or to try to introduce change (Barnes, 1948a; Timasheff, 1957; Martindale, 1960).

The second idea was that of organicism. On six important dimensions, societies were seen as being like biological organisms. Like the parts of the organism, there is an equilibrium between and within societies and between societies and their environments (Giddings, 1908).

This tradition linked with the evolutionary doctrines of Darwin created a massive intellectual movement that has been known as "social darwinism." Although this movement was found both in Europe and the United States, it was especially important in the United States. The basic proposition was that societies are organisms and that the differentiation of parts is determined by survival of the fittest. Any effort to ameliorate social conditions for the disadvantaged would lead to the deterioration of the human stock by facilitating the survival of the unfit (Hofstadter, 1955); (for an extreme statement, see Sumner, 1961). It is a theory calculated to appeal to the wealthy and powerful.

Although social darwinism as a major movement in sociology is dead, the organic model and the evolutionary perspective are still found in the contemporary work of Parsons. Both, however, are considerably modified. Organicism takes the form of thinking about society as a collection of parts, each of which contributes to the "on-goingness" of the whole. Evolution has lost its earlier connotation of progress (Bury, 1932; Parsons, 1937).

Socialism: from Marx to Marcuse. Sociology and socialism were in part born together. Karl Marx was simultaneously the most important nineteenth century individual in the development of socialist ideology (recognized as a founder by present-day socialists) and the most important figure in the nineteenth century development of sociology. He is the one with whom, more than any other, the field has been involved within a debate "acknowledged or unacknowledged" (Gerth and Mills, 1946). According to Maus (1962), "when sociology began to develop as a specialized science in [Germany] toward the end of the nineteenth century it immediately set itself, whether avowedly or not, to refute Marxian socialism."

In almost every respect, socialist doctrine runs counter to that of classical liberalism. Although there is an evolutionary process, it is in the form of a dialectic between those who control the society and those who are controlled. Control is manifested with respect to the means of production, the tools of economic output. In feudal times, this was the ownership of land, and the basic conflict was between the lords and the peasants. In capitalist society, it was the ownership of industry, and the conflict was between the bourgeois and the proletariat.

The key element is conflict. In fighting for their respective interests, the parties produce social change. Evolutionary movement comes from the synthesis of former conflicts and the generation of new ones. Political activity then is part of a dynamic of change. The state, serving the interests of the ruling class, is a foil for the revolutionary interests of the working class. Deliberate political action rather than being a spoiler of the evolutionary process becomes its essence. Societies are not at all like biological organisms (Marx and Engels, 1932; Marx, 1961).

Several key ideas have entered sociology from the Marxist tradition. Among these are interests, objectively preferable courses of political action based on position in the social structure; ideology, ideas serving class interests; the concept of class itself as an objective reality; and the fundamental dynamic of the means of production structuring social relationships.

In recent years, there has been a resurgence of academic interest in Marxian formulations in the critical sociology movement. A significant minority of sociologists are taking the position that sociological thought is fundamentally ideological and that theory should be criticized in terms of its ideological content. A key focus of this movement has been on the concept of alienation, in which people became progressively divorced from meaningful control over important aspects of their lives (Marcuse, 1964).

Conservative and radical sociology

Closely tied to the traditions of humanism and socialism on the one hand and positivism and classical liberalism on the other, Cohen (1968) has identified two models of sociological theory that are based on different assumptions about the nature of the social order. Although theories are more diverse and complex than suggested by these models, they do help to illustrate a range along which various theoretical positions can be arrayed. Model A is the conservative model, and Model B is the radical one.

Model A

1. Norms and values are the basic elements of social life.
2. Social life involves commitments.
3. Societies are necessarily cohesive.
4. Social life depends on solidarity.
5. Social life is based on reciprocity and cooperation.
6. Social systems rest on consensus.
7. Society recognizes legitimate authority.
8. Social systems are integrated.
9. Social systems tend to persist.

Model B

1. Interests are the basic elements of social life.
2. Social life involves inducement and coercion.
3. Social life is necessarily divisive.
4. Social life generates opposition, exclusion, and hostility.
5. Social life generates structured conflict.
6. Social life generates sectional interests.
7. Social differentiation involves power.
8. Social systems are malintegrated and beset by contradictions.
9. Social systems tend to change.

Metatheoretical positions

The differences among sociologists, which are substantial, can reasonably lead to the question of whether sociology can be said to exist as a discipline at all. That is, is there any common denominator that underlies the disparate positions relative to ideology, political philosophy, and the nature of social life? We think there is in the metatheoretical stance of the discipline. There are several propositions on which most sociologists would agree, be they radical or conservative.

The first of these propositions is that there is a social structure. Human activities are not random but patterned. Social behavior then is to some degree ordered, lending some degree of predictability to human behavior. The basis of this patterning and the processes through which it is manifest, however, are points of considerable disagreement. Some sociologists see the basis of social structure in language, norms, and values; others, in adaptation to the physical environment; and others, in the organization of economic activities. Furthermore, there is disagreement on the extent to which the social structure is a given that people must adjust to versus the extent to which it is continuously under negotiation.

A second proposition common to most sociologists is that the most fruitful explanations of human behavior must be sought in the study of collectivities rather than at the individual level. Whether the basis of social order is perceived as consensual or coerced, normative or negotiated, it is the group or larger collectivity that socially patterns behavior. However interesting individual behavior may be for other purposes, it cannot adequately explain the aggregate phenomenon called "social structure." Furthermore, characteristics of the collectivity influence (some say determine) individual behavior patterns.

A third proposition, closely related to the second, is that the social structure imposes a set of behavioral constraints on both individuals and groups. At any given point in time, people must take into account the existing patterns of social relationships. They will have some opportunities open to them to select some kinds of behavior and a lack of opportunity to select others. The same actions will have different consequences for people, depending on their location in the social structure.

Again there will be divergence in the ways in which these constraints are conceptualized. Some focus attention on social norms and the sanctions that others will impose on behaviors, whereas others look to the system of social class. Differences are found in the extent to which people are seen as being self-controlled versus coerced, but no sociologist sees humans as totally free from their own social arrangements.

Thus some degree of consensus on some basic propositions exists among sociologists, however much they disagree on how these are manifested (see Atkinson, 1971, who laments this degree of consensus).

SOCIOLOGICAL THEORIES

There have been almost as many frameworks for the discussion of sociological theories as there have been theories. Some have focused attention on the kinds of independent variables the theories have selected (Sorokin, 1928). Others have dealt with them historically (Timasheff, 1957) or in terms of contemporary schools of thought (Martindale, 1960). Most of these portrayals have focused, as we have to this point, on the conflicts between different theories and how they can be regarded as sharply distinct from one another in ways that are not resolvable.

Only recently has the approach been taken that different theories deal with different classes of events. Hence it is possible that they may be not mutually exclusive but additive. This approach has shifted the key question from one of selecting the theory that is best on the assumption that most have to be wrong to one of exploring the ways in which the various domains encompassed by different theories might be linked together. Important work has already begun to address this question (Blau, 1964; Buckley, 1967; Martel, 1971).

Theoretical domain

Martin U. Martel (Fig. 2-1) has made the most explicit, although least detailed, attempt to classify theories by domain. As he presents it (Martel, 1971), there are two

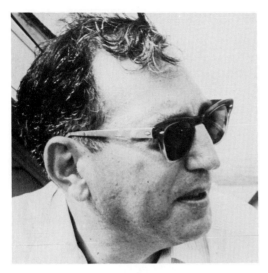

Fig. 2-1. *Martin U. Martel.*

major dimensions to be considered: the kinds of properties the theory deals with and the kinds of focal units to which it is applied. Properties are seen as physical or symbolic or some combination of the two, and focal units can range from societies taken as total entities to the individual. The core question is focused on the kinds of dependent variables that the theory treats as problematic.

The distinctions among types of properties relate primarily to the extent to which the theories take into account the problem of meaning. The physical theories are those in which meaning is excluded. That is, the variables to be explained are those which might be said to be a function of innate biological traits of the human species or the operations of impersonal social forces. How humans define reality or interpret events is simply irrelevant. Homans' exchange theory, for example, postulates innate needs that can be understood through the models of stimulus-response psychology (Homans, 1961), and human ecology is based on a darwinian model of interspecies competition (Hawley, 1950). Relatively speaking, physical theories seem to be those more narrowly based on biological assumptions and that seek to emulate the models of the physical sciences.

The symbolic theories are those which take the problem of meaning as central. How people define reality, interpret events, and construct meaning is the core problem.

On the other axis, theories differ in the focal units that are made problematic. Some theories are about societies; others are about communities, complex organizations, groups, interaction, or individuals. Any given theory tends to select a range of phenomena, or a level of organization, on which to focus.

Cross classifying on these two dimensions, Martel suggests that there are eight domains claimed by different theories (Fig. 2-2). Conceived in this way, each theory has taken a different "slice" of reality. It is hence likely that each one makes a valid contribution to knowledge. The central problem then becomes not selection of *the* theory to be used but to explore the ways in which different domains might be linked.

Paradigms

Another way of looking at theory is in terms of underlying paradigms (Friedrichs, 1970; Kuhn, 1970; Ritzer, 1975). Adhering to Masterman (1970), Ritzer (1975:7) defines a paradigm as follows:

A paradigm is a fundamental image of the subject matter within a science. It serves to define what should be studied, what questions should be asked, how they should be asked, and what rules should be followed in interpreting the answers obtained. The paradigm is the broadest unit of consensus within a science and serves to differentiate one scientific community *(or subcommunity)* from another.

Paradigms are both metatheories (basic assumptions about the nature of reality, the nature of man, etc., in short, epistemology) and methodological and theoretical achievements of science. Kuhn (1970) defines a paradigm as the theoretical and methodological achievements of a science. Examples of such achievements include aristotelian dynamics, newtonian mechanics, and others describing schools of thought or achievements within a science.

FOCAL UNITS (SUBUNITS)	DEPENDENT VARIABLES (MAIN TYPES)		
	Physical properties	*Physical and symbolic*	*Symbolic properties*
Societies	Ecosystem theory *(Duncan)*	Conflict theory *(Marxism and derivatives)*	Social systems *(Parsons)*
Communities	Human ecology *(Park, Hawley)*		
Subunits	Area subgroups, individuals	Interest groups, individuals	Institutions, norm patterns
Complex organizations		Organization science*	Latent-manifest functionalism *(Merton, Gouldner)*
Smaller groups			
Subunits	Task subgroups, specialists		Interest and reference groups, individuals
Interpersonal relations	Elementary social behavior *(Homans)*	Psychoanalytic theory *(Freud, Sullivan and derivatives)*	Symbolic interaction *(Mead, Blumer)*
Individuals			
Subunits	Response patterns	Needs, mechanisms	Defined acts

*No single "organization science" man quite typifies its chart placement, but some work of Conrad M. Arensberg, F. J. Roethlisberger, and William F. Whyte is illustrative.

Fig. 2-2. *Some current sociological frameworks, by focal domains. Domain refers to the main dependent properties whose variations a given approach seeks to explain, and the units these properties characterize. The selected approaches and named representatives are in some cases arbitrary; as may varyingly be said of their placements in the chart, which aims only to highlight overall, typical contrasts in use. Apart from Parsons and Homans, theorists named are Herbert Blumer, Otis Dudley Duncan, Sigmund Freud, Alvin W. Gouldner, Amos H. Hawley, George H. Mead, Karl Marx, Robert K. Merton, Robert E. Park, and Harry Stack Sullivan. (From Martel, M. In Turk, H., and Simpson, R. Institutions and exchange. Indianapolis: The Bobbs-Merrill Co., Inc., 1971.)*

According to Kuhn (1970), the principal function of paradigms is to guide research and theory construction within a science by proclaiming fields of endeavor as belonging properly to the science. Before paradigms develop, an early or immature science produces research that is scattered over a large, amorphous, conceptual map. All research problems appear equally interesting or relevant, and research is restricted almost to random fact gathering of easily obtained data.

The emerging science rapidly runs up against the problem of making sense out of what usually becomes a mass of unconnected data. At this point, if the particular discipline is to survive as a viable scientific endeavor, one or more paradigms emerge to unite the discipline. The paradigm frees the research and theoretician from the vast array of all sociological phenomena, for example, and one now can focus on selected phenomena in greater detail. First, principles, basic assumptions, primitive and defined concepts, and basic hypotheses are catalogued in a literature so that it is no longer necessary to build the field anew with each new study. Paradigms allow the researcher to take a lot for granted, which makes it easier to get on with research that builds on knowledge gained. Paradigms steer the researcher toward specific classes of facts to the exclusion of other facts as important for explaining why a certain problem exists. The objective is to use the paradigm to predict occurrences of a phenomenon and thereby to develop a more precise paradigm and ultimately to build a theory.

The second meaning of paradigm as metatheory is useful as well but much more difficult to study. The epistemology of the research is inextricably bound with the types of research problems chosen, the basic concepts employed, and the explanatory models advanced. In the discussion of the paradigms of sociology, both meanings of paradigm will be referred to. However, the elusive nature of epistemologies makes it difficult to describe particular research along this dimension. The following discussion of sociological theory is organized by centering attention on theoretical and methodological achievements as paradigms.

A paradigm is hence broader than a theory, and several theories may be subsumed under a single paradigm. Ritzer (1975) contends that it is the paradigm rather than the theory that defines schools of thought. Furthermore, sociology to a degree greater than almost any other discipline can be characterized as a multiple-paradigm science. Three competing paradigms have been identified: social facts, social definition, and social behavior.

According to Ritzer, the social facts paradigm is based on the centrality of social structures and social institutions, both of which are conceived as being real rather than simply convenient constructs. The efforts of the social factist are directed toward the nature of structures and their interrelationships. Preferred methods include the interview and questionnaire. Prime examples of this tradition, which derives from the work of Durkheim, are structural-functionalism and conflict theory.

The social definition paradigm derives from the work of Weber and focuses on intrasubjectivity and intersubjectivity. That is, how people define situations and act on them is central. Observation tends to be the preferred technique and action theory, symbolic interaction, and phenomenological sociology the main theoretical examples.

The social behavior paradigm is based on the stimulus-response psychology of B. F. Skinner, which emphasizes the effects of rewards and punishments in shaping subsequent behavior. According to Ritzer, "the behaviorist seeks to understand, predict, and even determine the behavior of man." Exchange theory is the leading example, and experimental methods are preferred by those of this persuasion.

These paradigms are presented as political positions within sociology. There is competition for dominance among adherents of these basic positions. Ritzer is careful to caution that the paradigms emphasize differences and have "ignored the common core of agreement within the discipline," although he nowhere indicates what that agreement is. Furthermore, he states that the great sociological thinkers have not restricted themselves to a single paradigm. Without claiming such lofy status for ourselves, we will be bridging paradigms in this text. First, it may be profitable to note a few major theories and their characteristics as identified by both Martel (1971) and Ritzer (1975).[1]

Some illustrative positions

Most of the variety of sociological theories are used sometimes explicitly but mostly implicitly in this text. It may be useful therefore to identify some of the major theories and to locate them with reference to Martel's and Ritzer's criteria as a way of sensitizing the student to the sources of various concepts used in this text.

Human ecology is a field that has focused on societies and communities using a physical model. Of the "macro" theories, it comes closest to being within the social behavior paradigm in that the basic concepts and assumptions are derived from biological theories, primarily the work of Darwin. Human ecologists have taken as their major problem the use of space by populations, with special emphasis on urban land use. This aspect of human ecology receives little emphasis in this text and is here limited to some studies of the location of services. Demography, which is the study of populations, is based on a statistical social fact paradigm. The chapter on disease and death draws mainly from the demographic tradition.

Conflict theory is a loosely defined field that has focused on societies using a mixed model within the social definition paradigm. Theories in this tradition are derived mainly from the seminal work of Marx. They emphasize conflict as a central dynamic of social change. Furthermore, they see the dominant mode of production as the central organizing feature of the society that structures power relationships between unequal people by virtue of their position in a social structure. The powerless are alienated from the social organizations in which they find themselves and from the products of those organizations. This perspective, especially the notions of class, power, alienation, and ideology (defined later), has had a major influence on the stance of this text.

Social systems theory has also focused on the society as the unit of analysis. As conceived by Ritzer (1975), it is partly in the social facts traditions (e.g., Parsons' four function schema for structural analysis) or the social definition paradigm (e.g., Parsons' action frame of reference). Either way, the emphasis is on the symbolic properties of systems, which are seen as culturally dependent. This tradition has also had a major influence on the stance of this text, especially through the concepts of norms, values, and role. The core issue addressed by these theories is the observed continuity of societies and the discovery of mechanisms by which an ongoing system is maintained. Some aspects of this approach will be found in most chapters of this text.

At the more "micro" level, *exchange theory* has focused on individual behavior and interaction, with almost exclusive attention to physical properties. This is the prototype theory of the social facts paradigm. In its clearest form, it is based on the models of stimulus-response psychology with an emphasis on the rewards and costs of alternative courses of action as these influence the likelihood of occurrence of any specific behaviors. In the form presented by Homans (1961), the influence of this theory on this text is minimal and indirect. Although we agree that rewards and costs are taken into account in selecting behaviors and that an exchange process is an important social dynamic, we also see the symbolic meaning of exchange as paramount.

In the past, there was a *psychoanalytic theory* of some importance in sociology, particularly in terms of the development of Freud's notion of the superego. This tradition has failed to demonstrate its utility and is of no importance to this text.

Symbolic interaction, as the name implies, focuses on the symbolic properties of interaction. Particularly important are the notion of the sense of self as a social product, the emphasis on the negotiation of meaning and action in individual and group encounters, and the emphasis on the perspectives of the various actors in defining the situation. These concerns are found throughout this text.

At the middle range of the theoretical spectrum and dealing with complex organizations and groups is *latent and manifest functionalism.* Particularly important is the focus on existing structures and changes with their differential impact on the interests of people at different locations in the social structure and the importance of location in the structure for demands made on others. Concepts from this tradition such as role sets, role strain, and reference groups are important underlying themes in this text. The symbolic and structural properties of social systems are important, as is the issue of negotiation and power.

Organization theory as presented in Martel's formulation is not sufficiently well defined. It seems to refer to any approach to the study of organizations that does not make problematic the symbolic dimensions. The famous Rothlisberger and Dixon discovery of the Hawthorne Effect in *Management and the Worker* (1939) is noted as falling into this category. To the extent that we use this perspective, it is largely unarticulated in this text.

Although most sociologists have worked within one of these traditions, some have begun to address the problems of linkage between them. Goode (1973), for example, is concerned with the symbolic properties of social behavior in a form consistent with latent and manifest functionalism but has taken as his basic model the exchange theories, making symbolization problematic in the process of exchange. Blau (1964) has linked exchange theory with organization theory and to some extent with social systems theory by postulating "emergent properties" in the exchange process as one moves from smaller to larger focal units. Buckley (1967) has looked to the cybernetic models of computer science to link lower order and higher order levels of organization. Although in our opinion a satisfactory approach still needs to be developed, the problem addressed is of central importance if a greater unification is to be possible in sociological perspectives. Still to be addressed is the issue of linking paradigms, which will probably come much later.

OUR POSITIONS

As the student may have guessed from the subtle cues discretely dropped up to this point, the stance of this text is eclectic with respect to sociological theory. It is our view that there is no general sociological theory in the sense of being all-encompassing (although several are general in the sense of being highly abstract). Moreover,

with reference to the understanding of any concrete social institution, organization, or group, all theories have value in that they have generated useful information through research that aids in constructing a picture of how these phenomena work. Each one, however, provides a partial picture. If the focus is on a phenomenon, as in this case health, then a variety of perspectives are needed.

We do not pretend, however, to present a fully balanced and objective summary of the sociology of health. Both as humans and as professional (whatever that means) sociologists, we carry strong biases. We are not neutral on issues of ideology, politics, or paradigm as they influence the field of sociology, nor are we without strong preferences and opinions about the state of medicine. Furthermore, we have strong beliefs about the nature of academic discourse. All these obviously influence our selection of materials and their presentation. It is important for the student to know "where we are coming from" to assess "where we are going."

Our views relative to sociology

With regard to the positivist-idealist traditions, we tend to favor the idealist with regard to subject matter and the positivist with regard to style. Humans actively work to make sense of what is happening to them and to exert control over their own lives. We think that the problem of meaning, central to the idealist-philosophical tradition, is key to understanding human behavior. At the same time, we reject the more extreme idealist assertions that human behavior is infinitely variable and unpredictable and therefore cannot be subjected to serious research. It is in fact patterned and researchable through intellectual procedures that derive from the positivist tradition. Largely implicitly, we are seeking a synthesis of these two traditions in which we can have the best of both worlds. That synthesis will not be accomplished in this book, and people committed to either of these philosophical traditions will find reason for dissatisfaction.

Our position with regard to the capitalist-socialist traditions is less ambivalent. Although we admire the expressed values of the capitalist with respect to freedom of choice and individual initiative, the notion that unbridled free enterprise leads to the realization of these values must be rejected on the evidence. Marx was right in observing that capitalism left to itself leads to the oppression of the many by the few, stifling both freedom and initiative. Some form of regulation of economic power by agencies responsible to the general public is required to keep freedom and initiative from being crushed. At the same time, the programs and practices of the Europeon socialist parties have not realized the ideal of socialism. In the European model, socialism has resulted in excessive bureaucratization of power, with extreme centralization of decision making. All that has happened is the shift of the capitalist drive to the state apparatus. We look to the development of a communist (not in the sense of official Communist parties but more in line with the ideology of the Yugoslavian praxis school of sociology) society modeled more after the societies of the Native-American tribes or modern China. This would be a system of public ownership and accountability with a decentralized system of power and decision making. Given the choice between capitalism (in either its free enterprise or European Communist forms) or socialism, we favor the latter.

With respect to the conservative-radical models as presented by Cohen, we again decline a choice, mostly because our sense of reality does not fit the models. Norms, values, and interests are all basic elements of social life, for example. Social life involves both commitments on the one hand and inducement and coercion on the other. Societies are both cohesive and divisive. Although Cohen's list does present several dimensions that underlie various theoretical stances, we are not impressed with the possibility of meaningful choice between the two models. In fact, it is the paradoxical existence of both models simultaneously in the empirical reality of living that most impresses us. We believe that we must accept both to preserve the human richness of experience and to reflect the reality of paradox.

With respect to paradigms, we have a dual commitment. Using Ritzer's definitions, we reject the social behavior paradigm as deficient in that it views much of what we regard as core issues as metaphysical. Particularly important to us is the social behaviorist's rejection of the problem of meaning as a relevant issue. To the behaviorist, how people define situations and decide on action is not important. Humans are reduced to cognitive processes derived from the study of pigeons. We do have a commitment to both the social facts and social definition paradigms. The first calls attention to the need to deal with social structures and institutions. These are useful conceptual constructs, a shorthand for aiding discourse about social realities. In some formulations, they closely reflect real contingencies of living. Social structures will be assumed to be real in this text, although we do not commit ourselves to any particular model of those structures. The social definition paradigm has the advantage of focusing on action. According to Ritzer (1975:27), the "crucial object of study is intrasubjectivity and intersubjectivity and the action that results. . . . Behavior is not seen as a simple stimulus-response phenomenon, but rather as a result of an evaluative process undertaken by the individual."

We see both paradigms as deficient. The social facts paradigm can reify social structures so that the acting individual is excluded. The degree to which the structures are negotiated and modified by behavior can be overlooked. Hence the social definition paradigm seems a necessary counterbalance. The social definition paradigm can reify the individual, seeing nothing but the process of defining and acting. The degree to which human action is constrained by the existing system of interrelationships and structures can be overlooked. Here the social facts paradigm provides a needed counterbalance. It is only in some combination of these paradigms that social realities can be appreciated.

Our paradigm preference is reflected in the text both in the selection of materials included and in the use of those materials. Social facts are parameters of action, things that must be responded to. The response is also of great interest because that is the determinant of subsequent action. For example, disease is real. It is an observable event that has predictable consequences. How diseases are defined and identified and responded to, however, is the core of sickness behavior, as discussed in the next section of the text. Our core problem is understanding. We are much less concerned with prediction.

Our views relative to medicine

Medicine is a necessary evil. So long as people normally prefer life over death and health over disease it is inevitable that people will try to intervene in the disease process and try to forestall death. It also seems inevitable that those who can hold out the promise of success in these ventures will be valued by other people. It makes no difference if the persons holding out this promise are shamans, sweat doctors, "scientific" physicians, or outright frauds. To this extent, medicine is necessary and honorable.

Even though necessary, medicine is also an evil. If people believe an individual has the power to heal, that individual is in a position to exercise power over others and to secure advantages at their expense. As it has developed in the European tradition, this power has resulted in physicians enjoying not only the highest prestige of any occupational group but also the highest incomes. Both as a result of a knowledge monopoly and high socioeconomic status, many physicians feel justified in treating patients as their social and intellectual inferiors, making the process of seeking help one of ritual humiliation on the part of

the patient. In short, the power to heal is the power to exploit, and this power has been used in Western medicine, particularly in the United States.

It would be an easy trap to conclude that physicians are all evil and that if different people practiced medicine this exploitation would not occur. This would not only be a distortion of reality (some are evil and some are not) but bad sociology as well. The major problem is one of social definitions and social arrangements, not one of personalities. The evils that we see are much more those of the system of ensuring health, treating disease, and forestalling death. There are many ways for societies to address these issues, some of which lead to greater exploitation (Waitzkin and Waterman, 1974). Physicians are as caught up in the system as anyone else. Few that we have encountered intend to humiliate patients or to aggravate their problems. Most desire a humane and efficient health care delivery system, but as Shaw observed, "The road to Hell is paved with good intentions." Untrained in economics or behavioral science, most physicians are unable to see alternatives to the way in which medicine is now practiced, and they have little understanding of the social circumstances of their patients.

The high socioeconomic status of the physician, for example, is taken for granted, yet it may be detrimental to health care. Lame Deer, a Sioux medicine man, has observed:

A medicine man shouldn't be a saint. He should experience and feel all the ups and downs, the despair and joy, the magic and the reality, the courage and the fear of his people. Unless he can experience both, he is no good as a medicine man.

Sickness, jail, poverty, getting drunk . . . Sinning makes the world go round. You can't be so stuck up, so inhuman that you want to be pure, your soul wrapped up in a plastic bag, all the time. You have to be God and the devil, both of them. Being a medicine man means being right in the midst of the turmoil, not shielding yourself from it. It means experiencing life in all of its phases. It means not being afraid of cutting up and playing the fool now and then. That's sacred too. (Lame Deer and Erdoes, 1972:79)

Isolated by a position of extreme wealth and power from the experience of most sick people, the modern physician has difficulty understanding the problems brought to him. Sickness becomes reduced to a technical denominator, and a system evolves that treats disease rather than people. To the symptomatic person the physician is an awesome figure, separated from ordinary mortals not only by technical expertise but also by such high status as to make him unapproachable. Another way of looking at this process is as one of alienation of the sick from the means of cure.

Again we emphasize that we are talking about the system of delivering health services, not the practitioners within that system. Physicians, nurses, social workers, technicians, and others involved in the production of health services are also trapped by the system. Many who work in the system see deficiencies and have labored hard to bring about changes. Even at the local level, their efforts have been stymied, and nary a dent has been made in the overall structure. In the 1960s it became fashionable in some medical circles to complain that the United States had a nonsystem for delivery of health services. Lecturing at Harvard College, John Knowles observed pungently, "If you think there is no system, just try and change it."

It is difficult to fault people for taking advantage of a position of power and prestige in a society that teaches its young from birth to "get ahead" even at the expense of others. Physicians are fortunate to be in a field where they can do what most members of their society would do if they could. Even if they prefer a different approach to life, the pressures for conformity are enormous.

Exploitation, alienation, and dehumanization are built into a system of providing services. We find these features deplorable, but change will not come from personalizing the issues. Making changes requires an understanding of the system qua system, and this text is aimed toward that task.

ORGANIZING THEMES

Given that we are taking the position that no one sociological theory contains all the answers and we are able to accept both the radical and conservative approaches to sociology, it necessarily follows that the approach taken in this text must be eclectic. What we have attempted in the following chapters is to put together a sociological portrait of the system of health care, taking information and perspectives from a variety of sources not confined to any given theory, ideological stance, political position, or paradigm. This does not mean that the text is without focus (at least we hope this is the case). We do have a perspective on the field of sociology and on its application to the study of medicine, but our perspective does not easily fit the conventional ways of describing sociological stances.[2]

The student will find the text loosely organized around four sets of themes that have informed our work: a conception of a social structure, a conception of culture, a focus on ideology, and a conception of the relationship of individuals to larger social structures.

Social structure

The basis for social structure is the differentiation of people into categories according to personal characteristics, tasks, or rewards. Most basic and widespread are differences by age and sex. Skin color, earlobe shape, or other inherited features are significant in some societies. These characteristics can serve to classify people within the context of specific societies so as to provide a basis for allocation of roles. Certain people are allowed to do some jobs but not others. These roles become the source of rewards in the society, including access to knowledge and income.[3]

The resulting system of social stratification is a framework for describing *opportunities* of various individuals and groups in the society. These opportunities include a range of phenomena from being treated with respect by others to commanding the necessary resources to gain access to goods and services. Those placed higher in the structure have more opportunities. They do work that carries with it a higher level of *rewards.* Their work is more likely to be clean, both physically and ritually. They are more likely to have high incomes and hence greater command of goods and services. They have more *power,* or capacity to induce or block change or to produce the outcomes they desire even in the face of opposition from others.

The social structure is also a framework for describing the *interests* of individuals and groups in the society. Any change in the social order will objectively benefit some groups and injure others. It is hence understandable that those who have more opportunities, rewards, and power will be reluctant to see changes in the structure, whereas those who have less will be more favorable to change. In other words, one group has an interest in maintaining the status quo, whereas the other has an interest in changing the social order. In this usage, we are following Marx by treating interest as an objective phenomenon. That is, it is built into the system and is not a function of what any group thinks or verbalizes at any given point in time. It is possible that people will not recognize their interests, a state Marx called "false consciousness."

Although social stratification has generally been applied to the analysis of societies and communities, it can also be applied to other focal units such as complex organizations or groups. The same issues can be found irrespective of focal unit.

At any given point in time, the particular social structure is historically derived from earlier structures. Hence we will be providing a historical context, albeit brief, for each topic covered in this text.

Culture

There is an important cognitive dimension that can be broadly subsumed under the concept of culture. People act not as automatons, responding mechanically to a location in a social structure, but in terms of what they think of as proper behavior. They have values that help them set priorities and resolve conflicts. These elements are bound in language and can be passed from one generation to another. They are a major component of learning. To some degree these elements are shared among members of a society or groups within a society.

The *norms* of a society or group constitute the standards for acceptable behavior. They are in effect rules of conduct that specify what people should do. Some norms are general in the sense of being widely shared, at least in abstract form, whereas others may be specific to certain groups. The *beliefs* of the society are its collective sense of what is real. Beliefs are descriptive statements. To the extent that they are shared (and they differ in generality along the same lines as norms) they constitute a distinctive world view for the group or society under consideration.

The importance of both norms and beliefs lies in their enforcement. Adherence to the belief system of the group and its standards of behavior will be rewarded, and deviations will be punished. These *sanctions* can vary in intensity from mild (e.g., a nod of approval or a shake of the head) to severe (e.g., a formal award of a title or honor on the one hand to the death penalty on the other). The intensity of sanctions is governed by seriousness with which the deviation is regarded, norms regarding the appropriateness of response by others, and beliefs in the effectiveness of the response in altering behavior.

Another component of culture is the *values,* or criteria used to order priorities and make choices in the event of conflict. Values are broad glittering generalities that postulate some ultimate good. Under the Protestant ethic (Weber, 1958), work is a value. It is good in and of itself. In societies with a strong work ethic, as in other societies, health is a value. Both are values in the sense that they can be appealed to in making a decision. They are also ranked. If a particular behavior is detrimental to health and necessary for work, how will the choice be made? The ranking of health and work relative to one another is likely to be the critical factor. One will be seen as more important. In other words, it will be more valued.

Differences in norms, beliefs, and values are what lie behind the concept of *ethnicity*. In different countries, different cultures have developed. Historically, these cultures have been expressed through different religious traditions. Hence nationality and religion have often been taken as indices of ethnic identity. In a multinational state such as the Soviet Union or the United States, there are substantial differences among groups in the society in cultural terms. Another way of expressing this is to say that there are different ethnic groups in the society. In popular usage, this is often taken to mean groups that are not fully assimilated, being the most recent immigrants historically. Some people are ethnics and hence distinct from others. Sociologically, however, all people are ethnic in the sense that they are carriers of an identifiable culture. The old Yankee is just as ethnic as the Chicano or Native American.

Ideology

Another theme employed in this text centers on the concept of ideology. As formulated by Marx, "ideology" refers to a set of ideas that derives from one's position in the class structure, that serves the interests of the class position, and that are part of the political process. Ideologies are the self-serving rhetoric of groups in the society that are used to either justify privilege and support the status quo or to attack privilege and to force social change.

Although we recognize class ideology as important and will deal with it at various points in the text, we prefer to take a somewhat broader view of ideology. Any social identity that is group linked, whether or not class linked, carries with it a set of

vested interests (Veblen, 1899). For example, the upper classes tend more often to adhere to a belief that the social system rewards merit and that those who are disadvantaged are so because of their innate inferiority. The poor tend to believe that the system is unfair and that advantages come from luck. Another example is that although no-fault automobile insurance will not affect the prestige or power of lawyers in the society nor will it significantly affect their incomes, lawyers nevertheless oppose no-fault insurance on the grounds that it is bad for the public and will drive up the costs of insurance in the long run. Left unstated is the fact that with no-fault insurance, lawyers are unnecessary. The rhetoric of opposition seems to be an ideology then, even though not class linked.

We also differ from the strict Marxian formulation by perceiving the basis of ideology as cultural and structural. To Marx, culture was a superstructure built on an economic base. Hence all ideology was rooted solely in the social structure. We see the structure as one base, whereas the culture has independent inputs. To take a simple example, university professors are all members of the same social class; however, there is polarization over some issues. Scientists, for example, see human progress as linked to the development of empirical knowledge that has been verified through experimentation. Work that furthers this end is more worthy and good than other kinds of investigation. Humanists see the capacity for appreciation of uniqueness as of primary importance. They see science as dehumanizing and mechanical, a process that degrades human values. These ideas serve the interests of each group by reinforcing a sense of worth in the members. They also serve to justify the importance of each enterprise to funding authorities. They hence engage a political process within a particular social class, seeking support in the general cultural norms.

In this text, ideology then will refer to any ideas that serve the interests of the group adhering to them and that play a part in a political process.

The individual

If the individual is thought of as a set of internal processes, as has been characteristic of psychological approaches, we have not taken a firm position on the nature of the individual. At this level, we prefer some of the work that is revising the classical psychoanalytic framework by discarding the positivist metaphysic. Much of the work of Fromm (1973), for example, is influenced by sociological thought and looks for interactional and external conflict as a dynamic of personality formation. However, we are more attracted to the existential and humanistic third force that is developing alternatives to both the psychoanalytic and behaviorist traditions (Yankelovitch and Barrett, 1970). One example is Maslow (1954) who rejects both the mechanical Freudian model of personality and the behaviorist stimulus-response model that ignores personality. He postulates a hierarchy of needs: body needs, safety, love, relationships, and self-actualization. His focus is on how human beings cope with the problem of meeting these needs (compare to Lindgren, 1959).

From a sociological viewpoint, however, we are less concerned with the internal dynamics of personalities than with the influence of external opportunities and constraints on behavior. Human behavior is situational. It takes place in settings in which rewards and deprivations are part of the situational logic. It takes place in interaction with others, and their interest must be taken into account and at least partially met. Human behavior is to some degree dependent on the availability of certain resources and access to them, and it is normatively constrained by notions of acceptability and morality. In short, social structures, culture, and ideologies are inextricably among the contingencies of human action. At the least, they must be taken into account by individuals seeking to satisfy their own internal needs.

This does not imply that the individual is a passive entity, a piece of flotsam on the social sea. It does mean that human behavior is not simply or even primarily an internal process. Differences in native abilities, family upbringing, group affiliation, ethnicity, past experience with particular organizational forms, objective interests, and priorities are sufficient to ensure that no two people will enter the same situation with identical perceptions about the nature of reality or fully compatible goals. Interactants must contend with each other in a given situation to realize desired outcomes. Hence self-presentation (Goffman, 1959) and negotiation are ongoing processes that characterize most encounters. Accommodations reached in each instance become part of the situational contingencies of future encounters. In this way and to some (undetermined) extent all social orders are negotiated. In any given encounter, to a greater extent, they are givens in the framework of interaction.

The use of organizing themes

This chapter has presented a brief and cursory overview of some key issues in sociology as a discipline. We hope that it is adequate for the experienced reader to gain some notion of our stance within the discipline and for the inexperienced reader to gain some sense of the key issues.

The organizing themes, built around conceptions of social structure, culture, ideology, and the individual, are intended to provide a map that can be used as one enters the forest of the sociology of health. These themes constitute ideas that have been in our minds in writing the subsequent chapters. For the most part, however, they are implicit rather than explicit in our presentation. From time to time, one or another will be highlighted. Generally, students will be relied on to recognize them on their own.

NOTES

1. In the most general sense, two distinct paradigms have been used by medical sociologists in the course of research and theory

construction. These are the phenomenological and the institutional paradigms.

The phenomenological paradigm is the most popular among modern medical sociologists. Studies that emanate from this paradigm generally are qualitative in nature. The unit of analysis or principal unit of observation includes the meanings shared by people interacting with one another, how individuals manage and are managed regarding self-identity, and the idea that social reality exists in the minds of the members of society. Accordingly there is no absolute reality but rather multiple realities created through the shared experiences and meanings of the members of society. A few examples of research in medical sociology that takes the phenomenological stance include New's study of the osteopathic student (1960), Roth's firsthand account of life on a tuberculosis ward (1963), Fox's research on the stresses produced within a metabolic research unit (1959), and Glaser and Strauss' analysis of the trajectory of dying (1968). These studies use qualitative research methods. Also they attempt to tease out of particular experiences in the health care arena what in fact is going on in the minds of the actors as realities are constructed and shared.

Phenomenological paradigms most frequently employ individual level variables such as physician and patient attitudes or medical student orientations toward practicing in rural areas. The problem or dependent variable usually is some form of behavior, either actual or anticipated.

The other major paradigm is what we have called the "institutional paradigm." In this paradigm, the focus is on differentiations or fundamental cleavages that exist between classes of people in the health care system. The two divisions of this paradigm are called the "distributive" and integument" paradigms.

The institutional paradigm is a stratification approach in the final analysis. For example, the researcher or theorist may seek to explain the distribution of medical resources, power, and control by identifying institutional or structural factors as causes.

Within this general framework, studies utilizing the distribution approach treat the health care system as a distributive system in which social and political power is viewed as a function of the background, training, and other pathways to social mobility within the system. Some examples of this approach include Parsons' analysis (1969) of the "competence gap" between providers and consumers of health care and Anderson's treatise (1972) on the distribution of health care services in the United States, Great Britain, and Sweden.

Medical sociologists who utilize the integument perspective attempt to identify what is believed to be the basic organizational structure or fabric that links classes of actors within the health care system. Classes are linked based on their positions within the system. Marx (1957) identifies the integument of institutions as the organizational bases for power, exploitation, and control over the opportunities to advance within the institutions. Studies using this perspective analyze the patterned conflicts that exist between unequal classes within the health care system. The distribution of power and resources is considered of lesser explanatory power than the institutional structures which contribute to the mutual interdependence of the powerful and the powerless, the providers and the consumers, and the owners and the laborers. These become the key explanatory variables. The importance of this level of analysis for explaining the relationships among classes of actors within the medical institution is described simply by Collins (1975) who wrote, "Why some people are poor is only one aspect of the same question as to why some people are rich."

To explain fully unequal distribution of power in any system or institution, one must analyze the institutional structures that are designed to keep the powerful going while restricting the opportunities for those seeking power to achieve it. Friedson's analysis (1970) of the autonomy of American physicians and the discussion in Chapter 12 of consumer participation in neighborhood health centers are examples of this focus.

Critical sociology has emerged recently to apply the integument paradigm of Marx toward an analysis of advanced industrial society (Habermas, 1968; Shroyer, 1970). Critical sociologists have developed reflective attempts to interpret how society is formed by uncovering organizational structures, such as modes of authority, repression, and exploitation, that form the bases for social organization. The objective of the critical sociologists, once these structures have been uncovered, is to inform members of society about the structures and their consequences. This has interesting implications for medical sociology should this paradigm become widely used. For the moment, critical sociology as applied to medical sociology has been confined to an analysis of the funding sources of medical sociological research as determinants of research questions, methods, and theories utilized. This has led to the criticism that medical sociology is a tool of the establishment de-

signed to implement the status quo by preserving the structure of the health care system.

2. We are tempted to call our approach phenomenological in the sense described by Yankelovitch and Barrett (1970) but hesitate to identify with the abstruseness of phenomenological sociology as currently defined within the discipline.

3. What we see as basic is the phenomenon generally dealt with under the headings social class, social stratification, and inequality (Mills, 1951; Harrington, 1963; Mayer, 1955; Bendix and Lipset, 1966; Tumin, 1967).

PART TWO

DISEASE AND THE SICK PERSON

Disease is an objective fact of life that is socially defined. The number and kinds of diseases recognized by any society is dependent on the state of knowledge in that society and on the nature of the culture. Equally the conditions under which people feel ill or become defined as sick is socially, historically, and culturally bound. This section considers the experience of "bad health" from objective, subjective, and social perspectives.

Chapter 3 focuses on disease and death, the dimensions of bad health that are least subject to human interpretation if the focus is on the presence or absence of the event. Neither, however, is a random phenomenon. Both disease and death strike more frequently at some populations and groups than at others. Furthermore, the ways in which the events are identified and classified are socially influenced and subject to change. Accordingly this chapter will explore the definitions of disease and death and provide a description of the ways in which both the definitions and events are socially patterned. It is these events that form the reality referent that people take as a base for making decisions about their own health.

Chapter 4 looks at the ways in which the health of individuals is assessed. Shifting from the biological realities of disease and death presented in the previous chapter, attention is given to the ways in which health and sickness are socially defined both in terms of social policy statements and with reference to discrete, individual decisions. There is a social process by which people become defined as sick, and the definition constitutes a social identity, or status. This process is described.

Chapter 5 looks at the process by which an episode of sickness is experienced. Sickness is treated as a kind of career, a sequence of social identities with particular expectations for behavior. Emphasis is placed on the ways in which decisions about sickness and the response to symptoms are made, including the decision to seek treatment and to cooperate with healing occupations.

Together these chapters treat disease and sickness as social problems as seen from the perspective of the patient or prospective patient. It is the results of the processes described here that form the raw material for the health specialists and the organized system of health care delivery.

CHAPTER 3

Disease and death

We are all mortal. Not only are we going to die, but unlike other forms of life, we know it. This knowledge is centrally important to humans, and it is a burden. Throughout recorded history, in all cultures, men have attempted to come to terms with the hard fact of mortality. The explanation of death is a central theme of religion, with some attempting to deny its importance and others attempting to give it meaning by defining it as a transitional stage from one form of existence to another. Attitudes toward mortality are ambivalent, so much so that it has been argued that humans share both a fear of death and a death wish (Dumont and Foss, 1972). The fear of death was expressed by the poet Thomas Nashe when he wrote the following in "In Time of Pestilence":

> Brightness falls from the air;
> Queens have died young and fair;
> Dust hath closed Helen's eye.
> I am sick, I must die.
> Lord have mercy on us.

Walt Whitman, in "When Lilacs Last in the Dooryard Bloomed," welcomed death thus:

> Come lovely and soothing death,
> Undulate round the world, serenely
> arriving, arriving,
> In the day, in the night, to all, to each.
> Sooner or later, delicate death.

Death is possibly the most important event in life (Borkenau, 1955). It is a taboo topic (Farberow, 1963) that is generally expressed in euphemisms such as "passing on," "going away," and "kicking the bucket."

Disease is closely linked with death. Perhaps because humans feel a need to explain death, they feel a need to say what people die of. In spite of the fact that everyone dies, people often take the position expressed by a physician that "nobody dies of old age," and they attribute the deaths of even the very aged to disease.

A preoccupation with disease is probably second only to that with death as a basic existential reality of life. In addition to being causes of death, diseases are of concern because they cripple, incapacitate, and cause pain to the point at which death is sometimes seen as preferable to the continuation of the disease. Such a viewpoint was expressed by Thomas Campbell in his poem "Absence":

> Tis Lethe's gloom, but not its quiet
> The pain without the peace of death!

Given the human significance of disease and death, it should not be surprising that societies have organized to both combat their occurrences and to interpret their significance. They are meaningful events, and both have become sociological concerns. The main thrust of this book is to review the social response to these events both as a form of social action and as a system of meanings. First, however, it is necessary to review the facts of disease and death. How frequently do they occur? Do populations differ in the frequency of these events and the ways in which they are manifested?

One of the oldest concerns of sociology has been the study of death from a statistical standpoint. For several centuries, efforts have been made to answer questions such as the following: At what rate do people die? Are some more vulnerable to untimely death than others? Do people die from different causes? How does the distribution of deaths affect the population of survivors?

More recently, health has become a more independent concern, and questions have been raised about disease patterns in societies. Are diseases more likely to be found in some population groups than others? Who gets what diseases? Do some population groups survive some diseases more than others? The answers to such questions are important not only from the standpoint of scientific curiosity, but also they are vital to public policy planning. Important changes have taken place that call for societies to shift their patterns of coping.

This chapter will review the highlights of what has been learned about disease and death from a sociological perspective. Attention will focus on the occurrence of first disease and then death, with the goal being to present the broad outlines of the rates at which these events occur, their distribution between and within societies, and changes that are occurring over time.

Before beginning, there are two important caveats. First, in any inquiry in which statistics are central, measurement is of prime importance. Careful attention must be paid to the definition of concepts, procedures for collecting data, and the process of analysis. In the interest of keeping this text relatively nontechnical, we have elected to ignore all but the most central of these issues and to provide references for the interested student, comforting ourselves with the idea that the motivated student will encounter them in demography and epidemiology courses. Second, the language used by sociologists to talk about health problems is more specific than that in common usage. Terms such as "disease," "illness," and "sickness" have distinct meanings in this text.

One contribution of the behavioral and social sciences to medical care is the recognition that nonhealth is multidimensional, having social, psychological, and cultural ramifications in addition to biological ones. The differentiation of commonly synonomous terms reflects this multidimensionality.

"Disease" as used by sociologists and in this text refers to the biological parameters of nonhealth. One organism invades another with predictable, negatively valued outcomes for the host, or there is a breakdown in the anatomical structure of an organism. Such events have been classified and called "diseases."

"Illness" refers to a subjectively defined state of an individual. It consists of what an individual feels about himself. If he feels unhealthy, he is ill, regardless of the presence or absence of a disease. Most of the time disease produces illness, and illness, it is increasingly thought, can bring on disease. The referent here is to a more psychological dimension of nonhealth.

"Sickness" in contrast is a social designation. It is a kind of social status that can be occupied by people who are socially defined as having a disease or being ill. The sick person is one who is treated as unhealthy by others. Such can occur whether or not illness or diseases are present.

In this chapter, the major focus will be on disease. In Chapters 4 and 5, attention will be more focused on sickness.

DISEASE

Although the notion that at times people "have something wrong with them" is universal, the concept of disease is a Western phenomenon. The conceptualizing of disease requires a rational model in which means and ends are separated and related, a cultural feature that developed in Europe during the eighteenth century in conjunction with the idea of progress and philosophical positivism.

To talk of disease suggests that the experience of nonhealth can be objectified. That is, it can be treated as an objective reality that exists independently of human thought or will. When people think of disease, they presume that it is not the figment of someone's imagination. It is real and can be observed, classified, explained, and acted on. How people respond to disease depends on what they think it is, and in this regard the way in which diseases are classified is of crucial importance.

This section will explicate why classification is important by reviewing the process and implications of medical diagnosis. Then the major types of disease concepts that are part of the Western tradition and the causes of disease that are imputed by a variety of cultures will be reviewed. With this background, the epidemiology of disease will be reviewed: its volume, trends, and distribution in societies. Finally, we will explore some alternatives to the disease concept as found in both Western and non-Western societies, demonstrating that the concept is culture-bound and raising some questions about its utility even for Western culture.

Classification of disease

Labels. No human society can afford to be mindless of disease, death, and the brief periods of glory prior to blowing out the candles for the final act. Every epidemic or widespread outbreak of disease produces substantial costs in services and social organization. To what extent can a society afford massive disruptions of its institutions and bear the impact that disease and mortality imposes on governmental routine, agriculture, industry, international politics, and trade? What in fact is disease's proper relation to morale, decision making, and human vitality?

Although these questions have not been answered and probably never will be, at least not definitively, we can put the problem in perspective by presenting the formation of types of disease concepts as a major societal activity, stimulated by disease and death's potential, real, and ubiquitous effects imposed on the social order. If in fact man cannot cure all disease and death, the least he can do is to attempt some definition. Thus societies advance epistemologies, classification systems, and other emendations based on speculation that if diseases are classified or conceptualized under some grand and scientific-like principles, the causes of disease will emerge and the society can take appropriate steps to cure illness, prevent the occurrence of disease, and hold death at bay. Perhaps one derives some comfort and ease knowing that disease concepts and theories about the causes of disease have and will continue to receive immense practical attention by clinicians, researchers, and the informed laity. The reality of these expedients, we believe, may lead to a reduction in the pain, suffering, fear, hysteria, and socioeconomic unrest that disease produces within a society. In all of this, we are reminded of a conversation between Everyman and his visitor, Death. Everyman beseeches

> O Death, thou comest when I had
>   thee least in mind.

After further exhortations, Death replies:

> Nay, thereto I will not consent,
> Nor no man will I respite,
> But to the heart suddenly I shall smite
> Without any advertisement.
> And now out of thy sight I will me hie;
> See thou make thee ready shortly,
> For thou mayst say this is the day
> That no man living may scape away.

Medical practice as a labeling process: diagnosis. The presentation of diseases as a set of social labels is not done lightly. Reflection on the tasks that occupy clinical practitioners in medicine shows that placing the proper label on a set of symptoms and signs is at the heart of medical practice, in which the process is known as "making a diagnosis" (Mechanic, 1968b).

Learning how to label properly is a large proportion of medical training.

The process of diagnosing is one of categorizing signs and symptoms: complaints of the patient, observations of patient behavior, investigation of the patient through physical examination, and laboratory findings (roughly in order of importance, although the emphasis in the training process is almost the reverse). Certain clusters of symptoms and findings have been given names. The physician identifies symptoms and names the disease, that is, makes a diagnosis. The main technical skill of the physician is the ability to remember a large number of these categorized clusters so as not to miss a diagnosis.

The reason for this emphasis on diagnosis is that once it is accomplished, the remainder of the task is thought to fall into place. By making a diagnosis, it is presumed to then follow that the cause of the complaint is known and a range of efficacious treatment is also known. To know the label is to know the cure. As Mechanic (1968b) stated, "Correct and reliable diagnosis is the basis of the sound practice of scientific medicine."

This of course is an idealized presentation that is limited to the case in which there is good confirmation of the theory of disease. In actual practice, some facts can be reliably inferred from diagnosis while others cannot. Continued research aims to increase the range of reliable inferences.

The process of diagnosis is not unique to Western medicine nor are the assumptions about the relationship between proper labeling and cause and cure. They are common in fact to all the practitioners reviewed in Chapter 6. Moreover, there is considerable controversy over the appropriateness of this model for the "management" of certain kinds of complaints.

One area in which this controversy rages currently is relative to mental illness. A large number of studies have shown that psychiatric diagnoses have low reliability. That is, two or more psychiatrists examining the same case are likely to place different labels on the "illness." Furthermore, the placing of a label tells little or nothing about either cause or treatment, the latter being similar regardless of diagnosis. This has lead some psychiatrists, notably Szasz (1961) and Torrey (1974), to argue that the disease model is inappropriate when applied to the "problems of living" that concern psychiatrists, especially since psychiatry treats many conditions that are not always considered to be disease (e.g., poverty, delinquency, drug abuse).

Torrey has gone so far as to suggest that the small proportion of problems that have a physiological base (he estimates 5%) should be treated by neurologists and the remainder handled with an educational rather than a medical model, allowing psychiatry to wither away and disappear.

Lest we overstate by implication the reliability of medical diagnosis of physical complaints, Fletcher (1952) has shown that the clinical diagnosis of emphysema varied according to the specialty of physicians. Also in a classic study, Bakwin (1945) took a sample of 1,000 schoolchildren and had their throats examined by a panel of physicians. Almost two thirds (611) had had their tonsils removed. Of the remainder, the physicians recommended tonsillectomy for over one third (174). Of the remaining 215 children, another panel of physicians recommended tonsillectomy for 99.

Concepts of disease. Specific theories of disease and its causes have developed among medical professionals and lay people alike. In tracing the history of these developments, one can argue for the position that the advent of particular theories was due less to scientific discovery than to physicians and lay people striving to explain the occurrence of disease within the context of medical practice and everyday life and to devise a better method of cure or, better still, prevention for the survival of society. In the words of an early physician, R. V. Pierce (1895:9):

Health and disease are physical conditions upon which pleasure and pain, success and failure, depend. Every individual gain increases public gain. Upon the health of its people is based the prosperity of a nation; by it every value is increased, every joy enhanced. Life is incomplete without the enjoyment of healthy organs and faculties, for these give rise to the delightful sensations of existence. Health is essential to the accomplishment of every purpose; while sickness thwarts the best intentions and loftiest aims. We are continually deciding upon those conditions which are either the source of joy and happiness or which occasion pain and disease. Prudence requires that we should meet the foes and obviate the dangers which threaten us, by turning all our philosophy, science, and art, into practical common sense.

Out of this kind of applied missionary zeal, at least three influential explanations of disease emerged to impress the patient that something active and technical was being done for him beyond the usual prayers, exhortation, and last requests. Pasteur's work blotted out any chance that anything but mechanistic, cellular, and germ theories would gain saliency. Medicine concentrated on microbes, or germs that one could see under the microscope. Furthermore, new drugs were developed to interdict germs, and the result was a saving of countless lives; proof enough, said the proponents, of the validity of this theory of disease. Of course, many of the drugs prescribed, such as tobacco were of questionable utility (Mullett, 1956).

The cellular concept of disease focused on biological changes in cellular structures as the culprit and not germs per se.

Mechanism grew out of a growing demand by patients for a system of cure that could give them relief from the sprains, dislocations, and other skeletal breakdowns associated with an upright posture. For this reason, the early mechanists were called "bonesetters," who suffered the wrath of members of the medical profession during the early 1900s. Osteopathy under the leadership of Andrew Taylor Still grew during the middle of the nineteenth century. Still lost three children in a meningitis epidemic which disillusioned him with orthodox medicine of the day—especially germ

theorists and their reliance on drugs. The mechanists defined the human body as a piece of complex machinery with interlocking parts. Disease was viewed simply as a breakdown in one or more parts of the machine, and depending on whether one subscribed to osteopathy, homeopathy, or chiropractic, the solution to disease lay in mechanical remedies applied to the broken part. Even cerebral physiology was defined in mechanical terms. In the words of Pierce (1895:119):

The organ representing fear sustains a special relation to the functions of the heart both in health and disease. Bright hopes characterize pulmonary complaints as certainly as cough. Exquisite susceptibility of mind indicates equally extreme sensibility of body, and those persons capable of fully expressing the highest emotions are especially susceptible to bodily sensations.

Leaving little to the imagination, Pierce provided the mechanical drawing of the emotive faculties shown in Fig. 3-1.

A few physicians, however, rejected this mechanistic attitude. Just before 1900 Sir William Osler noted that severe nervous strain, worry, and a sedentary life made people susceptible to disease. Thirty years later, Harvey Cushing suggested that ulcers were related to life-style and the state of the patient's mind. Yet the medical profession remained glued to the mechanistic approach to disease and the human body.

However, as time passed, this emphasis ran into a problem. General practitioners discovered that a goodly proportion of their patients did not have diseases with physical manifestations that could be considered organic and hence as real, objective, and the proper object of scientific medicine. Many problems presented by patients did not have physical causes that could be ascertained through physical, chemical, or bacteriological methods. Headaches, backaches, constipation, sleeplessness, and many more conditions rendered mechanistic or germ-oriented healers powerless to treat or cure. In the words of F. G. Crookshank, "Organic disease is what

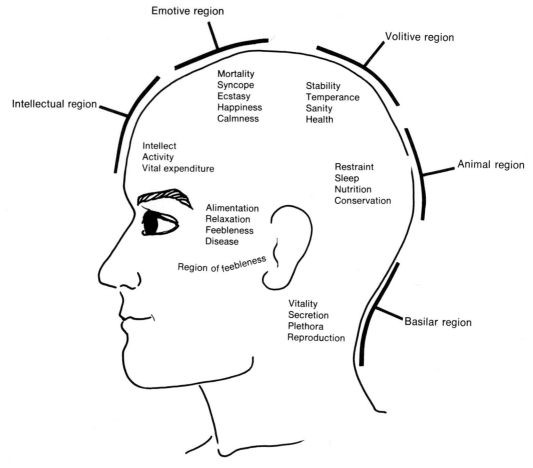

Emotive region

Volitive region

Intellectual region

Mortality
Syncope
Ecstasy
Happiness
Calmness

Stability
Temperance
Sanity
Health

Intellect
Activity
Vital expenditure

Restraint
Sleep
Nutrition
Conservation

Animal region

Alimentation
Relaxation
Feebleness
Disease

Region of feebleness

Vitality
Secretion
Plethora
Reproduction

Basilar region

Fig. 3-1. *Location of emotions as conceived by nineteenth-century physicians.* (From **Pierce, R. V.** *The people's common sense medical advisor.* **Buffalo: World's Dispensary Printing Office & Bindery, 1895.**)

we say we cure, but don't; functional disease is what quacks cure and we wish we could."

Out of this conflict developed what we call the "socioenvironmental theories of disease." Social epidemiology, one of the specific socioenvironmental theories, views disease as a process involving three interrelated units, the host, the noxious agent, and the sociocultural environment. The public health movement today is based in part on the epidemiological model of disease.

Wheeler (1914) in *The Case for Homeopathy* advances the concept that microbes or germs are agents of disease, not its cause.

According to this theory, germs affect only those who are susceptible, whose life forces or defense system have broken down.

The concept "stress" was introduced as an advance in the basic homeopathic concept. Selye (1956) used Claude Bernard's idea that humans possess a homeostatic mechanism that keeps one healthy. Selye argued that this mechanism can break down due to external pressures or internal problems such as worry or nervousness that prevent it from functioning at full efficiency. With the help of the homeostat, the body can meet most of the demands heaped on it, but if the homeostat breaks down, the individual gets sick. Thus disease is stress induced according to Selye's notions of stress. Whereas Selye concentrated on physical agents as stressors, other researchers have included psychogenic factors (personality traits seen as associated with the incidence of illnesses) and social situations. Divorce, death, and other major changes in the normal course of events are viewed as stressors that increase the odds that one will fall prey to some dreaded microbe or organ malfunction. According to these formulations, the level of health one maintains in great measure depends on the degree to which personality is congruent with the sociocultural environment.

Causes of disease. Besides the germ theory school, which posits germs as causal agents, other theories of disease refer to some combination of natural forces, human volition, and social factors as causes of disease.

It is intriguing that almost all these theories of disease explain the causes of disease in part by invoking one or more forces of nature. For example, *curanderismo,* the Mexican healing system, places the natural forces of heat and cold as basic principles of all life. As such, they play a major role in illness, and the forces must be kept in balance for health to prevail. *Curanderos(as)* will diagnose illness as hot or cold and prescribe a hot or cold herb to counteract the illness. Chinese medicine is based on four elements of nature: metal, wood, fire, and air. These natural forces flow through meridia in the body and achieve a balance in terms of heat and cold, *yin-yang.* Foods and herbs are characterized as hot or cold along with specific bodily disorders, and a balance of food and body is sought to cure or prevent illness. If one's body is too cold, one takes hot foods or herbs, such as *fong dong suin* or *bak hap,* great for keeping the lungs clear and in natural balance. Similarly, Navajo medicine men unite in themselves the three learned professions: theology, law, and medicine. Health is found when man is in absolute harmony with natural forces. For the Navajo, man cannot exist without

prayer, and every tree, every blade of grass has its prayer because that is what it means to be alive.

Human volition, or the willing of disease, is held as a cause of illness for most non–germ-oriented theories of disease. Other than the simple act of thinking sick and thereby becoming ill, many healing systems that posit natural forces as causes also hold that man can use these forces for evil purposes. There are *curanderos* who will use their skills to manipulate hot and cold natural forces to place a hex or curse on someone. Generally, this type of *curandera* (witch) specializes in killing people rather than curing them. Usually one pays the *curandera* who makes the curse out of some personal effects of the intended victim. The curse, perhaps represented by a wax figurine on black cloth, is placed in close proximity to the unsuspecting target, for example, in the pillow. Once placed, the curse draws the vital forces from the victim until death occurs or until the victim has the curse removed by a *curandera* who has enough control over the natural forces to subvert the original curse. Depending on the severity of the curse, an indication of which can usually be gathered from the physical signs representing the curse, the victim may suffer enormously. For the most severe curses, the victim usually dies within a few months if the curse is not removed.

Social factors such as social class, lifestyle, and social networks are important factors associated with the incidence of disease. These factors are most central to the socioenvironmental theories of disease. In its ultimate form, the human body is viewed as an individual planet (Montgomery, 1973) and the social environment as a field of magnetic force, and the trick is to manipulate the magnetic forces in such a fashion that each person is free to operate his own planet, unbound by any strings. Less radical perhaps but basically similar, the stress theories may present human habits of life as causes or at least factors associated with various entropic processes of the body. From this perspective, anger and fear can be considered as deadly as germs, since the effect on health can be devastating, and cure elusively rests in difficult-to-make changes in the patient's social environment or habits.

The move away from concentrating on germs per se as causes of disease has expanded our consciousness and put those concerned with the problem in a better position to discover meaningful cures. Unlike the germ theory, which in large measure is unicausal, the other theories of disease are multicausal. It can be misleading to claim the discovery of the single cause of disease. Such an ethos and mythos can have profound impact on a society, even to the point of controlling population mobility and the commerce between nations, which occurred during the many outbreaks of plague in Europe between 1348 and 1668 (Mullett, 1956).

Multicausal theories reflect the changes taking place in medicine today. Much of what is done in medicine under the guise of mechanistic or germ orientations will no longer be needed, partly because of preventive measures but also because diagnosis and treatment of that sort will be semiautomated, with technicians performing whatever treatment is necessary. The new frontier has emerged in the form of diseases that cannot be defined or even described in terms of specific germs, organ, or system breakdowns. Their causes lie somewhere in the community, perhaps in the stresses of everyday life, habits, patterns of human congress, crime, affluence, and other factors. Without multicausal theories, these diseases impress us as irreducible realities, as something one cannot hope to understand. If these so-called diseases of civilized man are to be conquered, theories of causality must be advanced that take the complexities of the social environment into consideration. Perhaps definitions of disease will change so that instead of diseases being defined in terms of the germ or the part of the body involved, one will turn to verified social environmental causes as the

units of these definitions. Thus in place of coronary artery disease, one would have low social support, diet deficiency, and low physical exertion disease, which would include heart, lungs, and several other connected organ systems. This conception leads one away from drugs designed to thin the blood and stimulate the heart to solutions that will hopefully change the several factors in the social environment which are responsible for the disease in the first place.

Disease patterns

At different times and places, different people have been vulnerable to different diseases. General patterns of disease have changed over time. The rate of change has been different for different societies, but all seem to be moving in the same direction. Within societies, diseases are distributed so that some population groups are sicker than others.

Our attention now turns to a description of disease patterns. We will present an overview of major trends in societies and major differentials within societies to find the populations at greater or lesser risk of disease. To do this, some highlights of the measurement process must be given.

Measurement issues. Although there are several ways of measuring disease patterns in societies, the health survey has become increasingly important in recent years. Other methods of data collection such as the reporting of notifiable communicable diseases to public authorities or the gathering of evidence through autopsy findings, for example, are important and may often be used to supplement survey findings. Such approaches are usually designed to answer other kinds of questions, however, and are not suited to describe the experience of entire populations. Although the health survey is a superior instrument for studying the incidence and prevalence of disease, it is deficient as a source of information because it is so recent. In fact, it was not until little more than a decade ago

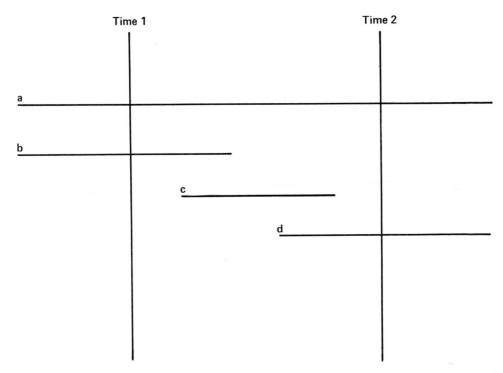

Fig. 3-2. *Disease patterns in relation to time, illustrating concepts of incidence and prevalence.*

that good national data were gathered on a regular basis for any country.

The key methodological issues then are the defintion of incidence and prevalance and the use of health surveys to gather information.

Incidence and prevalence. The terms "incidence" and "prevalence" refer to the way in which disease is measured relative to a specified period of observation. Incidence refers to the number of new cases of a particular disease (or group of diseases) during that time period. Prevalence refers to the number of cases present during that period. The time period used is almost always a year, but this can vary from one study to another.

These concepts may be more clearly visualized with the diagram shown in Fig. 3-2. Two upright bars represent the beginning and the end of a period of time. The horizontal lines represent discrete illness experiences, with the onset of symptoms at the left side of the line and the termina-

tion of symptoms at the right. As can be seen, disease experiences can relate to the time period in four ways: they can begin before the beginning of the time period and continue through to end after the time period is over *(a)*, they can begin before the time period starts and end during the time period *(b)*, they can begin and end within the time period *(c)*, or they can begin during the time period and end after the time period is over *(d)*. Diseases represented by all four lines would be counted to make a measure of prevalence because all existed during the time period being measured. An incidence measure, however, would count only those diseases represented by lines *c* and *d* because these are the only ones that show new diseases starting during the time period.

Several observations can be made regarding Fig. 3-2. First, measures of incidence and prevalence provide answers to different questions. If the question is how many people *are* sick during a period of time, the preferred measure is that of prevalence. If, on the other hand, the question is how many people *get* sick during that period, the incidence measure is preferred. Second, for both acute and chronic disease, and more so for the latter, prevalence rates tend to be accumulative. They reflect old cases plus new cases of the disease. Third, prevalence figures will always be higher than will incidence figures. Finally, the measures are probably appropriate for different types of disease. Chronic disease, because it is long-term, is better described with prevalence measures, whereas acute disease is better described with incidence measures.

Clearly it makes a difference whether the measure of disease is an incidence or a prevalence measure, and it is important for students to be always conscious of which they are examining. Much as we distrust statements that any research or interpretation procedure should "never" or "always" be done, we come close to being comfortable with saying that incidence figures must always be compared with other incidence figures and likewise for prevalence figures. Incidence figures cannot directly be compared with prevalence. That would be mixing apples and oranges.

Health surveys. In 1838 Chadwick (1842) surveyed the working class population of Great Britain to find the "chief removable circumstances affecting the health of the poorer classes of the population." His survey was of expert witnesses, but it attempted statistical summaries with an eye to influencing national legislation. In 1850 Lemuel Shattuck surveyed the records of the Commonwealth of Massachusetts. His report reviewed developments in public health and reported on a sanitary survey. Calling attention to the progress made in the state, he opined, "Cleanliness may be next to Godliness, but it is often its rival; we have built drains instead of cathedrals."

These efforts aside, the first modern health survey was not carried out until 1926 when the United States Public Health Service (USPHS) studied 7,500 families in Hagerstown, Maryland (Sydenstricker,

1926). An attempt was made to determine the amount of sickness over the preceding five-year period. Since this was the first use of modern sampling methods, it was the first study to produce reliable estimates of morbidity.

In the 1930s Johns Hopkins University surveyed the Eastern Health District of Baltimore, and between 1935 and 1937 the USPHS surveyed a national sample of 40,000 individuals in what has come to be known as the First National Health Survey (Perrot et al., 1939; Downes and Collins, 1940).

Great Britain carried out a sickness survey between 1944 and 1951 and began a program for regular sampling of hospital inpatients in 1949 and a national cancer registration program in 1945. Between 1951 and 1954 Denmark carried out a national morbidity survey (Lindhardt, 1959).

With the exception of the hospital inpatient and cancer registration programs in Great Britain, all these efforts were one-shot surveys. Each provided valuable snapshots of patterns of disease at single points of time; none was devised in a way that allowed for the examination of disease trends over time. However, for both the data generated and the refinement of methods, these surveys were valuable in their own rights. Equally important, they provided information that led to the establishment of a continuous National Health Survey in the United States beginning in 1956.

The National Health Survey conducted by the USPHS is the source for almost all the information that has been obtained about trends in disease. It is the first and only continuous survey of a population. It deserves some comment.

The National Health Survey was legislated into existence on July 3, 1956, in response to a felt need for better information to be used in planning and evaluating health services in the United States. In the language of the act passed by Congress (National Center for Health Statistics, 1963):

The Congress hereby finds and declares—
1. that the latest information on the num-

ber and relevant characteristics of persons in the country suffering from heart disease, cancer, diabetes, arthritis, and rheumatism, and other diseases, injuries, and handicapping conditions is now seriously out of date; and

2. that periodic inventories providing reasonably current information on these matters are urgently needed for purposes such as (a) appraisal of the true state of health of our population (including both adults and children), (b) adequate planning of any programs to improve their health, (c) research in the field of chronic diseases, and (d) measurement of the numbers of persons in the working ages so disabled as to be unable to perform gainful work.

This legislation created three major data collection activities. A *health interview survey* was launched on July 1, 1957, collecting data from a national household sample on illness and disability. In April, 1961, a *health examination survey* began physical examinations on a subsample of the interview respondents, providing the first national data on measured disease and allowing comparison of interview with examination findings. A year later, in April, 1962, a *health records survey* was started, which abstracted information from hospitals and nursing homes on length of stay, costs, and

the characteristics of patients receiving institutionalized care. These three surveys have been conducted on a monthly basis since their inception, providing a source of information for assessing levels and trends in illness and disease and sickness in the United States. Unless otherwise identified, the following findings come from these surveys.

Distribution of disease in populations. Because of the short time period for which data have been collected, it is not possible to say with certainty whether there have been any significant long-range trends in either the incidence or prevalence of disease in general. At the same time, it is certain that disease does not strike at random in any society. Some people are more vulnerable to disease than others. Age, sex, race, socioeconomic status, and place of residence are among the factors that influence the incidence and prevalence of disease.

Differential incidence and prevalence. Data collected in the National Health Survey and from other sources support the following propositions:

1. *The older people get the less likely they are to catch an acute disease and the more likely they are to have a chronic disease.* The incidence of acute disease is high

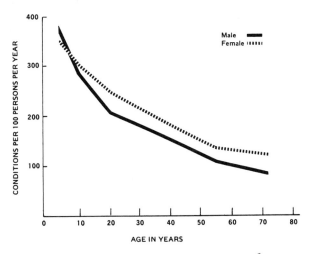

Fig. 3-3. *Incidence of acute conditions per 100 persons per year by age and sex: United States, 1970-1971.* (From USPHS, publication 1000, series 10, no. 82, p. 5, 1973.)

Table 3-1. Extent of chronic illness and activity limitation among persons age 17+ years in labor force, by occupational category, age and sex: United States, July, 1961–June, 1963*

| Occupational category, age, and sex | Number per 1,000 persons in labor force | | | | |
| | Persons with 1+ chronic conditions | | Persons with limitation due to | | |
	Total	With limitation of activity	Heart conditions	Arthritis or rheumatism	Orthopedic impairment
All occupations	523.9	109.9	14.5	12.1	26.5
All persons in labor force					
White-collar workers	529.2	92.0	14.7	8.7	19.9
Blue-collar workers	503.2	104.9	11.3	11.0	28.8
Service workers	550.7	138.5	17.7	17.4	30.6
Farm workers	589.9	213.4	27.6	33.3	52.4
Age					
17-44 years					
White-collar workers	476.9	62.1	5.1	3.1	17.5
Blue-collar workers	444.2	72.0	3.9	4.3	24.8
Service workers	465.7	91.1	6.2	5.4	23.7
Farm workers	447.1	105.8	8.6	4.8	33.8
45-64 years					
White-collar workers	595.5	122.8	24.7	14.9	22.7
Blue-collar workers	592.7	149.5	21.6	20.3	34.7
Service workers	639.3	181.2	30.2	29.6	40.9
Farm workers	697.1	261.8	37.6	47.9	63.9
65+ years					
White-collar workers	712.4	267.9	66.1	33.1	30.9
Blue-collar workers	715.8	282.9	49.1	45.2	45.2
Service workers	722.6	268.6	38.0	45.3	29.2
Farm workers	809.1	491.1	69.6	101.4	89.5
Sex					
Male					
White-collar workers	537.3	106.9	19.9	8.1	24.6
Blue-collar workers	499.8	106.1	11.8	10.6	31.7
Service workers	498.1	142.6	21.6	10.2	35.6
Farm workers	590.0	219.0	28.3	34.1	54.8
Female					
White-collar workers	518.8	73.1	8.1	9.4	14.1
Blue-collar workers	519.7	98.6	8.8	13.4	15.0
Service workers	578.1	136.2	15.4	21.3	27.9
Farm workers	589.6	175.4	20.5	29.9	35.4

*From USPHS, publication 1000, series 10, no. 21, p. 13, 1965.

at the younger ages and declines with advancing age (Fig. 3-3). The converse is true of the prevalence of chronic disease, which increases with advancing age (Table 3-1). Although it is true that anyone can get either an acute or chronic disease at any age, the notion that disease is no respecter of age is statistically untrue. Relatively speaking, different kinds of disease are respecters of different ages. This means that different age groups have different kinds of experience with disease. The young are

Table 3-2. Unadjusted and age-adjusted percent of persons with chronic conditions and with associated limitation of activity by color and family income: United States, July, 1965–June, 1967*

Family income, chronic conditions, and limitation of activity	Unadjusted (percent) White	Unadjusted (percent) Non-white	Age-adjusted (percent) White	Age-adjusted (percent) Non-white
All incomes†				
1+ chronic conditions	50.8	39.9	50.2	44.4
3+ chronic conditions	14.7	10.5	14.3	13.1
Limitation of activity	11.5	11.2	11.2	13.8
Under $3,000				
1+ chronic conditions	66.7	46.5	53.3	49.1
3+ chronic conditions	31.7	16.9	19.3	17.7
Limitation of activity	29.6	18.1	18.2	18.6
$3,000-$6,999				
1+ chronic conditions	48.8	35.9	49.5	42.6
3+ chronic conditions	13.6	7.2	14.1	10.6
Limitation of activity	11.0	7.8	11.4	11.6
$7,000 and over				
1+ chronic conditions	48.4	36.6	50.5	40.4
3+ chronic conditions	11.0	6.0	12.6	8.0
Limitation of activity	7.1	5.8	9.1	8.5

*From U.S. Public Health Service, publication 1000, series 10, no. 56.
†Includes unknown family income.

more likely to experience short, intense episodes of acute conditions that may be incapacitating but are quickly over. The elderly have long-drawn-out chronic diseases, many of which can be controlled but not cured.

2. *Women have more acute and less chronic disease than men.* Females 10 years of age have consistently reported a larger number of acute conditions than have males of comparable ages (Fig. 3-3), and men over the age of 17 years have reported a higher prevalence of disabling chronic disease (Table 3-1). However, some controversy about these figures exists, which should be noted.

Wilson (1970) suggests that the data may reflect only a tendency of women to report more illness in an interview. He contends that the macho ethic of males leads them to downplay symptoms and to underreport disease. Although there are no data to test

Table 3-3. Leading notifiable diseases among Native Americans,* 1962†

Disease	Rate per 100,000 population Native American†	Rate per 100,000 population All races (United States)
Gastroenteritis	4,988	—
Otitis media	4,007	—
Pneumonia	3,107	—
Measles	1,418	262
Strep throat	1,185	170
Influenza	1,143	—
Trachoma	1,060	—
Gonorrhea	797	142
Dysentery‡	292	8
Chickenpox	458	155
Tuberculosis (United States rate for 1961)	263	37

*Excludes Alaska native.
†From United States Department of Health, Education, and Welfare: Indian poverty and Indian health. *Indicators,* March, 1964.
‡Comparable data for Native Americans and all races available only for bacillary and amebic dysentery. Total Native-American rate of 706 includes "all other forms" of dysentery.

this notion completely, results of the health examination survey are not subject to differential reporting, and those data show higher rates among women for the following chronic conditions: definite heart disease, definite hypertension, definite and probable rheumatoid arthritis, moderate or severe osteoarthritis, poor visual acuity, poor hearing sensitivity, and so-called nervous breakdowns.[1] The only disease entity reported from the examination survey that shows higher rates among men is definite coronary heart disease.[2] Our conclusion is that the sex differential is real.

3. *Nonwhite populations have less but more serious disease than white populations.* With statistical controls on income and age, nonwhites have a higher prevalence of activity limitation from chronic disease (Table 3-2). This means that the differences are not simply an artifact of the fact that nonwhites, 90% of whom are black, tend to be both younger and poorer than whites. No comparable figures have been published for acute disease.

A special survey of Native American reservations carried out by the USPHS in 1962 found an incidence of acute illness many times greater than for the United States population at large (Table 3-3). The high disease rate was related to overcrowding, poor water supply, and poor sewage treatment on the Native American reservations. Over half the Native Americans lived in one- or two-room homes, almost three fourths used potentially contaminated water supplies, and 8 out of 10 were without adequate sewage treatment facilities.

The race differentials probably reflect two factors: (1) for some illnesses there is a genetic component that is linked to race, and (2) minority status is associated with discrimination in areas related to health. In general, the second factor is more important, since similar patterns can be found relative to white Appalachian minorities in United States cities and Asian minorities in Great Britain.

4. *The higher the socioeconomic status of a population the higher the incidence of acute disease and the lower the prevalence of chronic disease.* The major exception to this generalization is for those in extreme poverty, most of whom are not in the labor force and hence do not show up in the statistics on occupational differentials. When the data are adjusted for age differences, those with higher income have a higher incidence of acute conditions, except for those making less than $2,000 per year (Fig. 3-4); and white-collar workers have a higher incidence than do blue-collar workers, with the highest incidence among service workers (Fig. 3-5).

Chronic conditions severe enough to limit normal activities show the reverse association, whether one looks at income, education, or occupation (Tables 3-1, 3-4, and 3-5).

There is reason to treat the data on acute illness and socioeconomic status with some caution, since there are grounds for suspecting that symptoms are more likely to be treated as "normal" among low status populations and are less likely to be reported as diseases. The reasons for this caution will be elaborated in the next chapter.

5. *The more rural the place of residence the lower the incidence of acute disease and the higher the prevalence of chronic disease.* Incidence rates for acute disease are highest among persons living in large cities and become progressively lower approaching the farm populations (Table 3-6). The percentage of persons with activity limitation due to chronic disease is highest in nonfarm areas outside metropolitan regions and lowest in suburbs of central cities (Table 3-5).

6. *In the United States, both the incidence of acute disease and the prevalence of chronic disease are higher in the South and West than in the Northeast and North Central regions* (Tables 3-5 and 3-6).

7. *International comparisons of the United States with Sweden and England suggest that disease rates are roughly comparable among European countries, but no reliable data are available from other parts of the world.*

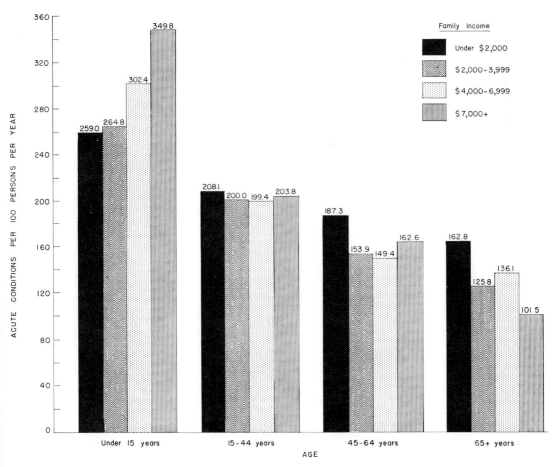

Fig. 3-4. *Incidence of acute conditions per 100 persons per year by family income and age: United States, 1962-1963. Excluded from these statistics are all conditions involving neither restricted activity nor medical attention.* (From USPHS, publication 1000, series 10, no. 9, p. 67, 1964.)

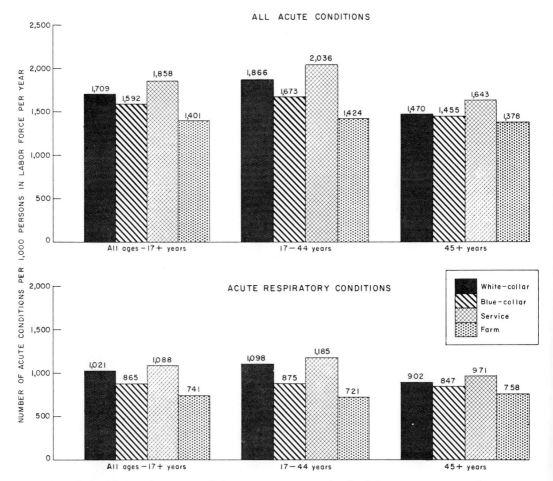

Fig. 3-5. *Incidence of acute conditions among persons in the labor force per year by oc-cupational category and age: United States, 1961-1963.* (From **USPHS**, publication 1000, series 10, no. 21, p. 14, 1965.)

Table 3-4. Age-adjusted* percent distribution of persons 17 years and over by degree of chronic activity limitation according to selected characteristics: United States, 1969-1970†

Selected characteristics	Percent distribution				
	All persons 17 years and over	*With no limitation of activity*	*With limitation, but not in major activity‡*	*With limitation in amount or kind of major activity*	*Unable to carry on major activity*
Population 17 years and over	100.0	83.7	3.3	8.7	4.2
Educational attainment					
Less than 5 years	100.0	65.7	4.0	15.2	15.1
5-8 years	100.0	79.1	3.2	11.6	6.2
9-11 years	100.0	83.9	3.3	9.5	3.4
12 years	100.0	87.2	3.1	7.2	2.5
13-15 years	100.0	86.5	3.9	7.3	2.3
16 years or more	100.0	88.2	4.1	5.8	1.9
Usual activity status					
Usually working	100.0	89.3	2.9	7.3	0.5
Usually keeping house	100.0	83.1	3.8	12.5	0.6

*Adjusted to the age distribution of persons 17 years and over in the civilian, noninstitutionalized population of the United States.
†From USPHS, publication 1000, series 10, no. 80.
‡Major activity refers to ability to work, keep house, or engage in school or preschool activities.

Trends. Although clear differences exist in the distribution of disease within societies and there are groups with greater or lesser risk of disease, it is difficult to say with certainty whether any long-range trends have occurred in the general levels of incidence and prevalence. At the same time, there are important shifts in the levels of several specific disease entities. Cognizant that fools rush in where angels (i.e., data) fear to tread, we nevertheless suggest the following as propositions:

1. *There have been no trends in the general levels of acute disease incidence or severity.* Data collected by the National Health Survey between 1964 and 1971 show no trends in the incidence of the major classes of acute disease, although there were marked seasonal variations in incidence (Fig. 3-6). The generally higher rates for the winter months are explained by the rise of upper respiratory infections during that period of the year.

During the same period, there were fluctuations in the severity of acute disease, but again there were no long-range trends. Data on the number of days on which activities were restricted because of acute conditions show differences from year to year, with no evident trend (Table 3-7). The lower severity in 1966 to 1967 and the higher severity in 1968 to 1969, for example, reflect greater incidence of influenza-like illness in the latter period.

For the longer run, however, there are no data. The earlier surveys did not collect information on acute disease but concentrated on chronic conditions. Evidence from examination of the remains of persons who died many centuries ago, including Egyptian mummies, suggests that the same basic types of illness have existed for

Text continued on p. 70.

Table 3-5. Aged-adjusted* percent distribution of persons by degree of chronic activity limitation, according to selected characteristics: United States, 1969-1970†

Selected characteristics	All persons	Percent distribution			
		With no limitation of activity	With limitation, but not in major activity‡	With limitation in amount or kind of major activity	Unable to carry on major activity
Population, all ages	100.0	88.3	2.6	6.2	2.9
Sex					
Male	100.0	87.2	2.8	5.4	4.6
Female	100.0	89.3	2.5	6.8	1.5
Family income					
Less than $3,000	100.0	79.9	3.5	10.1	6.5
$3,000-$4,999	100.0	85.2	2.8	7.7	4.3
$5,000-$6,999	100.0	88.6	2.5	6.2	2.7
$7,000-$9,999	100.0	89.9	2.5	5.5	2.1
$10,000-$14,999	100.0	90.7	2.5	4.9	1.8
$15,000 or more	100.0	91.5	2.5	4.3	1.6
Family income and color					
All incomes					
White	100.0	88.5	2.7	6.1	2.7
All other	100.0	86.2	2.1	7.0	4.8
Less than $5,000					
White	100.0	82.5	3.3	9.0	5.2
All other	100.0	81.9	2.7	9.0	6.5
$5,000 or more					
White	100.0	90.2	2.6	5.2	2.0
All other	100.0	90.1	1.6	4.9	3.3
Geographic region					
Northeast	100.0	89.3	2.4	5.7	2.5
North Central	100.0	89.1	2.6	6.0	2.3
South	100.0	86.9	2.6	6.7	3.7
West	100.0	87.9	3.2	6.2	2.7
Place of residence					
All SMSA	100.0	88.9	2.6	5.9	2.6
Central city of SMSA	100.0	88.6	2.5	6.1	2.8
Not central city of SMSA	100.0	89.2	2.7	5.7	2.4
Outside SMSA					
Nonfarm	100.0	87.1	2.7	6.6	3.5
Farm	100.0	87.6	2.5	7.0	2.9

*Adjusted to the age distribution of the total civilian, noninstitutionalized population of the United States.
†From USPHS, publication 1000, series 10, no. 82, p. 4, 1973.
‡Major activity refers to ability to work, keep house, or engage in school or preschool activities.

Table 3-6. Incidence of acute conditions per 100 persons per year and average duration of days of restricted activity and bed disability per condition, by selected characteristics: United States, July, 1970–June, 1971*

Characteristic	Incidence of acute conditions per 100 persons per year	Average duration of disability (days per condition)	
		Restricted activity	Bed disability
All acute conditions	210.1	4.1	1.8
Condition group			
Infective and parasitic diseases	27.0	4.2	2.3
Respiratory conditions	110.3	3.3	1.7
Upper respiratory conditions	65.2	2.7	1.1
Influenza	39.0	3.7	2.2
Other respiratory conditions	6.1	8.0	4.2
Digestive system conditions	11.5	3.6	1.7
Injuries	31.8	5.7	1.8
All other acute conditions	29.4	5.1	2.1
Sex			
Male	200.0	3.8	1.6
Female	219.5	4.3	2.0
Age			
Under 6 years	361.5	3.1	1.4
6-16 years	286.4	3.0	1.5
17-44 years	194.2	4.1	1.8
45 years and over	119.1	6.9	2.9
45-64 years	125.3	5.8	2.5
65 years and over	105.6	9.8	3.8
Place of residence			
All SMSA	214.0	4.0	1.8
Outside SMSA:			
Nonfarm	208.2	4.1	1.8
Farm	163.8	4.6	1.8
Geographic region			
Northeast	212.0	4.1	1.8
North Central	197.1	3.8	1.7
South	196.3	4.3	1.9
West	253.3	4.0	1.7

*From USPHS, publication 1000, series 10, no. 82, p. 3, 1973.

Table 3-7. Comparative incidence and disability-day rates per 100 persons per year for selected statistics on acute conditions: United States, each year July, 1963–June, 1971*

Characteristic	July 1963–June 1964	July 1964–June 1965	July 1965–June 1966	July 1966–June 1967	July 1967–June 1968	July 1968–June 1969	July 1969–June 1970	July 1970–June 1971
	Incidence per 100 persons per year							
All acute conditions	208.5	212.7	212.0	190.2	189.4	206.8	204.8	210.1
Condition group								
Infective and parasitic diseases	29.8	27.5	25.1	23.7	21.9	23.0	24.5	27.0
Respiratory conditions	110.0	116.4	125.9	104.5	106.2	121.6	113.0	110.3
Upper respiratory conditions	72.0	77.7	77.1	72.2	61.0	63.1	65.8	65.2
Influenza	33.4	33.9	43.7	28.8	41.3	54.7	41.1	39.0
Other respiratory conditions	4.6	4.8	5.1	3.5	3.9	3.8	6.1	6.1
Digestive system conditions	11.1	11.2	10.4	9.0	8.9	10.2	11.0	11.5
Injuries	29.7	29.9	25.4	28.1	28.9	24.2	27.7	31.8
All other acute conditions	28.0	27.7	25.2	24.9	23.5	27.9	28.7	29.4
Sex								
Male	200.0	202.9	203.4	185.4	182.5	202.4	196.9	200.0
Female	216.4	222.0	220.1	194.7	195.8	210.9	212.2	219.5
Age								
Under 6 years	360.5	377.1	335.3	335.3	327.9	317.3	346.6	361.5
6-16 years	253.4	258.7	251.4	232.6	232.6	267.8	263.1	286.4

17-44 years	186.2	182.1	197.8	173.5	176.9	199.6	193.2	194.2
45-64 years	139.7	145.8	138.3	124.5	125.5	139.5	132.8	125.3
65 years and over	114.8	132.6	127.1	103.4	97.4	100.6	103.0	105.6
Place of residence								
All SMSA	212.3	217.9	216.0	194.4	192.3	217.5	209.4	214.0
Outside of SMSA:								
Nonfarm	208.5	209.3	209.0	188.4	186.4	194.3	199.9	208.2
Farm	169.7	175.6	183.5	150.7	170.5	143.6	167.3	163.8
Geographic region								
Northeast	192.2	210.2	202.7	194.9	188.9	210.3	199.2	212.0
North Central	208.9	212.8	208.8	187.1	174.1	197.4	193.6	197.1
South	198.7	201.4	209.8	180.7	194.9	193.1	204.6	196.3
West	252.1	237.6	235.9	206.1	206.2	242.7	233.1	253.3

Number of disability days per 100 persons per year

Type of disability day								
Days of restricted activity	811.5	832.2	819.5	716.6	786.9	915.7	850.6	855.9
Days of bed disability	345.9	349.3	365.6	297.4	337.2	419.4	377.1	381.2
Days lost from work among currently employed persons	325.4	341.3	370.3	312.4	339.1	392.3	379.0	329.6
Days lost from school among children age 6-16 years	442.0	455.6	462.7	394.2	401.6	487.7	451.6	482.9

*From USPHS, publication 1000, series 10, no. 82, p. 3, 1973.

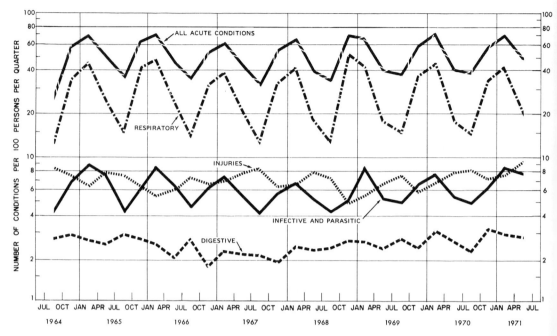

Fig. 3-6. *Incidence of acute conditions per 100 persons per year: United States, 1964-1971.* (From USPHS, publication 1000, series 10, no. 82, p. 8, 1973.)

a long time, and infectious agents have not changed in their virulence (their capacity to produce disease of a given degree). People get just as sick now and from the same types of organism as was the case in ancient times (Sigerist, 1951).

2. *Both the incidence and severity of many specific acute diseases have been reduced,* although there seem to be no trends in the general incidence and severity of acute disease in general. This is one area in which medicine has made an apparent impact. Diseases that were once major scourges have been eliminated or are in the process of being eliminated. These include smallpox, polio, mumps, measles, rubella, tetanus, and diphtheria. In addition, most infectious, parasitic, and nutritional diseases are to some extent controllable by medical praxis. Hence, it is generally true that when diseases are contracted, they tend to be less severe than in past times. These are major changes, the impact of which will be clearly seen in the discussion of mortality.

3. *It is probable that the prevalence of chronic disease has risen as acute disease came under greater control.* Data on the proportion of the population with one or more chronic conditions, collected by the National Health Survey for the years 1959 to 1966, show a small annual rise in the prevalence of chronic disease in general (Table 3-8). The collection of these data was discontinued on the assumption that the trends reflected mainly increased skill in data collection.[3] There is, however, reason to suspect that the increases are real.

First, the population of the United States is getting older. Larger proportions of the population are above the age of 65 years, with the greatest proportional increase being in the population over 75 years of age. It is well established that the prevalence of chronic disease increases with age. Based on Census Bureau population projections and on the age-specific prevalence of chronic disease in 1959 to 1961, the increase in chronic disease attributable to the aging process alone should exceed 20% be-

Table 3-8. Increases in proportion of population with one or more chronic diseases: United States, 1962-1966*

Age	Year			
	1962–1963	*1963–1964*	*1964–1965*	*1965–1966*
Under 17	20.1	20.6	21.4	22.4
17–24 years	37.7	38.8	39.5	43.2
25–44 years	52.4	53.1	55.2	59.2
45–64 years	64.3	65.4	66.2	70.6
65+ years	81.2	82.3	83.4	85.2

*From USPHS, publication 1000, series 10, nos. 5, 13, 25, 37.

Table 3-9. Total population and percent distribution of persons by degree of chronic activity limitation: United States, July, 1957–December, 1970*

Year†	Percent distribution					
	Total population		With no limitation of activity	With limitation but not in major activity‡	With limitation in amount or kind of major activity	Unable to carry on major activity
	Number in thousands	*Percent*				
July, 1957–June, 1958	168,369	100.0	89.9	2.7	5.2	2.1
July, 1958–June, 1959	171,300	100.0	90.2	2.5	5.2	2.1
July, 1959–June, 1960	174,621	100.0	89.5	2.8	5.5	2.2
July, 1960–June, 1961	177,984	100.0	88.7	2.9	6.1	2.3
July, 1961–June, 1962	180,790	100.0	88.0	3.3	6.5	2.2
July, 1962–June, 1963	183,146	100.0	87.6	3.4	6.7	2.3
July, 1963–June, 1964	185,797	100.0	87.9	3.4	6.5	2.2
July, 1964–June, 1965	188,430	100.0	88.0	3.1	6.7	2.2
July, 1965–June, 1966	190,710	100.0	88.8	2.8	6.3	2.1
July, 1966–June, 1967	192,359	100.0	88.3	3.0	6.5	2.2
1967	193,403	100.0	88.5	2.8	6.3	2.3
1968	195,392	100.0	89.1	1.8	6.4	2.8
1969	197,422	100.0	88.4	2.4	6.4	2.8
1970	199,843	100.0	88.2	2.9	6.0	2.9
Average for July, 1963– June, 1967	191,537	100.0	88.5	2.9	6.4	2.1
Average for 1969-1970	198,636	100.0	88.3	2.6	6.2	2.9

*From USPHS, publication 1000, series 10, no. 80.
†The data for the period July, 1957, through June, 1967, were collected by means of the "condition approach." The data for calendar years 1967 and 1968 or a mixture of the "condition" and "person" approaches, since half-samples using each approach were employed from July, 1967, through June, 1968. The information on limited persons for 1969 and 1970 is derived entirely from the "person approach."
‡Major activity refers to ability to work, keep house, or engage in school or preschool activities.

tween 1960 and 1985 (Twaddle, 1968a). Second, chronic disease has been linked with urbanization, and as larger proportions of the population live in urban environments, chronic disease should increase. Epidemiological and clinical studies have linked many chronic diseases with environmental pollution, crowding, and the interpersonal stress of urban life (Gordon, 1963).

Although the prevalence of chronic disease is probably rising, there is no evidence to suggest that the same is true for its severity. Data from the National Health Survey show no significant change in the percentage of the population with restricted activities attributable to chronic diseases between 1957 and 1970. This holds whether one looks at all activity limitations or limitations of major activities (Table 3-9).

Unfortunately, earlier surveys do not help answer the question because of differences in method and data collection procedures. Although there is reason to believe that chronic disease should be rising, the data are inconclusive at this point.

Disease as an ethnocentric concept

The concept of disease is a uniquely Western phenomenon. In other cultures, the orientation is often toward health rather than disease. Although such cultures recognize organic malfunctions, they conceptualize and respond to them differently. Both for its comparative value and for an appreciation of alternatives to Western traditions, a few of these alternatives are briefly illustrated in Chapter 6.

Recognition that the concept of disease is part of our culture and that thinking about health and illness exclusively in disease terms represents a cultural bias is important for another reason. Some sociologists have come to question the usefulness of the concept of disease for an understanding of health and illness. It has been argued that even for specifically medical concerns, the concept is too limited and needs to be supplemented with nondisease concepts. Because this is an important argument that

may well be the wave of the future for sociological study, one of these arguments is reviewed in some detail.

The concept of brokenness. The concept of disease is central to medicine. As discussed previously, the major intellectual task of a physician is to make a diagnosis, from which a course of action follows. It is often presumed that a diagnosis, that is, identifying a particular disease entity, also implies a cause. This assumption has been challenged by Leonard Syme, an epidemiologist at the University of California.

Syme (1966) contends that epidemiology has suffered from an uncritical use of medical disease concepts that are *not* useful in studying the cause of illness. He bases this claim on the observation that much has been made of the differences in disease rates, although the similarities are of at least equal importance. For example, there is great variation from state to state in the death rate from coronary heart disease, which is higher in the United States than anywhere else in the world and is higher on the East and West Coasts than in the middle western states. Lost in this observation is the fact that the proportion of deaths from coronary heart disease is almost the same from one state to another. Similar observations can be made for many cancers.

What has to be explained therefore is not the rates of different diseases, but rather the incidence of disease in general. Syme suggests that all diseases are related to similar variables in the same ways. On investigation, all diseases are related to cigarette smoking and marital status. Migration from farm to urban locations is associated with a wide range of diseases. Hence disease-specific explanations of cause may be missing important aspects of the central problem.

Clinical approaches rest "on the assumption that disease states are manifestations of basic and fundamental derangements of biological functioning," which leads to a "molecular level of explanation" (Syme, 1966). Against this, Syme suggests that we should attempt "to achieve understanding by developing a more general and comprehensive level of understanding . . . it might be preferable in a situation where we have a mass disease being produced by forces in our environment to describe those forces and act at this level. In this sense, the causative constellation may be viewed as residing at the environmental, not molecular level."

The wide range of diseases related to features of the social environment and the theory that disease is a response to stress have led to the hypothesis that under situations of stress, people "break." How they break and to what extent is a matter of great variability from one individual to another. For one, it may be a mental breakdown and for another a physical one. Within each category there may be a variety of different ways in which brokenness can be manifested. It is brokenness that needs to be understood, not disease (Syme, 1966).

In a seemingly independent development, Antonovsky (1972, 1973) has proposed a similar viewpoint. Working empirically with populations in Israel, he proposed that the time had come to "add to— though not to supplant—this focus (on the etiology of diseases) by the serious consideration of the etiology of disease, in the singular." He proposed the concept of "breakdown" to refer to this "global concept of disease" (1972). His attention turned to "those facets which seem to be common to all diseases," among which are the following:

1. A disease always has at least one of two socially undesirable consequences: it is painful to the individual; and/or
2. It handicaps him in the exercise of his faculties or performance of social roles;
3. It is characterized by a kind and degree of acuteness-chronicity with a given degree of threat to life; and
4. It is recognized by the medical institution of a society as requiring care under its direction (1972:539).

Analyzing ethnic groups in Israel, each of these facets was broken down into several categories. Pain was divided as follows: no painful condition, mild pain, moderate pain, and severe pain; functional limitation: no limiting condition, mild limitation, moderate limitation, and severe limitation; condition: no acute or chronic, mild chronic but not degenerative, serious chronic degenerative, and acute life-threatening; and medical treatment: no particular medical attention, medical observation or supervision, and active medical treatment. Combining categories, there were 288 possible profiles ($4 \times 4 \times 6 \times 3$) of which ninety-seven were empirically found. It was possible to rank different groups in terms of general levels of health and to show that different groups had different breakdown profiles (1973). Furthermore, six of the profiles encompassed almost half of the population.

It should be emphasized that the approach suggested by Syme and Antonovsky is not typical of social epidemiologists at the present time, most of whom focus on the concept of disease. Some variant on the theme of brokenness or breakdown, however, is likely to be the wave of the future, in which epidemiology will stake out its own questions independently of medical sector concerns. It shows one area in which traditional notions of disease are coming to be challenged.

The concept of disease is at the same time a rather precise way of approaching the problem of health and illness and an ambiguous idea leading to great variability in definition and application. Death is less conceptually ambiguous but retains many problems of definition and explanation.

DEATH

Although little evidence exists that there have been marked changes in the patterns of disease in the recent past as measured by incidence and prevalence, the evidence is strong that disease has different consequences, which are reflected in the incidence and distribution of deaths in societies. There are good data on mortality going back several centuries, and given the relative clarity of the event, there are good grounds for cross-national comparisons.

Measurements

To make comparisons, it is necessary to make measurements. Conventions for measuring the incidence of death have been developed in demography that have become universal, facilitating comparisons in different nations and cultures. These are largely a matter of definitions, which will be reviewed. At the same time, the clinical criteria for defining (pronouncing) death are in some disarray because of technological advances in medicine, making it less clear when any given death has occurred.

Clinical criteria

Marley was dead: to begin with. There was no doubt whatever about that. . . . Old Marley was dead as a door nail.

Dickens—A Christmas Carol

For many people the days of such certainty are over. The following scene is more frequently found in modern hospitals:

"What do you think?"
"I don't know. Why don't we wait until tomorrow. If the tracings are still flat, we can pull the plug then."

Consider what has happened. In the Middle Ages in Europe, people were considered alive and treated as such until the onset of rigor mortis, a stiffening of muscles that occurs many hours after the cessation of heartbeat and respiration. Sometime before the thirteenth century it was observed that rigor mortis inevitably followed when heartbeat and breathing ceased. Since that time, the clinical criteria for pronouncing death have been (1) the absence of any heartbeat or pulse and (2) the absence of breathing activity. These criteria are not simply medical norms. They have been incorporated into the legal code as the only permissible criteria to use.

The past few decades have seen some dramatic changes in medical technology

that have made the clinical criteria for pronouncing death obsolescent in some cases. Machinery has been built that can take over the functions of the heart and lungs. The most sophisticated is the heart-lung machine, which is used during some forms of surgery where the heart is temporarily stopped as part of the operative procedure. Using traditional criteria, the patient is first killed and then brought back to life, and during the interim a machine keeps the rest of his body functioning. Also intermittent positive pressure breathing (IPPB) machines can keep lungs working, and cardiac pacemakers deliver intermittent shocks to the heart, which serve to keep it beating at a regular pace. Large numbers of patients in and out of hospitals are connected to one or both of these machines at any given time.

The result has been a form of cultural lag (Chapter 1), in which the normative system (clinical criteria) has failed to keep up with technological change. The task of certifying that a death has occurred must frequently be accomplished under conditions in which the legally acceptable signs are mechanically obscured. In response to this situation, the medical community is searching for criteria that can be measured independently of heartbeat and respiration yet is as nearly as possible perfectly correlated with both. The dilemmas raised are one factor explaining the growth of interest in death research in recent years.

An emerging consensus is turning attention from the heart and lungs to the brain. At the Cape Town Conference on Heart Transplants in August, 1968, thirteen transplant surgeons agreed that "neurological examination and electroencephalic tracings should show no signs of cerebral activity" (Denton Cooley quoted in R. Glaser, 1970) but did not agree on the length of time these signs should be present. In the same year, the Ad Hoc Committee of the Harvard Medical School proposed a set of clinical criteria for defining the "brain death syndrome." These included (1) the absence of response to painful stimuli, (2) the absence of spontaneous movements or breathing, (3) the absence of reflexes, (4) the presence of fixed dilated pupils, and (5) the failure of spontaneous breathing when the respirator is turned off for 3 minutes (Beecher et al., 1968).

These criteria, with the addition of a "flat" electroencephalogram lasting at least 24 hours, are a matter of active debate in the medical community. The issues are ethical, as well as technical (Ramsey, 1970).

Mortality measures. As important as the clinical criteria are as legal and ethical questions and as an influence on outcomes in individual cases, it is unlikely that they will affect the distribution of deaths in societies or the measurement of long-range trends. On an individual level, deaths come one to a customer, and death is a dichotomous event. On the aggregate level, however, there are differences in the frequency at which people die during any given time period (death rate) and the probability of living any given length of time (life expectancy). These aggregate events are capable of being measured rather precisely.

Crude death rates. The simplest measure of aggregate deaths is the crude death rate, which is defined as follows:

$$\frac{\text{Total number of deaths}}{\text{Population size}} \times 1,000$$

The crude death rate refers to a specific period of time, usually a year, and gives a picture of the overall rate at which people die in the population unit under consideration. Combined with the crude birth rate, the crude death rate is used to determine the rate of population growth.

Large differences in the crude death rate probably reflect real differences in the mortality experience of populations. Unfortunately many other factors also affect the crude death rate. The age, sex, race, and marital status distribution of the population are examples of factors that can conceal real differences or show differences which do not exist. Consequently the crude death rate is almost never used for comparative purposes.

Specific death rates. Various aspects of the structure of a population can affect death rates irrespective of the risks of individuals. People 70 years of age are much more likely to die during the course of any given year than are those age 20 years. It follows that a population with a large proportion of elderly people will have a higher crude death rate than one with a large proportion of young people, even when the risk of death is identical at every specific age. Accordingly it is often useful to calculate an age-specific death rate to compare directly the experience of two populations at each age. This procedure is much more precise than the crude rate. A similar procedure can be carried out for any population characteristic on which data are available.

The form of the specific death rate is as follows:

$$\frac{\text{Number of deaths within specific category}}{\text{Population size of category}} \times 1,000$$

Adjusted or standardized death rates. For direct comparison of two or more populations taken as wholes, rather than making the comparisons within categories, it is more common to compute adjusted or standardized rates. To do this, one or more characteristics known to be associated with death rates are identified, and death rates are computed for each category. This produces a list of specific death rates. Standardization involves the additional step of applying the specific rates of different populations to the same population, computing the number of deaths that would occur in each category, summing the deaths, and computing a new overall death rate. The result is two or more death rates that can be compared, controlling for differences in the structure of the population itself.

Life expectancy. It is also possible to apply age-specific death rates to a hypothetical population and to calculate the average length of life remaining at any given age. The technique is complicated, involving the construction of a life table, which is a basic actuarial tool for the setting of life insurance premiums. The procedure for constructing life tables is beyond the scope of this text, and the interested student is referred to the references at the end of the text.

With this brief background, the aggregate patterns of death can be examined both in general and a particularly sensitive groups, infants.

General mortality

To describe mortality in general, major trends over time and major differences within populations must be identified.

Trends. In the long run death rates have gradually declined, slowing or leveling off in the most highly industrialized countries in the past two decades. As a result of research on available records, tombstones, and physical remains, it has been estimated that during the Bronze Age in Greece, life expectancy at birth averaged approximately 18 years. At the beginning of the Christian era in Rome, life expectancy had increased to about 22 years, increasing to about 33 years in the seventeenth century. In the early eighteenth century in England

and Wales, average length of life was 40.9 years during the period from 1838 to 1854, and in the United States between 1900 and 1902 it was 49.2 years (Dublin et al., 1949; Peterson, 1969).

The most dramatic increase in life expectancy occurred during the middle part of the twentieth century. By 1960 life expectancy was 70.6 years in Czechoslovakia, and by 1970 it was 66.6 years for males in the United States as compared with 71.8 in Sweden, 68.4 in New Zealand, and 66.7 in Hong Kong (United Nations, 1971).

The age-adjusted death rate in the United States was 17.8 per 1,000 in 1900. It declined slowly and regularly until 1936, with the exception of a marked peak in 1918 attributable to the influenza epidemic of that year. Beginning in 1937 the death rate dropped more rapidly because of the introduction of sulfa and antibiotic drugs to the civilian market. This decline lasted until 1954, as shown in Fig. 3-7. Since 1954 the death rate has held steady.

Basically similar patterns are found in most industrialized countries, with historical differences such as the timing of epi-

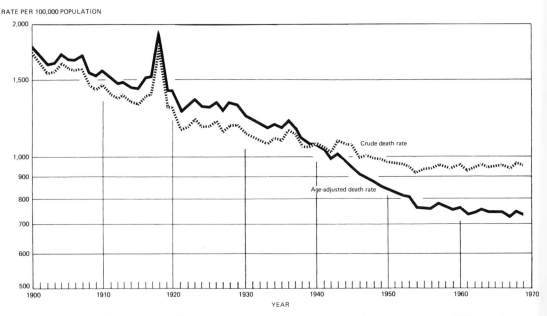

RATE PER 100,000 POPULATION

YEAR

Fig. 3-7. *Crude and age-adjusted death rates: death-registration states, 1900-1932, and United States, 1933-1969.* (From USPHS, publication 1000, series 20, no. 15, p. 1, 1973.)

demics and the impact of warfare producing variations from one country to another. England showed a high crude death rate, especially for males, during World War II and a relatively flat slope otherwise (Fig. 3-8). In Fig. 3-8, the crude death rate is converted to a standardized mortality ratio, which controls for the effects of age and sex composition changes. A similar curve for Czechoslovakia is shown in Fig. 3-9.

Mortality decline is a world-wide phenomenon that developed gradually as a re-

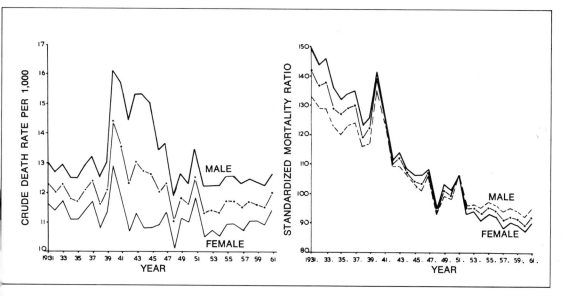

Fig. 3-8. *Death rates per 1,000 population and standardized mortality ratios (1950-1952 standard): England, 1931-1961.* (From USPHS, publication 1000, series 3, no. 3, p. 10, 1965.)

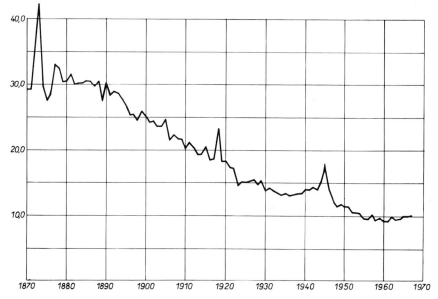

Fig. 3-9. *Crude death rate per 1,000 population: Czechoslovakia, 1870-1967.* (From USPHS, publication 1000, series 3, no. 13, p. 2, 1969.)

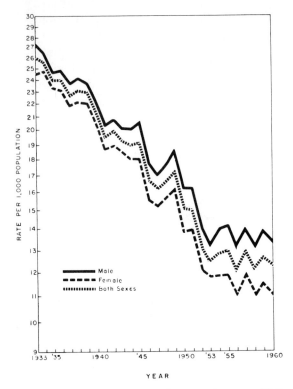

Fig. 3-10. *Total crude death rate and death rates by sex: Chile, 1933-1960.* (From **USPHS,** publication 1000, series 3, no. 2, p. 2, 1964.)

sult of improved nutrition and transportation, which in turn relieved localized famines. In recent years, there has been an impact from medicine and public health programs. The result has been that relatively underdeveloped countries with high death rates have the opportunity to decrease mortality much more rapidly than has been the historical case. The case of Chile is illustrative (Fig. 3-10). The rapidly rising standard of living and improvements in medical care between 1930 and 1960 resulted in a mortality decline much more rapid than that of the United States during the same period. An especially dramatic case is that of Ceylon, where a malaria control program resulted in a nine-year increase in life expectancy between 1946 and 1947 (Peterson, 1969).

Differentials within societies. Many factors influence mortality: inheritance, nutrition, public health, medical care, and environmental risks. A large number of vari-

ables would have to be covered to provide a complete picture, a task which is beyond the scope of this text. What follows is a few items known to have a major impact on mortality and that have to be taken into account in any minimally adequate analysis. Among these are age, sex, marital status, socioeconomic status, and race.

Age and sex. Death rates are high during the first year of life. After that, they drop to a low point until approximately the age of 40 years. Beginning at that point, the death rate rises geometrically. At every age, the death rate for males is higher than that for females (Fig. 3-11).

Disregarding infant mortality (deaths under 1 year of age), the age differential seems straightforward. After a certain point in life, the risk of death increases with increasing age, and the death rates are strongly biologically based.

The sex differential is less clear. It has been argued that it reflects the different so-

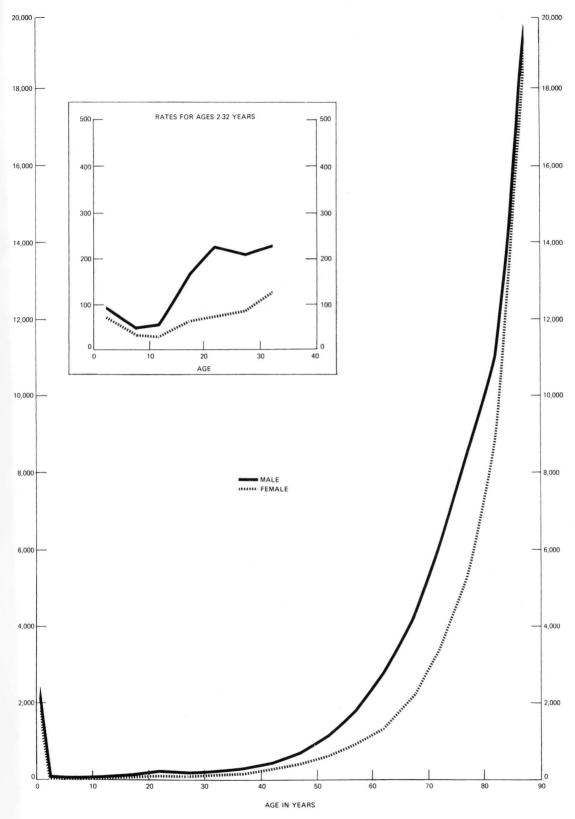

Fig. 3-11. *Death rates by ages and sex: United States, 1969.* (From USPHS, publication 1000, series 20, no. 15, p. 9, 1973.)

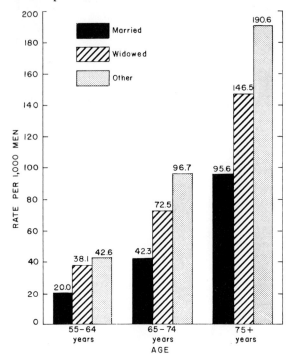

Fig. 3-12. *Death rates for men age 55 years and over by marital status: United States, 1962-1963.* (From USPHS, publication 1000, series 22, no. 9, p. 6, 1969.)

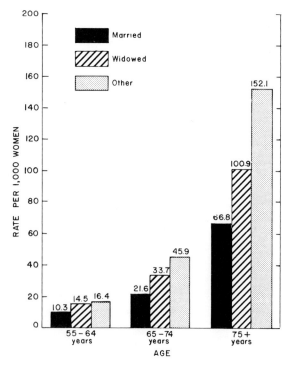

Fig. 3-13. *Death rates for women age 55 years and over by marital status: United States, 1962-1963.* (From USPHS, publication 1000, series 22, no. 9, p. 6, 1969.)

cial risks faced by men and women, primarily in the occupational sphere. However, there seems to be an inherently biological base to the sex differential. Males die at a higher rate at all points in the life cycle, including prenatal deaths. The differential is not limited to the working years. An interesting study by Madigan (1957) explored male-female differences in an attempt to sort out social and biological factors. He compared two Roman Catholic teaching orders with similar life-styles and found (1) that the sex differential was reduced as compared with the general population, indicating that some of the differential is social, and (2) the differential was still present, indicating a biological component. In his review of literature, he found that the sex differential is not limited to humans but is found in other mammal populations as well. For the present, it seems best to consider sex differentials in mortality as biosocial.

Marital status. The lowest death rates at any age are found among the married; they are higher among the widowed and highest among those neither married nor widowed (Figs. 3-12 and 3-13). It is not known why this is the case, although it is presumed that married people lead more orderly lives and have relationships with others that help to diffuse the impact of stress. For whatever reason, being married improves life expectancy.

Socioeconomic status. There is a tendency for death rates to vary inversely with socioeconomic status. That is, the higher the level of occupation or education (there are no reliable data by income) the lower the death rate. This relationship is more clearly demonstrated relative to education (Table 3-10) than in the case of occupation (Table 3-11).

Because socioeconomic status is related to so many factors, it is almost impossible to specify the causes for this relationship.

Table 3-10. Average annual number of decedents* and age-specific death rate for persons age 25 years and over, by education and sex: United States, 1962-1963†

Sex and age	Decedents 25 years and over (number in thousands)	Education (rate per 1,000 population)			
		Total	Elementary or none	High school	College plus
Both sexes (25 years and over)	1,623	16.1	28.7	9.0	9.1
25-44 years	106	2.3	3.6	2.1	1.6
45-54 years	159	7.6	9.8	6.5	5.9
55-64 years	278	17.4	20.0	15.0	13.6
65 years and over	1,079	62.6	66.8	53.8	55.1
Male (25 years and over)	914	18.9	33.0	10.9	9.5
25-44 years	65	2.9	4.5	2.9	1.7
45-54 years	102	9.9	12.8	8.6	7.3
55-64 years	180	23.3	26.2	21.2	17.0
65 years and over	568	73.5	78.5	61.7	63.1
Female (25 years and over)	709	13.5	24.4	7.5	8.6
25-44 years	41	1.7	2.6	1.5	1.5
45-54 years	57	5.3	6.5	4.8	4.3
55-64 years	98	11.9	13.9	9.8	10.3
65 years and over	513	53.8	56.7	48.6	48.3

*Population is the estimated "civilian" population for March, 1962; decedents are the estimated average annual number of deaths occurring in 1962 and 1963.
†From USPHS, publication 1000, series 22, no. 9, p. 13, 1969.

Table 3-11. Death rates for men 20 to 64 years old with work experience by occupation, age, and color: United States, 1950*

	Age							SMR
	20-24	*25-29*	*30-31*	*35-44*	*45-54*	*55-59*	*60-64*	*20-64*
White								
Professional, technical, and kindred workers	124.7	115.7	153.8	315.7	937.8	1893.5	2919.7	85
Managers, officials, and proprietors, except farm	147.7	131.5	153.0	331.4	949.7	1893.7	2894.6	89
Clerical and kindred workers	93.3	128.8	153.0	334.4	961.6	1817.1	2689.6	83
Sales workers	107.0	109.4	166.0	362.7	1097.8	2167.2	3177.1	96
Craftsmen, foremen, and kindred workers	176.7	160.6	199.5	395.2	1013.6	2076.7	3208.3	98
Operative and kindred workers	181.5	178.4	215.9	411.5	1034.6	1942.7	2865.6	95
Service workers except private household	123.6	162.5	235.4	514.1	1378.0	2240.2	2915.8	109
Laborers, except farm and mine	256.6	283.1	358.4	646.3	1451.9	2380.5	3491.5	127
Farmers and farm laborers	249.3	233.9	245.5	363.2	836.4	1631.9	2452.4	83
All occupations	171.9	165.5	201.6	387.7	1010.7	1936.8	2881.0	92
Nonwhite								
Professional, technical, and kindred workers†	246.0	320.4	318.4	618.6	2015.2	4367.9	6038.4	183
Managers, officials, and proprietors, except farm	170.8	189.8	317.6	612.5	1114.6	2179.7	3399.9	112
Clerical and kindred workers	210.2	179.7	221.4	360.5	953.1	1928.3	2336.3	88
Sales workers	185.3	190.3	383.6	544.7	1240.0	2839.0	4401.8	127
Craftsmen, foreman, and kindred workers	184.7	284.0	419.2	630.4	1459.1	2948.9	4169.4	140
Operatives and kindred workers	242.3	296.6	388.2	573.3	1250.7	1869.8	2145.2	110
Service workers except private household	288.3	390.8	533.2	836.4	1802.1	3253.5	3791.6	161
Laborers, except farm and mine	591.6	697.0	954.5	1513.7	2917.6	4983.7	6170.9	276
Farmers and farm laborers	471.8	558.0	701.8	904.9	2014.7	3638.1	5040.9	190
All occupations	371.1	439.9	589.6	874.7	1872.2	3323.3	4276.5	174

*From Mechanic, D. *Medical sociology: a selective view.* New York: The Free Press, 1968, pp. 250-251. Modified from National Vital Statistics Division. *Mortality by occupation and industry among men 20 to 64 years of age, U.S.,* 1950. Special Reports, **53**(2), Sept., 1962.
†Data for the nonwhite professional class are based on very small numbers. The degree of possible error in this category is large.

Table 3-12. Average annual number of decedents and age-specific death rates for persons age 25 years and over, by education and color: United States, 1962-1963*

Color and age	Decedents 25 years and over (number in thousands)	Education (rate per 1,000 population)			
		Total	Elementary or none	High school	College plus
All persons (25 years and over)	1,623	16.1	28.7	9.0	9.1
25-44 years	106	2.3	3.6	2.1	1.6
45-54 years	159	7.6	9.8	6.5	5.9
55-64 years	278	17.4	20.0	15.0	13.6
65 years and over	1,079	62.6	66.8	53.8	55.1
White (25 years and over)	1,443	15.9	28.6	9.2	9.0
25-44 years	81	2.0	2.7	2.0	1.5
45-54 years	131	6.9	9.0	6.1	5.4
55-64 years	237	16.3	18.4	14.6	13.4
65 years and over	993	62.5	66.6	54.5	55.0
Nonwhite (25 years and over)	180	17.9	25.9	7.7	10.7
25-44 years	25	4.8	6.7	3.6	3.8
45-54 years	28	13.5	13.7	12.2	16.8
55-64 years	41	28.6	30.8	21.4	21.6
65 years and over	86	64.6	68.7	34.3	58.9

*From USPHS, publication 1000, series 22, no. 9, p. 13, 1969.

Table 3-13. Expectation of life at selected ages, by color and sex: United States, 1971*

Age	Total			White			All other		
	Both sexes	Male	Female	Both sexes	Male	Female	Both sexes	Male	Female
0	71.0	67.4	74.8	71.9	68.3	75.6	65.2	61.2	69.3
1	71.4	67.9	75.1	72.1	68.6	75.8	66.2	62.3	70.2
5	67.6	64.1	71.3	68.3	64.8	72.0	62.5	58.6	66.5
10	62.8	59.2	66.4	63.5	60.0	67.1	57.6	53.7	61.6
15	57.9	54.4	61.5	58.6	55.1	62.2	52.8	48.9	56.7
20	53.2	49.8	56.7	53.9	50.5	57.3	48.2	44.4	52.0
25	48.6	45.3	51.9	49.2	46.0	52.5	43.8	40.3	47.3
30	43.9	40.8	47.1	44.5	41.3	47.7	39.4	36.2	42.7
35	39.3	36.2	42.4	39.8	36.7	42.9	35.2	32.2	38.3
40	34.7	31.7	37.7	35.1	32.1	38.2	31.2	28.3	34.0
45	30.3	27.4	32.2	30.6	27.7	33.6	27.3	24.6	30.0
50	26.1	23.3	28.9	26.4	23.6	29.2	23.6	21.2	26.1
55	22.1	19.5	24.7	22.3	19.7	24.9	20.3	18.1	22.5
60	18.5	16.1	20.6	18.6	16.2	20.8	17.1	15.2	19.0
65	15.1	13.2	16.9	15.2	13.2	17.0	14.6	12.9	16.1
70	12.1	10.6	13.4	12.1	10.5	13.4	12.4	10.9	13.7
75	9.5	8.4	10.4	9.4	8.3	10.2	11.7	10.6	12.6
80	7.3	6.7	7.7	7.1	6.5	7.5	10.5	10.2	10.8
85	5.3	5.2	5.4	5.1	4.9	5.2	9.2	9.5	9.0

*From National Center for Health Statistics. Vital statistics of the United States, 1971. *Life Tables,* **2** (5), 5-11.

Low socioeconomic status is associated with occupational risk, poor housing, poor nutrition, exposure to violence, poor access to medical services, crowded living conditions, and a reduced likelihood of recognizing medically important symptoms, all of which have been linked with high death rates. It is a stark fact of life that chances of dying are linked with location in a social structure.

Race. Race is not separate from socioeconomic status. In most Western societies, including the United States, nonwhites disproportionately suffer low income, education, and occupation. In general, death rates are higher for nonwhites than whites. Controlling for education and age reduces but does not eliminate this fact (Table 3-12). Life expectancy at birth in 1967 was 71.3 years for whites and 64.6 years for nonwhites, a difference of almost seven years. The white advantage is found at all ages from birth until the age of 68 years (Table 3-13). Life expectancy at the older ages is somewhat greater for nonwhites, reflecting

the earlier elimination of weaker members from deaths at earlier ages.

Causes of death. The most dramatic changes have been in the shifting causes of death in this country. In general, there has been a marked drop in deaths from acute illness and a slight increase in deaths from chronic disease (Fig. 3-14). If the ten leading causes of death in 1900 and 1967 are ranked in order of frequency, the shift is apparent:

1900	*1967*
Influenza and pneumonia	Heart disease
Tuberculosis	Cancer
Gastroenteritis	Strokes
Heart disease	Accidents
Strokes	Influenza and pneumonia
Chronic nephritis	Diseases of early infancy
Accidents	Arteriosclerosis
Cancer	Diabetes mellitus
Diseases of early infancy	Other diseases of circulatory system
Diphtheria	Other bronchopulmonic diseases

Half of the ten leading causes in 1900 are no longer on the list in 1967. Tuber-

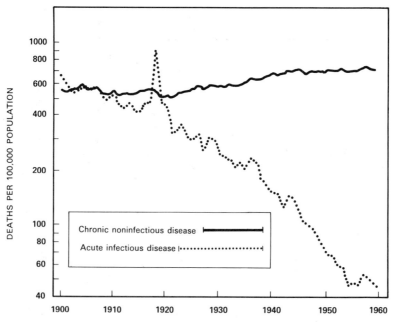

Fig. 3-14. *Death rates attributable to acute and chronic diseases: United States, 1900-1960.* (**From USPHS,** *Chart book on health status and health manpower,* **Sept., 1961.**)

culosis, which killed nearly 200 out of every 100,000 people in 1900 was reduced to a rate of only 3.5 in 1967. Gastroenteritis killed nearly 150 per 100,000 people in 1900 and less than 3.8 in 1967. Chronic nephritis dropped from approximately 90 to less than 0.5 out of every 100,000 people, and there have been no deaths from diphtheria in many years.

By contrast, the death rate from heart disease has increased by almost 500%; the cancer death rate has almost doubled; stroke has held constant; accidents have dropped as have influenza and pneumonia. The four new leading causes are all chronic diseases.

With two exceptions, accidents and diseases of early infancy, the leading killers are diseases associated with aging. The major impact of improved housing, nutrition, and medical care has been to virtually eliminate deaths in the early years of life from acute disease and to replace these with deaths in the later years from chronic disease. In the advanced years of life, the mortality experience of the United States is favorable. In comparison with other countries, rates for this country's leading causes of death are low, and major improvements are to be found elsewhere (Burgess et al., 1965). Accidents, which are a leading cause of death among young adults, show much higher rates in the United States than in Sweden or the United Kingdom, and this country's infant mortality experience is a national disgrace.

Infant mortality

Infant mortality, deaths to people in the first year of life, is regarded as a sensitive indicator of health and economic development (Stockwell, 1961). It is also the largest contributor to life expectancy and hence deserves special attention.

The measurement of infant mortality differs from other death rates. Instead of using midyear population as a denominator, it is based on the number of live births according to the following formula:

$$\frac{\text{Deaths under 1 year of age}}{\text{Live births}} \times 1,000$$

Infant mortality rates are usually divided into the following two periods: neonatal, referring to deaths in the first month of life; and postneonatal, deaths between 1 month and 1 year of age. Neonatal deaths are frequently subdivided to isolate those deaths occurring in the first 24 hours of life.

Trends. The decline in the crude death rate has been concentrated at the earliest stages of life. Accordingly, the decline in infant mortality was much more rapid than for death rates at any other point in the life cycle (Fig. 3-15). The rapid decline lasted until 1955, at which time the curve leveld off. Since 1955, infant mortality in the United States has remained relatively constant, reaching a level of 19.8 per 1,000 live births in 1970.

It has been argued that the leveling of the infant mortality rate is the result of the United States reaching a point near an irreducible minimum. However, a comparison with other countries establishes that this is not the whole story. Several other countries have achieved rates considerably below that of the United States (Fig. 3-16). In fact, figures reported in the United Nations *Demographic Yearbook* for 1970 identify at least nineteen countries with infant mortality rates lower than that of the United States, ranging from a low in Iceland of 11.7 to New Zealand with 16.7 to Hong Kong with 19.6. Although some of the figures may reflect undercounting of live births (especially in Lebanon, 13.6, and Iraq, 16.2) many of the remaining countries have registration systems notably more complete than that of the United States. Against systems in the Netherlands (12.7), Sweden (13.1), and Denmark (14.8), infant mortality in the United States is probably underestimated.

Since infant mortality is the major component of life expectancy, a comparison of the United States with other countries may be instructive. It shows that the relative

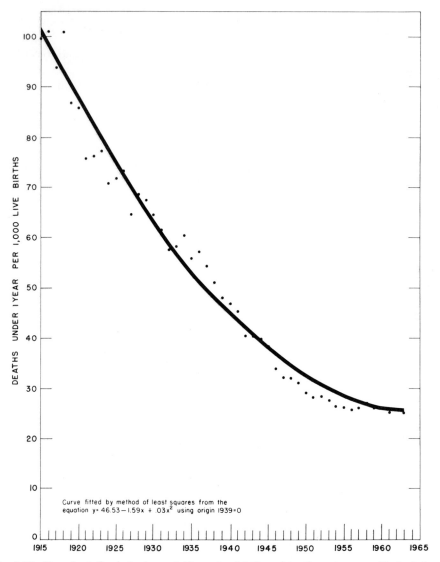

Fig. 3-15. *Trend of the infant mortality rate: birth-registration states or United States, 1915-1963.* (From USPHS, publication 1000, series 20, no. 3, p. 5, 1966.)

rank of the United States regarding life expectancy for males has fallen from thirteenth place in 1959 to thirtieth in 1970. For females, the ranking in life expectancy has fallen from seventh place to twelfth during the same period (Table 3-14).

Distribution of infant deaths. As with the case of general mortality, infant mortality levels vary with age, sex, socioeconomic status, and race. Among infants, however, these differences are much more pronounced. Since survival of the first year of life usually means a long life expectancy, differentials at this age are more consequential.

Age and sex. In general, infant deaths are concentrated at the earliest period of infancy, and at all ages during the first

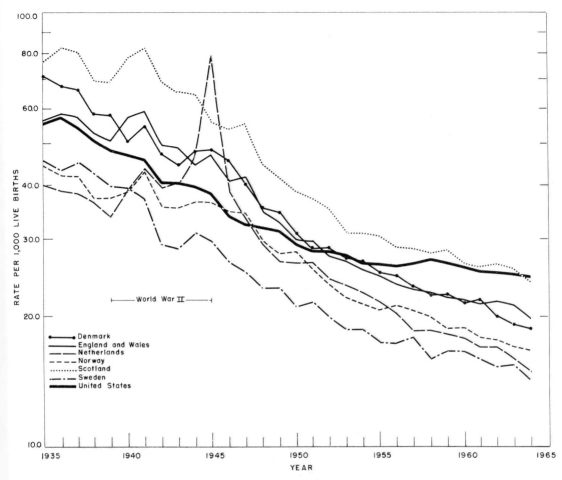

Fig. 3-16. *Infant mortality rates: selected countries, 1935-1964.* (**From USPHS,** publication 1000, series 3, no. 6, p. 22, 1967.)

year of life the death rate for males is higher than for females (Fig. 3-17). In the United States in 1967, for example, there were 79,028 infant deaths. Of these, 43% occurred during the first 24 hours of life, 24% occurred between 1 day and 1 week of age, 7% occurred between 1 week and 1 month, 20% occurred between 1 and 6 months, and only 6% occurred in the second six months of life.

The death rate for infant males in the same year was more than 12% higher than the rate for females (25.2 per 1,000 live births and 19.6 per 1,000 live births, re-

spectively). This ratio was fairly constant during the first year.

Socioeconomic status and race. Low income and low parental education are associated with high infant mortality. In part because of its relationship with socioeconomic status, racial minority status is also associated with high infant mortality (Table 3-15). A study of infant mortality in the United States between the years 1964 and 1966 found that infant mortality was about 140% of the national average when family income was under $3,000, and the education of the parents was limited to

Table 3-14. Life expectancy at birth*

	Males				Females		
	Country	*Latest year reported*	*Years of life*		*Country*	*Latest year reported*	*Years of life*
			1959†				
1.	Norway	1951-1955	71.11	1.	Norway	1951-1955	74.70
2.	Netherlands	1953-1955	71.0	2.	Sweden	1957	74.29
3.	Sweden	1957	70.82	3.	Netherlands	1953-1955	73.9
4.	Israel (Jewish			4.	England and Wales	1959	73.8
	population)	1959	70.23	5.	Canada	1955	72.92
5.	Denmark	1951-1955	69.87	6.	Australia	1953-1955	72.75
6.	New Zealand			7.	United States	1958	72.7
	(European						
	population)	1950-1952	68.29				
7.	England and Wales	1959	68.1				
8.	Canada	1955-1957	67.61				
9.	Northern Ireland	1957-1959	67.44				
10.	Czechoslovakia	1958	67.23				
11.	Australia	1953-1955	67.14				
12.	West Germany	1958-1959	66.67				
13.	United States	1958	66.4				
			1965†				
1.	Netherlands	1956-1960	71.4	1.	Sweden	1962	75.4
2.	Sweden	1962	71.3	2.	Iceland	1951-1960	75.0
3.	Norway	1951-1955	71.1	3.	Netherlands	1956-1960	74.8
4.	Israel (Jewish			4.	Switzerland	1959-1961	74.8
	population)	1963	70.9	5.	Norway	1951-1955	74.7
5.	Iceland	1951-1960	70.7	6.	Canada	1960-1962	74.2
6.	Denmark	1956-1960	70.4	7.	France	1963	74.1
7.	Switzerland	1959-1961	69.5	8.	England and Wales	1961-1963	73.9
8.	Canada	1960-1962	68.4	9.	Denmark	1956-1960	73.8
9.	New Zealand			10.	United States	1963	73.4
	(European						
	population)	1955-1957	68.2				
10.	England and Wales	1961-1963	68.0				
11.	Northern Ireland	1961-1963	67.6				
12.	Greece	1960-1962	67.5				
13.	Eastern Germany	1960-1961	67.3				
14.	Spain	1960	67.3				
15.	Czechoslovakia	1962	67.2				
16.	France	1963	67.2				

*1959 and 1965 from Rutstein, D. D. *The coming revolution in medicine.* Cambridge, Mass.: Massachusetts Institute of Technology Press, 1967, pp. 15-17; 1970 from United Nations: *Demographic yearbook.* New York: United Nations, 1971.
†Year of tabulation.

Table 3-14. Life expectancy at birth—cont'd

Males			Females		
Country	*Latest year reported*	*Years of life*	*Country*	*Latest year reported*	*Years of life*
		1965—cont'd			
17. Japan	1963	67.2			
18. Australia	1953-1955	67.1			
19. Puerto Rico	1959-1961	67.1			
20. Malta	1961-1963	67.0			
21. West Germany	1960-1962	66.9			
22. United States	1963	66.6			
		1970†			
1. Sweden		71.85	1. Sweden		76.5
2. Norway		71.03	2. Netherlands		76.4
3. Netherlands		71.0	3. Iceland		76.2
4. Iceland		70.8	4. Norway		75.97
5. Denmark		70.6	5. France		75.5
6. Israel		69.19	6. Denmark		75.4
7. Japan		69.05	7. Canada		75.18
8. Bulgaria		68.81	8. United Kingdom		74.9
9. Canada		68.75	9. Japan		74.30
10. German Dem. Rep. (E)		68.72	10. Australia		74.18
11. Switzerland		68.72	11. Switzerland		74.13
12. United Kingdom		68.7	12. United States		74.0
13. Malta		68.45			
14. New Zealand		68.44			
15. Ireland		68.13			
16. France		68.0			
17. Australia		67.92			
18. Belgium		67.73			
19. German Fed. Rep. (W)		67.55			
20. Greece		67.46			
21. Czechoslovakia		67.33			
22. Spain		67.32			
23. Italy		67.24			
24. Puerto Rico		67.14			
25. Scotland		67.06			
26. Hungary		67.00			
27. Southern Rhodesia (white)		66.9			
28. Poland		66.85			
29. Hong Kong		66.74			
30. United States		66.6			

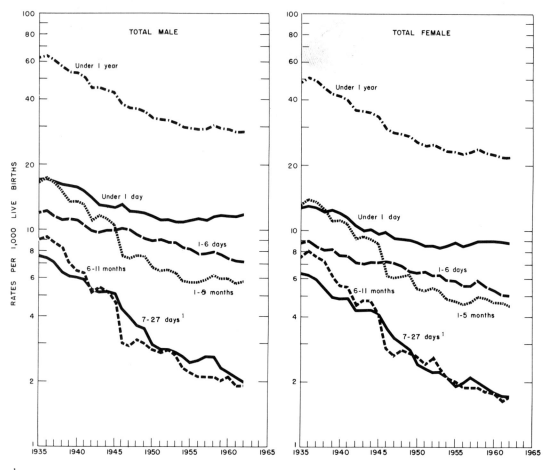

[1]From 1935 to 1948 this category refers to deaths at ages 7-29 days.

Fig. 3-17. *Infant mortality rates by age and sex: United States, 1935-1962 (beginning in 1959 include Alaska and Hawaii).* (**From USPHS, publication 1000, series 3, no. 4, p. 4, 1965.**)

eight years or less. At every income and education level, the mortality of black infants was higher than that for white infants by a factor of more than 50% (Table 3-15).

The relationship between social stratification and infant mortality holds for countries with highly developed national health programs as well. Morris (1963) shows that the higher the social class (measured by the Registrar General's classification of occupations) the lower the infant mortality in Scotland, for example (Fig. 3-18).

A survey of Native-American reservations in the United States, published in 1964,

clearly shows some reasons for the linkage between socioeconomic status and infant mortality. As a group, Native Americans are woefully poverty stricken, and between 1954 and 1962 their infant mortality averaged out to be double that of the white population (Table 3-16). Rates of notifiable infectious diseases were many times higher among the Indians. In addition, they were subject to extreme overcrowding (an average of 5.4 persons per home), almost three fourths got water from potentially contaminated sources, and more than 8 out of 10 had no facilities or unsatisfactory facilities for disposal of human wastes.

Table 3-15. Estimated average annual number of legitimate live births and infant deaths per 1,000 live births by race, sex, family income, and parental education: United States, 1964-1966*

Family income and parental education	Deaths per 1,000 live births					
	All races		White		Black	
	Male	Female	Male	Female	Male	Female
All incomes	25.6	20.3	23.1	18.2	43.5	35.1
Family income						
Under $3,000	36.2	27.9	32.0	22.4	44.3	40.7
$3,000-$4,999	28.1	21.9	24.7	19.2	53.7	38.9
$5,000-$6,999	20.3	15.9	19.5	16.1	29.8	15.1
$7,000-$9,999	21.3	18.2	20.8	17.4	—	—
$10,000 and over	22.1	17.6	21.4	17.4	—	—
Father's education						
8 years or less	36.3	29.7	33.8	26.8	44.7	39.9
9-11 years	29.6	25.1	24.8	22.8	55.3	35.3
12 years	21.6	16.2	20.1	14.8	34.9	28.9
13-15 years	23.4	17.8	22.1	15.8	—	—
16 years or more	20.2	14.5	19.7	14.2	—	—
Mother's education						
8 years or less	37.6	32.9	34.8	29.2	48.0	44.0
9-11 years	31.0	24.2	27.2	21.8	47.2	35.6
12 years	22.6	16.1	20.8	14.9	41.1	27.2
13-15 years	14.9	16.9	14.6	15.3	—	—
16 years or more	24.0	16.0	23.2	16.0	—	—

*From USPHS, publication 1000, series 22, no. 14.

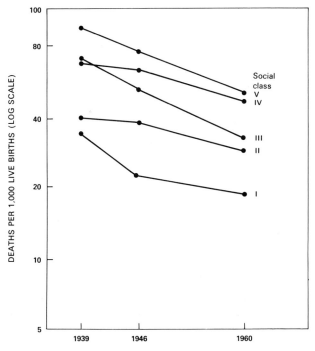

Fig. 3-18. *Infant mortality in Scotland by social class, 1939-1960.* (From Morris, J. N. Some current trends in public health. *Proceedings of the Royal Society,* 1963, 159B, 66.)

Table 3-16. Infant death rates: Native American* and all races, United States†

	Rate per 1,000 live births	
Year	Native American	All races (United States)
1954	65.5	26.6
1955	61.0	26.4
1956	56.0	26.0
1957	58.0	26.3
1958	57.0	27.1
1959	47.0	26.4
1960	47.0	26.0
1961	42.5	25.3
1962	41.8	25.3 (est.)

*Excludes Alaska native.
†From United States Department of Health, Education, and Welfare. Indian poverty and Indian health. *Indicators,* March, 1964.

Causes of death. The concentration of infant mortality in the period of early infancy suggests a relationship between the health of the mother and infant death. Those deaths further removed from the time of birth increasingly reflect environmental conditions that influence the infant in a way more divorced from maternal health.

Maternal health. Two strong predictors of infant mortality during the neonatal period are weight at birth and age of the mother. Birth weight is regarded as being a function of maternal nutrition. Inadequate diet of the mother during pregnancy is associated with low birth weight, which in turn is associated with high infant mor-

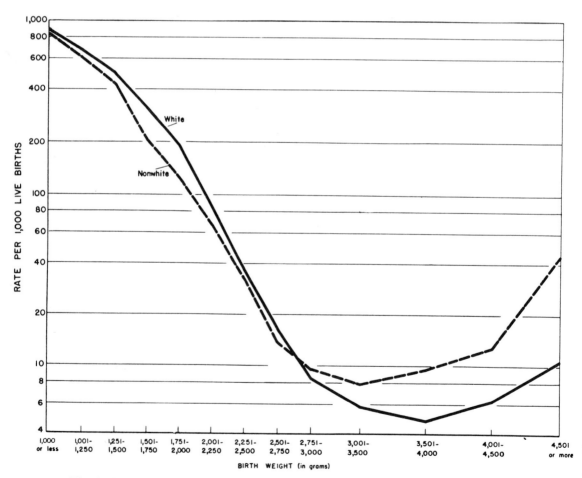

Fig. 3-19. *Neonatal mortality rates among single births in hospitals by detailed birth weight and race: United States, January 1 to March 31, 1950. Weight scale may be viewed as being continuous with the rates plotted at midpoints of the weight intervals.* (From USPHS, publication 1000, series 21, no. 3, p. 23, 1965.)

tality (Fig. 3-19). The optimal age for delivering children, especially for first births, is between ages 20 and 34 years. Women much younger or older at the time of delivery are more likely to be faced with an infant death (Fig. 3-20).

Both maternal nutrition and age at birth of first child are related to socioeconomic status. Low income families tend to have poorer nutrition and earlier age at first birth.

Disease. The leading causes of infant mortality are remarkably similar in the industrialized world. A comparison of the United States, Denmark, England and Wales, Scotland, Netherlands, Norway, and Sweden reveals that the following diseases are among the top five causes of infant mortality in all of these countries: congenital malformations (ranging between 14%

and 27% of all infant deaths); birth injuries (ranging between 9% and 20%); postnatal asphyxia and atelectasis (between 7% and 22%); and immaturity, unqualified (between 11% and 20%). All these causes are related to birth weight and nutrition.

DISEASE, DEATH, AND SOCIETY

It should be apparent that disease and death cannot be treated simply as biological events. Although their biological component is undeniable, the rate at which they occur and the patterned differences in those rates lead inevitably to the conclusion that their explanation requires an understanding of social events as well. Disease and death are thus biosocial events that sociologists and other behavioral scientists can help to understand.

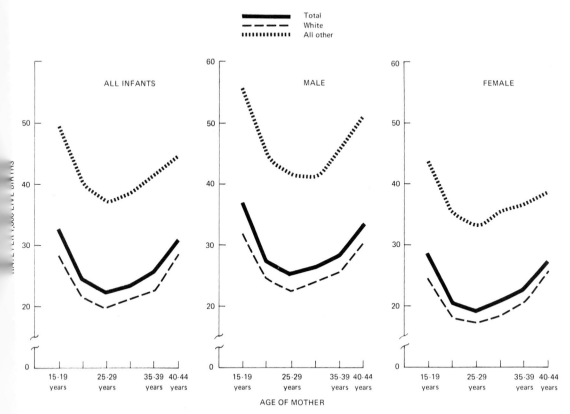

Fig. 3-20. *Infant mortality rates by sex and race of infant and age of mother: United States, 1960 live-birth cohort. Rates for women under age 15 years and 45 years and over were omitted because there were too few cases.* (**From USPHS, publication 1000, series 20, no. 14, p. 4, 1973.**)

Social epidemiology

The sociological discipline that examines disease and death rates is demography, the field of population study. The demographic tradition has as its primary interest the understanding and prediction of population size and composition. As a major component of this concern, along with fertility and migration, mortality study has been a long-standing commitment of sociologists. More recently, disease patterns have come to be a focus, first because of their contribution to death rates and later in their own right.

Modern demographic interests have parallelled some long-standing concerns of a branch of medical investigation, variously labeled public health, preventive medicine, and community medicine. This concern has also been interested in death rates, primarily as an index of the health of populations under study. It has also had as a primary focus the study of disease in populations, especially epidemics.

As social patterns have been demonstrated to influence disease and death rate patterns, the measurement of social structures and identities has been incorporated into traditional epidemiology, producing what has come to be known as social epidemiology. A large scale investigation of social factors in the etiology of disease and death is now underway, the scope of which is beyond the range of this text.

Health and the impact of medicine

Data presented in this chapter are important in providing (1) a picture of the health levels of various populations and a base for estimating the impact of medical care on health and (2) as a baseline of background information for understanding illness behavior and the organization of medical services.

To summarize the first point, there is little to indicate that medicine has had a major impact on disease patterns in general. Although certain specific diseases have been eradicated or reduced, the incidence of acute disease seems constant, with regu-

lar seasonal fluctuations, and the prevalence of chronic disease may be rising slightly. Furthermore, the death rate has been falling for at least two centuries largely because of the improvement of transportation and food storage systems, which has allowed relief of localized famines. The only demonstrable impact of medicine on the death rate occurred between the late 1930s and the middle 1950s, corresponding to the introduction of sulfa and antibiotic drugs.

The major impact of medicine has been to markedly shift the causes of death from infectious, parasitic, and nutritional conditions to chronic and debilitating diseases. The new causes last over a longer period of time and generally occur at older ages. The impact of this shift will become apparent when we discuss the organization of medical services. Suffice it to say for the present that the system as now constituted is well tuned to meeting the needs of those with acute disease and poorly organized to cope with chronic disease.

Disease and death as background for understanding illness behavior and medical care

In following chapters it will be seen that the objective experience of groups and collectivities is an important influence on the ways in which they define health and illness, seek treatment, and organize procedures for promoting health and caring for those defined as sick. An important dimension of this objective experience is their exposure to disease and death, both their own and those of people they encounter frequently. Disease and death rates are an index of this kind of experience. Hence to understand social class differences in the use of medical services, for example, it is necessary to be able to refer to the incidence and prevalence of disease and its consequences for that group.

Disease and death patterns, then, provide a baseline from which we can build, first by exploring the process by which people become defined as sick, the topic of Chapter 4.

NOTES

1. Data are reported in USPHS, publication 1000, series 11. For each disease see respective issues 6, 13, 17, 20, 30, 32, and 37.
2. See USPHS, publication 1000, series 11, no. 10.
3. This is based on a conversation between one of us (A. C. T.) and Robert Wilson of of the National Center for Health Statistics. His claim was that the interviewing skill and sophistication of the center had improved over time and that the data reflected its ability to uncover more conditions rather than any real change in prevalence. If this were the case, we would expect that the trend line would level off in the near future and that this proposition would be testable. Also we suspect that this conclusion was in error. For both reasons, we regret the discontinuation of data collection in this area. Some of The Center's reasoning can be found in USPHS, publication 1000, series 2, no. 48.

CHAPTER 4

Health, illness, and sickness as social identities

A healthy person is someone who has been inadequately studied.

Alexander Burgess, M.D.

Health is a state of complete physical, mental and social well being, and not merely the absence of disease or infirmity.

World Health Organization

Health and illness are primarily sociological concepts . . .

Winton and Bayliss (1955)

We all know what health and illness are. Or do we? A review of the quotations at the beginning of this chapter suggests that many definitions have been offered and several distinct positions have been taken by persons in the health field. Is health a residual category to be applied whenever no disease process is evident, or is it an optimum condition when biological, social, and psychological functioning reaches a state of perfection? Is it a medical definition or is it something that can be defined by anyone, depending on how they feel and how much they can do? What kinds of people are defined as healthy and what kinds as ill or sick? How do healthy people become redefined as sick people? These are fascinating questions, and they are the subject of this chapter.

To address these questions it is necessary to briefly review the concept of social identity and to outline a field of sociological concern that has become known as "label-

ing theory." Against this background we will explore the kinds of definitions that have been offered for health, illness, and sickness as general criteria that can be employed in labeling people as sick. Our attention will then turn to social and personal characteristics that influence whether and to what extent different health and illness labels are applied. Finally, we will look at the process by which labeling takes place in such a way as to convert healthy people into sick people and vice versa.

SOCIAL IDENTITY AND LABELING THEORY

Social behavior is greatly influenced by social identities. How people behave toward another person depends to a great extent on who they think that person is. Who they think a person is often depends on how they or others have labeled him. That is, there is a tendency for people to apply names to others that purport to describe that person, and much subsequent interaction is based more on the kind of label applied than on the nature of the persons involved. One of the more penetrating insights of researchers in the sociology of deviant behavior is that the process of labeling can itself alter behavior, often producing deviance (Lemert, 1951).

Terms such as "health," "illness," and "sickness" constitute social labels. The application of these labels to people becomes a social identity that others take into account in deciding how they should behave, and, as outlined in the next chapter, they are important influences on the kinds of behaviors people engage in. Accordingly it is important to know how such labels are applied, including the kinds of criteria employed in making decisions and the conditions under which these criteria are employed.

DISEASE, ILLNESS, AND SICKNESS REVISITED

In everyday language, "disease," "illness," and "sickness" are interchangeable terms, as noted in Chapter 3. Because the experience of unhealthy states has several dimensions and there is a need for clarity as to which dimensions are being discussed, it has become conventional among sociologists to attach different meanings to each of these terms.

Disease

Being unhealthy frequently has biological dimensions in which there is some alteration of bodily functions that results in a reduction of capacities or a shortening of the normal life span. These events are to varying degrees objectively measurable and can be said to exist whether or not they are recognized by anybody. Such events will be called "disease." By definition, the concept of disease is most consistent with the positivist philosophical tradition, and it is the dimension of nonhealth most central to medical practice. Its identification and labeling are most often the province of specialized roles, the most prominent in Western societies being that of the physician.

Illness

People frequently define themselves as unhealthy because of subjective feelings, and reporting these feelings can result in others defining them as unhealthy. Experiences such as pain, weakness, dizziness, nausea, and anxiety fall into this category. Such events will be called "illness." By definition, the more subjective state of illness is more consistent with the philosophical tradition of idealism than is the case with disease, and it is the dimension of nonhealth most frequently recognized by the sick people themselves. Illness is usually assumed to be caused by disease, and it is frequently the trigger that initiates the seeking of medical care. It is not, however, the same as disease, since feelings of illness can take place in the absence of disease, and disease can take place, at least at some stages, in the absence of illness.

Sickness

When people are defined by others as being unhealthy or they publicly define themselves as unhealthy, a shift in social identity takes place. The people in question carry a new label, such as "sick," "ill," "diseased," or "sickly." Under these conditions, they are treated in a manner that differentiates them from people defined as healthy. Such a social identity will be called "sickness." Whereas disease is a sociobiological status and illness is a sociopsychological status, sickness is a social status. The events that lead to the definition of sickness may be either disease or illness or functioning in the social order. Furthermore, whereas the investigation of disease is the province of biology and medicine and that of illness is the province of psychology, sickness is the unique province of sociology. Also it must be said that sickness is usually presumed to reflect disease or illness, although it can occur independently of both.

DEFINITIONS OF HEALTH AND SICKNESS

Although biological, psychological, and social criteria are of importance and are being recognized increasingly by all disciplines concerned with health, different disciplines tend to emphasize one or another set of criteria and to downplay others. Kaplan (1964) identified this situation as the "Law of the Instrument," formulated as follows: "Give a small boy a hammer and he soon discovers that everything he encounters needs pounding." This means that the more one is trained in one technique of investigation or the more one is trained to look at problems from one perspective the less able one is to think in terms of other perspectives or other techniques. Accordingly, physicians tend to think of nonhealth as disease, psychologists think of nonhealth as illness, and sociologists regard it as sickness.

Although sickness will be our major concern (after all, we should not be expected to break with the pack entirely), one must be aware that not only do these other perspectives have merit, but also they are not unrelated to sickness. We must therefore build toward a conception that does not exclude any valid viewpoint by starting with disease-oriented definitions and building in the psychological and social dimensions.

Medical definitions: sickness as disease and illness

The traditional focus of medicine has been on disease, a label applied to biological malfunctioning. From this perspective, health is a residual category defined by the absence of disease. In recent years, some physicians have become interested in mental functioning, expanding their interest to include disturbances in thought patterns, behavior, and emotional states. By analogy with the disease model, such events have been labeled "mental illness." Mental health has been defined as the absence of symptoms and is also a residual category. The criteria provided by these perspectives are important as core guidelines used by the medical profession for deciding who is healthy and who is sick.

Physical disease. The concept of disease focuses on man as an organism composed of cells, tissues, and organs that must function adequately and in reasonable harmony to ensure biological continuity. Like any other organism, man can play host to other organisms in ways that may enhance or jeopardize biological functioning, resulting in reduced capacity or death.

Given the volume of research and clinical experience in medicine, it might be expected that criteria for evaluating health status are settled issues. There are, however, at least four different perspectives in modern medicine that are associated with different medical concerns. The *germ theory of disease,* which provided the intellectual base for the treatment of infectious disease, focuses on the invasion of a host organism by microorganisms. *Epidemiological theory* focuses on environmental factors in disease and is the basis for public health. The *mechanistic concept* views the body by analogy with a machine and seeks out mechanical obstructions, providing the base for surgery. The *cellular concept* provides a perspective important for current research into the causes of chronic and degenerative disease (Kosa and Robertson, 1969).

The pragmatic resolution of potential conflicts emerging from these perspectives has been the position widely held among medical people that disease is any state that has been diagnosed as such by a competent professional. In addition, the consensus is that criteria should be consistent with the philosophical tradition of positivism. This assumes that there are objective standards against which the functioning of an organism can be measured, the significance of deviations assessed, and health status assigned. Making a diagnosis consists of placing the proper label on the individual. With the patient properly categorized, notions of cause and proper treatment automatically follow.

Even under these conditions, criteria are not unambiguous. Not only are there many parameters of measurable biological functioning that may not be consistent with one another, but also standards of normality are not necessarily fixed for any one of these measures. The life cycle of growth, development, and deterioration provides a case in point in that the same measures often mean different things at different ages. For example, blood pressure tends to increase with age not only statistically but also relative to standards of acceptability. As a result, the measurement of any parameter is often related to age as part of the process of interpretation.

Mental illness. Psychiatry began as a medical specialty using a disease model in which mental problems were seen as directly analogous to physical disease. In part, this was because Freud was a physician who began his work with patients who demonstrated physical symptoms of paralysis. Hence the overt problems to be solved were not immediately differentiated from those traditional to medical practice. It was Freud's genius that he demonstrated that physical symptoms could be caused by mental processes. One result was the emergence of the concept of psychogenic disease and the "tacking on" of mental causes to a physical nomenclature. Another was that the handling of psychological problems became the province of medicine (Offer and Sabshin, 1966).

The human personality was conceptualized by analogy with physical forces. At the base were a set of relatively undifferentiated urges (the id) focused on sexuality and destructiveness. These exerted pressures to act in a manner analogous to fluid mechanics because of the restraint exerted by the ego (rational calculus of results) and the superego (the incorporation of community standards into the ego). The basic model was that of Newtonian physics rooted in radical positivism (Yankelovitch and Barrett, 1970).

Since impulse control is a universal problem that no person handles perfectly, one position taken by some psychiatrists is that all people are in need of treatment. Most take a somewhat less extreme position and argue that the population can be differentiated into those in need of treatment and those who do not need treatment. Although

criteria vary, there is a broad consensus that objective criteria do exist that can be employed accurately by trained observers. These criteria focus more on how people feel, the kinds of thoughts they have, and behavior patterns that may be injurious to themselves or to others (Offer and Sabshin, 1966). These criteria differ sharply from those concerned with physical disease, in which the reliance is much more on objective evidence rather than the reports of patients.

Signs and symptoms. We have overemphasized the distinction of criteria for defining physical disease and mental illness to highlight differences. In practice, the recognized evidence in support of the definition of health status is not unitary for either side. Two types of evidence are generally recognized by physicians.

The first type, called "signs," consists of directly observable events such as fevers, palpable masses, measurements of blood pressure, the results of laboratory analysis, and behavior patterns that threaten others (e.g., assault) or the patient (e.g., a suicide attempt). These signs are seen as objective evidence of disease or illness that fit the positivistic criteria of being independent of human thought or will. They are therefore seen as more definitive of health status than are symptoms.

Symptoms differ from signs in that they are not always directly observable by physicians but rather become known through the reporting of the patient. Symptoms include changes in feeling states (e.g., pain, weakness) or capacities or other changes noted by the patient and causing him concern. Symptoms are seen as "softer" forms of evidence by most physicians than are signs. In the absence of corroborating signs, symptoms are often not held as in themselves defining health status (Twaddle, 1974).

Physicians differ, however, in the relative emphasis they place on signs and symptoms, and these differences correspond to the differences between the definition of sickness as an event defined by the diagnosis of a physician and sickness defined by the reported self-designation of the patient (Kosa and Robertson, 1969). In a later chapter we will show that these differences in orientation have a marked influence on the quality of interaction between professionals and clients. For the present, it is a description of medical thinking against which we can compare other kinds of definitions.

A sociological perspective: sickness as deviance

The medical definition of sickness as disease or illness was for a long time adopted by sociologists, who concentrated their efforts on finding antecedent causes in the social order for biological events. Although this approach has some practical utility, the contribution of such research to the development of sociology was limited until such time as the dependent variable was defined in sociological terms. With a sociological definition of sickness, it would be possible to relate health to other aspects of the social order and to expand the depth and range of understanding of this event.

The breakthrough came with the observation that some important changes had occurred in the social response to deviant behavior. Acts that in the past would have been defined as sin (and controlled by religious sanctions) or crime (and controlled by the legal system) are increasingly defined as sickness and controlled through the agency of medical care (Fox, 1968; Pitts, 1968; Freidson, 1970; Coe, 1970; Twaddle, 1973b; Zola, 1975). The result was to conceptualize sickness as a form of deviant behavior that was directly related to other forms such as sin, disloyalty, and crime (Parsons, 1951, 1958; Freidson, 1966; Twaddle, 1974).[1]

From the deviance perspective, health and sickness are defined with reference to social norms (Parsons, 1951, 1958, 1964; Lewis, 1953). According to Parsons (1958), health becomes "the state of optimum capacity of an individual for the effective performance of the roles and tasks for which he has been socialized. It is thus defined

with reference to the individual's participation in the social system." In a like manner, sickness becomes "a socially institutionalized role type. It is most generally characterized by some imputed disturbance of the capacity of the individual in normally expected role or task performance which is not specific to his commitment to any specific task role, collectivity norm or value."

What this suggests is the following. When any individual fails to conform to a range of behaviors defined as acceptable (i.e., violates a norm), his failure may be interpreted as being attributable to one of two causes: (1) he may not want to conform, or (2) he may not be able to conform. In the first instance, he is likely to be defined as criminal, and the response of others will be to punish him so as to raise the costs of nonconformity and to increase motivation toward conformity. In the second instance, he is likely to be defined as sick, and the response of others will be to treat him so as to increase his capacity to conform.

Health is thus equated with conformity to norms of physical and mental capacity for adequate participation in social activities. Sickness is a definition applied to incapacities, or nonconformity to such norms. Sickness becomes that class of deviant behavior attributed to disease and illness. On this basis, health and sickness become sociological variables and subject to full sociological analysis.

This conceptualization has been somewhat controversial, particularly among those who wish to study the relationship between social structures and disease and those who wish to confine the study of deviance to motivated departures from norms. It has been, however, highly influential in sociological thinking about health and calls attention to a range of new problems for research, including the relationship between crime and illness and between hospitals and prisons. To date, however, no such empirical studies have been published (Aubert and Messinger, 1958; Twaddle, 1973b; Zola, 1975). Most important, this perspective has resulted in the conceptualization of sickness as a social role, which will be discussed in the next chapter.

The main strength of the deviance perspective is that it calls attention to some aspects of sickness that have often been overlooked, particularly the social and psychological components of disease and illness. At the same time, it does not allow a full appreciation of the biological aspects of disease, which have been central to traditional medical thought. It shares with medical perspectives the limitation of being a partial perspective; instead what is needed is a framework that allows simultaneous consideration of both biological and social aspects.

A systems perspective: sickness as maladaptation

Workers from several different theoretical orientations have recently begun to think of health and sickness as a form of adaptation of "actors" to an environment within which action occurs. The variety of perspectives that have chosen to focus on adaptation suggests possibilities for linkages among disciplines broadly consistent with the principles of general systems theory.

General systems theory has three major premises:

1. There is a hierarchy of organization running from small and simple to large and complex, for example, cells, organs, organisms, groups, societies.

2. At each level a system consists of the organization of smaller and simpler systems.

3. The actions of any system interact with an environment that includes higher and lower order systems in such a way that action modifies the environment and the environment, in turn, provides an altered set of conditions and possibilities for further action. These changes produce changes in the structure of the initial system and in its behavior.

Through this system of action and feedback, organization at all levels is in a state of continuous modification and change as each level continuously adapts to its environment (Buckley, 1967).

The application of general systems theory to the definition of health and sickness has not been fully developed. Relative to the medical and deviance perspectives therefore it is not possible to provide a definitive statement of how the perspective works. The work of Dubos (Chapter 1) and recent developments in Parsons' social systems theory, however, suggest some important dimensions of what may well become a dominant viewpoint in the next decade.

According to Dubos (1959, 1965, 1968), disease results from the maladaptation of organisms to their environment. Humans, for example, can adapt to almost any environment without immediate negative consequences, as in the case of pollution. Or a change may result in immediate manifestation of disease that in the long run is one that can be accommodated. A microorganism that is new to a species, for example, can cause disease of epidemic proportions. The disease, however, results from the newness of the relationship between the host and the microorganism. A continued association generally results in an accommodation in which the microorganism can inhabit the host without causing disease (Zinsser, 1935).

With every change in environment, new diseases develop because there are new adaptations to be made. From this perspective, disease is a stage in the accommodation of organisms to environmental change. Since each accommodation changes the environment and each change produces new needs for accommodation, the utopian future of a disease-free life is necessarily a myth (Dubos, 1959).

With respect to infectious disease, accommodations are fairly rapid. The adjustment to changes in the microorganic environment are usually accommodated in a few generations. New manmade changes such as air pollution, food additives, and overcrowding seem to be introduced with little short-run dislocation. In the long run, however, accommodation may be more difficult, and many chronic diseases take many years to show up after the environment has changed. In Dubos' latest book (1968) he expresses his concern that although man can probably adapt biologically to the current course of change, it is likely to be at the sacrifice of much that brings joy and meaning to life.

Parsons' work has moved in a similar direction, albeit in a more abstract vein. In his search for some of the types of problems faced in common by all societies, he has posited that any society must provide for (1) adaptation to the external environment, (2) goal attainment with reference to the allocation of resources, (3) interunit integration, and (4) pattern maintenance at the level of some degree of shared meaning. His earlier concept of sickness as a form of deviant behavior (Parsons, 1958) becomes a concern with adaptation.[2] Although this development has not been exploited (Twaddle, 1973b), it promises several opportunities for advances.

Most important, the concept of adaptation is not limited to social systems, and the relationship between biological, psychological, and social systems is now problematic. Also concerns such as those expressed by Dubos can be incorporated into sociological theory, providing a meeting place between sociologists and workers in other disciplines. For these reasons, we expect that the concept of adaptation will become increasingly influential.

Perfect health, normal health, and sickness

It is apparent that many frames of reference can be employed in the assessment of health status, but underlying these are some common dimensions. Health can be defined in terms of disease, deviant behavior, or adaptation. Paralleling these dimensions, it has been shown that different groups of people define themselves as "sick" in response to different classes of symptoms. For some, sickness is defined in terms of changes in feeling states such as pain,

weakness, and nausea. For others, the important symptoms are changes in capacities such as paralysis or weakness but including the inability to do anything they are used to doing. Others respond to symptoms such as unusual lumps, or changes in bowel movement patterns or skin texture that involve neither feeling state nor capacity changes (Baumann, 1961; Twaddle, 1969). Extrapolating, it seems that those oriented toward feeling states have a psychological frame of reference, those oriented toward capacities have a social frame of reference, and those oriented toward other symptoms have a more biological frame of reference.

Given that there are a wide variety of criteria for defining health and sickness, that different groups tend to respond to different symptoms, and that some people may respond to different symptoms at different times, it is evident that universal consensus on who is healthy and who is sick must be difficult to achieve. Nevertheless, almost everyone would agree that some people are well and others are sick and that there are differences in the degree to which people get sick (i.e., some are sicker than others).

Keeping this variety in mind, it has been argued that a state of perfect health can be conceptualized as an ideal toward which people are oriented but not one they expect to achieve. From a biological standpoint, this might be a state in which every cell of the body is functioning at optimum capacity and in perfect harmony with every other cell or one in which each organ functions at optimum capacity and in perfect harmony with every other organ. From a psychological standpoint, it may be a state in which the individual feels that he is in perfect harmony with his environment and capable of meeting any contingencies while at the same time others regard him as happy and easy to get along with. From a social standpoint, it may be a state in which an individual's capacities for participation in the social system are optimal. This orientation is reflected in the Burgess quotation at the beginning of the chapter. It is axiomatic that by any accepted standards,

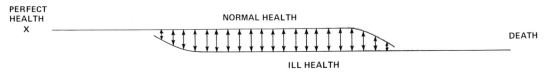

Fig. 4-1. *Relationships among perfect health, normal health, ill health, and death.* (From Twaddle, A. *Social Science and Medicine*, 1974, 8(1), 29-38.)

individuals never achieve perfect health.

Disease, illness, and sickness, on the other hand, can be defined in terms of signs, symptoms, capacities for social participation, and feeling states that fall within the experience of most individuals.

Since nobody attains perfect health and not everyone is defined as sick, there must be a range of less than perfect health that is defined as normal (Fig. 4-1). What is normal for one individual may be abnormal for another, so that there may be considerable overlap among behaviors, symptoms, or other clues considered as normal from those defining sickness. Depending on the number of cultural traditions, groups, and definitions involved, this overlap will increase or decrease.

The two most important points that influence the designation of health identities are as follows: First, to the extent that one must talk about normal health within the context of group and cultural definition rather than perfect health or any other fixed definition, health becomes a social norm. Second, there is a substantial area in which the definition of health and illness is subject to variability both within and among societies, as compared with a smaller range at either extreme in which nonsocial clues are sufficiently strong to preclude the need for social definition.

FACTORS INFLUENCING HEALTH IDENTITIES

The formal definitions of health and sickness offered earlier are abstract, and although they represent some important intellectual orientations, they do not relate directly to observations of behaviors oriented toward defining health identities. Nevertheless, they serve to alert us to some important problem areas. First, health is not easily defined, contrary to first common sense impressions. Second, health and sickness are defined with reference to social norms no matter what specific definitions are used. Finally, a variety of cues may be used to start the process of redefining healthy people as sick. Keeping these dimensions in mind will help to organize observations drawn from research.

Several factors influence health identity, the most important being the presence or absence of disease or illness, various demographic characteristics constituting other social identities, ethnicity, social stratification, and organizational context. It is worth reviewing a few studies in some detail so as to pick up the "flavor" of the research findings, identify additional factors, and appreciate the weaknesses in the research process.

Disease and illness

The process of redefining health identities usually begins with the discovery of a symptom. A person experiences a change in the way he feels, in capacity level or some other change that is defined as possibly indicating the presence of a disease. In a large proportion of the instances where such changes occur, a disease or illness is actually present. If the costs of such a decision are not too high relative to benefits, a problem to be discussed in the next chapter, the emergence of symptoms will result in the person being redefined as sick.

That sickness is related to disease and illness is a commonplace and even trite observation. After all, sickness is presumed to be the result of disease and illness. However, to have a disease is not sufficient to be treated as sick. A person can be sick on his own authority for only a limited period of time, especially if his symptoms are not obvious to others. At some point, the sick person must be seen by someone with the authority to make the declaration that the sickness is legitimate and is in fact the result of disease. In Western societies, the person with such authority is *generally* the physician.

The degree of sickness thought of as legitimate depends on the kind of disease thought to be causing it. It makes a difference how many and what kinds of diseases are recognized by the culture, society, or group in question. For example, in Apache society only two diseases are recognized: snake disease in which the patient wastes away and bear disease in which the patient bloats up. If symptoms do not fit one or the other of these categories, there is little opportunity for the patient to be legitimately sick. In Western societies based on so-called scientific medicine there are over 1,000 recognized disease categories, and people have many more opportunities to fit a legitimate cause for sickness. The influence of these differences has never been ascertained. The potential for significant influence is large, however, and the case for a relationship between disease categories and the rate of sickness is plausible.

Not only is the classification of types of disease important but the presumed nature and severity of the disease are also significant. Is it dangerous to others, is it likely to result in death, or will it "go away by itself" if given enough time? The more dangerous the disease to the person or to others the greater the likelihood that sickness can be legitimately claimed.

All this assumes that sick people are those with diseases. However, as noted, disease, illness, and sickness are not the same. It is possible for a person to be defined as sick or to feel ill in the absence of disease. To the extent that disease is what gives legitimacy to sickness, there is a problem of reality orientation. To what extent are symptoms or other claims to sickness the result of disease processes? The

absence of such a correspondence may deny legitimacy to the claim of sickness. For this reason, some legitimating agent often serves to pronounce disease. Most sickness, however, is related to disease processes that are short term and familiar, and the stage of formal legitimation occurs in only a minority of cases.

Although disease is presumed to underlie sickness, this relationship is assumed rather than demonstrated in most instances. Since sickness can result from factors other than disease, the two are not equivalent, and disease is only one factor that can predict sickness.

Demographic characteristics

Criteria employed in assessing health identities have some general common parameters and are limited by conceptions of the disease processes present in any given culture. There are also important variations within cultures. Criteria may be specified differently depending on the characteristics of the people under consideration. Differences in the distribution of disease by sex, age, and marital status discussed in Chapter 3 probably reflect both the incidence and prevalence of disease and the differential process of definition.

Age. There are different norms as to what constitutes a reasonable level of health at different points in the life cycle. The physical and emotional capacities expected of 8-year-olds are different from those expected of 40-year-olds or 80-year-olds. Eight-year-olds are expected to be more energetic, less coordinated, and less emotionally controlled than 40-year-olds. In our society, 40-year-olds are expected to be more energetic, more coordinated, and equally emotionally controlled than 80-year-olds.

Virtually all standards for health identity shift with age. If a person is being evaluated for having temper tantrums, for example, different conclusions might be reached depending on whether the person is 6 or 60 years of age. A blood pressure reading of 140/90 is not only normal but "good" for a 50-year-old person, whereas the same reading would be indicative of a problem in a 10-year-old. The point is obvious, but it should not be overlooked.

Sex. Men and women are presumed to be different biological entities in many societies and hence require different standards for assessing health identities. Norms for many laboratory tests are sex specific. In many societies, women are thought to have magical properties, and some psychological symptoms are presumed to relate to this special status rather than being indicators of illness. In many tribes and in some isolated rural areas of the United States, women are expected to have "visions" and to be able to predict events. Comparable behavior among men would be seen as hallucinations worthy of treatment.

Gender typing, the assigning of characteristics to one sex or the other, can influence health identity. In our society, for example, aggressiveness, strength, and emotional control are seen as masculine characteristics, whereas passivity, weakness, and emotionality are seen as feminine. Characteristics inconsistent with gender type, such as a large female or an emotional male, tend to be negatively valued. Gender-typed behaviors engaged in by the wrong sex (e.g., a boy who plays with dolls or a girl who is a bully) are more likely to be seen as indicative of a problem needing treatment.

Data on the relationship between sex and disease such as that reported in Chapter 3 may partially reflect the cultural presumption that women are delicate creatures which in turn results in a greater presumption of illness for women than would be the case for men (Ehrenreich and English, 1973). In our society, men are socialized to more stoic patterns and are less likely to report symptoms or to seek treatment (Lennane and Lennane, 1973).

Marital status. Although there is little question that being married is associated with having good health, it is not clear why this is so. There is some opinion that the married population tends to be selective of healthy people and that the relatively un-

healthy are less likely to get married. It has also been suggested that marriage is conducive to good health in that it leads to more regular life-styles, less risk taking, and the like.

The most likely explanation is that living intimately with others leads to more rational health care practices. Especially if children are present, meals are likely to be better balanced and sleep patterns more regular. Equally important, people who live with others are more likely to notice symptoms and to seek attention early in the course of disease, resulting in less disability and lower mortality. Hence married people are more likely to recognize symptoms and are less likely to develop serious disease.[3]

Norms

Within almost all societies and especially within those historically created by migrants from several other countries, there are a variety of cultural systems. Each of these groups has its own system of norms and values that over time merges with other normative systems. Even after several generations, however, differences are detectable at least as variations on the general cultural system. Different ethnic groups are definable by nationality identification and religion, and these vary in the criteria employed to assess health identity (Mechanic, 1969).

The literature on ethnicity and health identity has focused on the response to symptoms, particularly pain. Two studies have dealt exclusively with pain, and two others have included other symptoms.

The most detailed investigation of responses to pain was carried out by Zborowski (1952, 1969). He focused on a group of hospitalized patients who all had the same diagnosis and presumably equivalent levels of objective pain. He then compared the responses of "Old American," Italian, Irish, and Jewish patients. Italians and Jews were characterized by emotionally "open" responses to pain and were likely to vocalize their discomfort. The reasons for their emotional responses differed, however. The pain itself was most significant to the Italians, whereas the implications of the pain for the future was more significant for the Jews. By contrast, the Old Americans and the Irish did not vocalize or complain of their discomfort and took a more stoical attitude. Details of their responses differed in that the Irish seemed to deny the pain, whereas the Old Americans would report the pain experience in detail while maintaining a detached "scientific" attitude.

In a review of literature, Wolff (1954) noted that different ethnic groups were similar regarding the threshold at which pain was perceived. Responses to pain, however, were highly variable. He related this variability to differences in traditions of stoicism or emotionalism and to the meaning assigned to the painful experience.

Another study was carried out by Zola (1966) with patients in the outpatient clinic of the Massachusetts General Hospital in Boston. He also focused on a limited set of medical diagnoses but included a wider range of symptoms, paying particular attention to the way in which Italian and Irish patients presented their complaints. He found that the Italians presented a significantly more elaborate description of their symptoms than did the Irish. Furthermore, the Irish denied that their symptoms had any effect on their relationships with other people, whereas the Italians characteristically reported the disruption of interpersonal relationships as a major part of their complaint.

Drawing on a classification of symptoms proposed by Baumann (1961), Twaddle (1969) studied the first symptoms of illness reported by a sample of older married males in Providence, Rhode Island. In that study, it was found that feeling state changes, predominantly pain and weakness, were the most important for all ethnic groups studied. Italian Catholics, Protestants, and Jews, however, did show characteristic differences. Feeling state changes were the only sign of illness reported by the Italians. When the first sign of illness

was not a feeling state change, however, the Protestants reported changes in capacities (e.g., inability to do something they were used to doing), whereas the Jews reported changes which involved neither capacity change nor feeling state changes (e.g., lumps, bleeding).

To date these are the only studies to focus on the norms of subsocietal population groupings as they relate to health identities. Much work remains to be done not only to validate these findings but also to extend the knowledge to other ethnic groups. For the present, it seems clear that different groups have different orientations that create different criteria for deciding that a health problem exists.

Opportunities

As discussed in the next chapter, the designation of a person as sick carries with it the implication that something will be done about the sickness. The capacity to respond to symptoms, then, should influence the likelihood of defining sickness. If for any reason it becomes difficult or impossible to respond to symptoms, it should be less likely that the symptoms will be regarded as important.

The major tool for measuring the distribution of opportunities is socioeconomic status. The capacity to respond is structured by income and wealth, occupational prestige, and education and knowledge. Two studies have focused on the relationship between socioeconomic status and health identity.

In 1954 Koos studied the health and illness behavior patterns of inhabitants of a small town in upstate New York. As part of his study he presented a household sample with a list of medically important symptoms. The respondents were asked to report whether each symptom warranted the attention of a physician. For each symptom listed, the highest status respondents were uniformly more likely to report a need for medical attention than were the lowest status repondents. For all but two symptoms, loss of appetite and persistent backache, at least 75% of the highest class respondents reported a need for medical attention. In only three instances, each involving bleeding, did more than half of the lowest class respondents report such a need.

Drawing on earlier studies by Apple (1960) and Mechanic (1962), Gordon (1966) identified four criteria that could be used to "validate the occupancy of the status sick." These were prognosis, symptoms, being under the care of a physician, and functional incapacity. He presented a list of twelve descriptions of illness to a sample in New York City and found that prognosis was the most important factor in designating someone as sick. The poorer or more uncertain the prognosis the greater the tendency to define someone as sick. This held across class lines with no significant difference between low status and high status respondents. With functional capacity controlled, the presence of symptoms and being under the care of a physician were more likely to be important criteria to high class respondents than to low class respondents. Functional incapacity was more important the lower the social status of the respondent.

A similar pattern has been found with respect to mental health. Both Hollingshead and Redlich (1958) and Langner and Michael (1963) have suggested that feeling state changes such as depression are relatively more important signs of mental illness among higher status populations, whereas behavior problems such as overt aggression are more important among lower status populations. Furthermore, higher status respondents are more likely to be referred directly to psychiatrists, whereas lower status respondents are more likely to be referred first to the police or courts and from there to the psychiatrist.

Organizational context

Although little has been written about the relationship between organizational contexts and health identities, there is reason to believe that both the type and specificity of health identity should vary with the type of social organization under consideration.

Studies of sickness rates aboard different ships in the United States Navy show that the proportion defined as sick varied widely from one ship to another. Variation was greater within classes of ship (cruisers and aircraft carriers were compared) than between classes. It was thought, although not demonstrated, that specific organizational characteristics were important (McDonald et al., 1973).

The level of organization or focal units (Chapter 2) and the type of organization can influence the specificity of health identity. For general focal units, general designations such as healthy or sick may be adequate. For a hospital at the administrative level, it would be important to know not only that a person is sick but also whether it is a medical or a surgical case. At the treatment level, it may be important to know the specific diagnosis. Hence designations such as "sick," "infectious disease," and "type A beta hemolytic streptococcus" may be adequate health identities for different social units. Given that the problem is relevant to the type of organization, any identity designation has to be more specific to be minimally adequate for smaller units within the organization. For organizations in which the particular identity is not as relevant (health identities, for example, would be less relevant in an educational as compared with a health care organization) more general identities may be acceptable irrespective of the focal unit.

THE PROCESS OF LABELING HEALTH IDENTITIES

It should be clear that not only are there many kinds of criteria that may be employed to assess health identities but also many factors influence the selection and application of those criteria. It should also be clear that investigation of these criteria and factors has barely begun, and what has been presented is likely to be only a partial listing of what will ultimately be considered relevant.

When one looks at the ways in which individuals become defined as sick, it is apparent that the criteria and factors discussed so far are best treated as contingencies that influence a process of negotiation in which specific people immersed in specific social situations bargain with others regarding the meaning of more or less ambiguous events. The variety of ways in which persons can be defined as sick and the specific combinations of criteria and factors that can be taken into account are vast, producing a degree of variability that cannot be fully encompassed in any formal presentation. The well roles that define the meaning of being healthy to given individuals and groups, the specific nature of signs and symptoms that intrude into well roles, the process of negotiation or bargaining, and the rewards and costs attached to different outcomes are parameters that must be taken into account in understanding any particular outcome for given individuals. These are the primary considerations that guide the process by which healthy individuals become redefined as sick.

Well roles

The kinds of cues that an individual is likely to respond to in making the judgment that he might be sick are influenced by and assessed against the background of what is normal for that individual. The kinds of physical and emotional capacities required for feeling right and for carrying out normal daily activities serve to structure the kinds of incapacities that are likely to be noticed and defined as important.

The inability to run a mile in less than 6 minutes may be inconsequential to most males, for example, but to an athlete specialized in long distance running, this limitation may be seen as a serious disability. To the average male, this capacity level is well within the normal range but to the athlete it may be a sign of illness. To give another example, a strained back may be incapacitating to someone whose job consists of loading trucks, whereas it may be relatively trivial to an executive. By the same token, a headache may be trivial to the truck loader, whereas it might be incapacitating to an intellectual.

Specific incapacities must be evaluated therefore relative to the specific tasks and roles they affect. *If a specific biological or psychological capacity is not required for the performance of normal "well" activities it is less likely to be regarded as significant* than would be the case if it impaired normal activities. Also the greater the importance attached to the capacity affected the more likely a specific biological or psychological change will be noticed and seen as important.

The nature and severity of symptoms

The extent to which symptoms are noticed and the degree of importance attached to them are likely to be related to their expected present or future impact on normal activities. In addition, several features of the illness are generally taken into account, since they affect people's presumptions about the nature of the disease or illness and its severity.

Factors related to the nature of the symptoms include the following:

1. *Assumptions of causality.* The extent to which the disease or illness is seen as voluntary, the result of natural causes, or "sin." The key question is the degree to which the individual is seen as having brought the illness onto himself, ranging from self-inflicted wounds to carelessness in personal behavior.

2. *Assumptions of treatability.* The degree to which the person is expected to recover from the condition either spontaneously or with proper care. An untreatable condition is less likely to be classified as sickness and more likely to be seen as a handicap or as a condition associated with a normal process such as aging.

3. *Assumptions of prognosis.* The length of time the condition is expected to last, the degree of impairment it is expected to cause, and the likelihood of death presumed to be associated with the condition. The poorer or more uncertain the prognosis the more likely the condition will be treated as sickness.

The more a condition is seen as resulting from voluntary behavior, especially that which is disapproved (e.g., venereal disease), the more it is regarded as incurable (e.g., paralysis), and the more it is associated with death (e.g., cancer), the more the individual with that condition will be stigmatized (Goffman, 1963). That is, the more the individual is set apart as being different from others the more he will have to contend with the prejudice of others, in addition to the factors inherent in his condition. This has implications for medical care that will be explored in subsequent chapters.

Factors related to the presumed severity of symptoms include the following:

1. *Physical manifestations.* The clarity of symptoms to the individual concerned and to others. Comas, facial lesions, and other visual symptoms are immediately apparent to others, whereas vague discomforts, unusual discharges, and other similar symptoms may not be. Assuming that the factors associated with the nature of the condition are equal, the more visible the condition the more it will be seen as severe.

2. *Impression management.* Complaints, grimaces, and similar visible signs from the affected individual that communicate discomfort or direct information about the condition. The more the individual is seen as involuntarily communicating discomfort the more serious his condition will be taken to be.

3. *Familiarity of the condition.* The frequency with which the disease occurs in the group, conceptions about the degree of medical risk to others, and the specific symptoms and disabilities. The more familiar the condition the less likely it is to be seen as serious (Mechanic, 1962). A condition that is familiar, is regarded as minor, and does not significantly interfere with everyday behavior is less likely to be regarded as sickness, even when its presence is known.

Rewards and costs

In the discussion of perfect health we indicated that it is a state toward which people are oriented rather than one they expect to attain. In a broader sense, being healthy is a goal that most people would define as desirable no matter their culture or social circumstances. It does not follow that people will always behave in ways consistent with maintaining good health. As with any of life's objectives, the goal of good health sometimes must compete with other goals such as social standing, self-esteem, and the maintenance of satisfactory interpersonal relationships. The importance of being healthy is part of a calculus, rational or otherwise, in which the value of keeping healthy or of restoring impaired health must be weighed against perceived rewards and costs relative to attaining other goals.

People who place a high value on independence and self-reliance, for example, are less able to cope with the dependency implied by becoming sick. Such people are more resistant to acknowledging any symptoms and are committed to maintaining an image of being healthy (Phillips, 1965). Restoration of health through expensive treatment may be rejected if the patient perceives the cost to his family as being too high. Treatment that may result in disfigurement or incapacitation may also be rejected for similar reasons (Barker et al., 1953).

Taking risks of disease or injury may be an important part of self-esteem for many people. The cost of being thought of as "chicken" or unmasculine may outweigh the cost of putting safety first. To run in front of a moving car risks injury or death, yet is commonly understandable if the objective is to remove a child from the path of danger.

Suicides at examination time, especially in schools that have infrequent examinations, are one indicator that there are fates worse than death.

Negotiation

Several theories in social psychology suggest that there is a pressure toward consistency in human orientations. When one discovers that he holds opinions that are

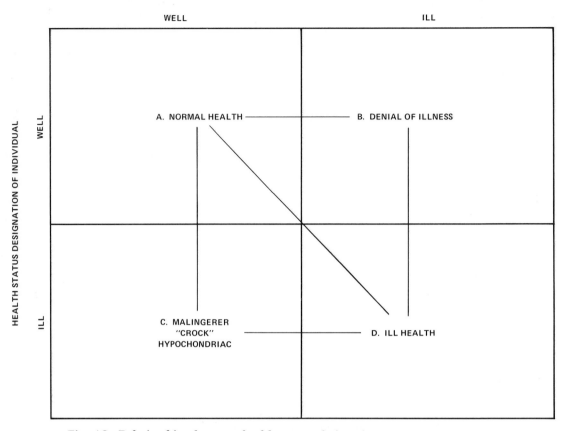

Fig. 4-2. *Relationships between health status designations of the individual and his status definers.* (From Twaddle, A. *Social Science and Medicine,* 1974, 8(1), 29-38.)

contradictory or conflicting with those of others in the social environment, there is a tendency to either adjust one's own opinion or that of others so as to achieve a common definition of the situation. There is a language in medical care settings that seems to fit this general model.

Health identities are almost always created in a process of interaction and negotiation between an individual whose identity is in question and others whose opinions are important. To state an idealized case, we can conceive a point in time at which both the individual in question and others are in agreement that he is well, and visualize a process by which he becomes defined as sick (Fig. 4-2). If there is consensus throughout the process of redefinition,

health identity will be unambiguous. In many cases, probably most, the process of redefinition begins with either the individual or others, and one side must be convinced before a consensus can be reached. In these cases, the others may either define the individual as denying his illness (a designation with overtones of a psychiatric problem) or see him as a "crock" or hypochondriac (with overtones of malingering). In these conflict situations, there is pressure to agree on either "well" or "sick" as appropriate labels.

In actuality the process is much more complicated, since the others may not be in agreement among themselves. This, of course, leaves the individual much more negotiating room. The others will differ in

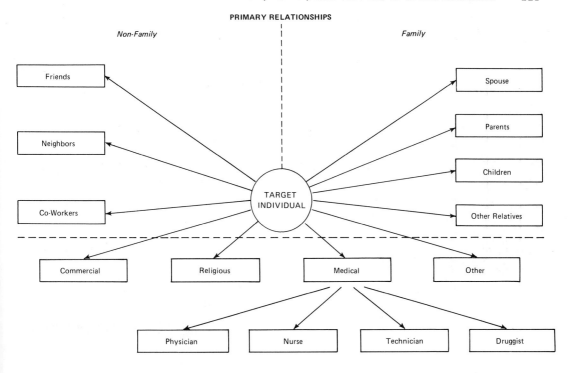

Fig. 4-3. *Role set of sick or potentially sick person.* (From Twaddle, A. *Social Science and Medicine,* 1974, 8(1), 29-38.)

the degree to which they can influence the outcome, depending on the degree of expertise they are presumed to have and on the nature of their relationship with the individual in question (Fig. 4-3).

One issue is that different people have different stakes in the outcome of symptoms for the individual in question. Any given outcome has different consequences for different people. Impairment of emotional behavior, for example, may be of critical importance to family members while having little or no importance for an employer. Inability to carry out specific work obligations would be more important to the employer than to the family (Mechanic, 1962). What capacities are affected will influence who notices symptoms and what kinds of meanings are attached to them.

The documentation of the influence of negotiation on health identities is far from complete, but there are several studies that point in the same direction. In 1965, for

example, Knutson observed that the actual performed role of the sick person differed according to with whom he interacted. People were expected to behave differently in relation to physicians, spouses, children, bosses, nurses, and others. Each of these others had expectations drawn from a different framework of interaction.

Mechanic (1965) showed that college students tended to define themselves as sick and to seek medical care in ways that were oriented toward parental expectations. Although they did not conform exactly to the expectations of either parent, behavior approximated that of one parent most of the time.

Looking at the recovery process, Roth (1963) showed that hospitalized tuberculosis patients developed a system of norms for assessing the state of their health as a method of structuring the passage of time in the course of recovery. With a population of working class people in the Bronx,

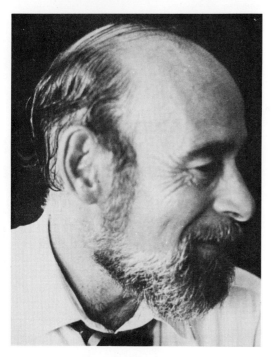

Fig. 4-4. *Eliot Freidson.*

Freidson (1961) (Fig. 4-4) demonstrated the importance of both culture and interpersonal influence in deciding health identities and in selecting a treatment agent. He proposed the existence of a "lay referral system" in which people are guided from one person to another in seeking to interpret symptoms. We will return to this formulation in the next chapter.

In a study of older married males in Providence, Rhode Island, Twaddle (1969) found that with the first appearance of a symptom, the man usually consulted with his spouse. If there was agreement that an important deviation from normal health had occurred, a physician was usually contacted immediately. If, on the other hand, there was disagreement between the man and his wife, or the wife's opinion was not taken seriously, consultation with other family members, neighbors, friends, and coworkers was initiated. When someone who was regarded as authoritative, either because of a similar prior illness or special training, suggested seeing a physician, a physician was consulted with little delay.

Taken together, this literature suggests that most changes in biological and psychological functioning are inherently ambiguous. Except in their most extreme manifestations, changes in feeling states, capacities and physiological processes are not necessarily definitive of health identity changes. Such changes are signals that raise questions as to their meaning.

Mechanic (1968b) has suggested that people typically respond to symptoms by first attempting to interpret them as normal. It is only when they are unable to cope with symptoms within the framework of normality that the question of sickness is seriously entertained. Again health and sickness are assessed within a framework of norms that form a "bounded rationality" (Simon, 1951) for assessing health status.

A person's identity as sick may be approached from the standpoint of a starting time before there is any question to the individual or anyone else of there being a condition having implications for present or future role disability or both. In his well identity, the individual can be considered to have a set of rights and obligations that may be placed in jeopardy if he is defined as sick. The imposition of any change in the definition of his capabilities may affect various rights, demands, or both in the eyes of various others.

If a more or less ambiguous biological or psychological change has been produced, questions may be raised relative to the state of his health. If the signs of sickness are relatively unambiguous and severe, the individual may have little say about his health identity. If, for example he becomes paralyzed, unconscious, or unable to communicate, a change in health identity may be defined and acted on by others. In the more general case, however, signs of illness are characterized by ambiguity, and the designation of health identity is negotiated between the individual and other people around him. Depending on presumptions of expertise, power, and good will, the influence of any particular other person varies in strength.

HEALTH STATUS INDICES: ARE WE READY?

There is considerable interest in developing procedures for measuring health identities. Government agencies want to be able to define the number of people who are sick and the degree of sickness to plan health care programs. Behavioral scientists interested in health and illness want to gain precision of definition sufficient to study large populations. There is little question that the ability to construct a simple quantitative index of health would make both these tasks simpler, and considerable effort is being expended toward that end. In our opinion, such efforts are at best premature, however laudable the aim. To present our case, we will briefly review the nature of health identity and compare it to the current measurement efforts.

The nature of health identities

To summarize the major features of health identities, the following points seem essential:

1. Health and illness are normatively defined. Norms provide standards of adequacy relative to capacities, feeling states, and biological functioning needed for the performance of those activities expected of members of the society. These normal expectations vary with disease and illness patterns in the society, demographic characteristics, group norms, opportunities, and organizational context.

2. Disease and illness have biological and psychological parameters, respectively. They are identities given with reference to norms of biological and psychological functioning irrespective of whether medical or nonmedical criteria are employed.

3. Except in extreme cases, deviations from normality are inherently ambiguous. Health identity changes do not follow automatically from biological and psychological changes. Rather such changes are events requiring interpretation. Depending on the extent to which a deviation is assessed and the significance attached to it, health identity changes may or may not follow it. The skillful use of medical criteria serves to reduce but not eliminate this ambiguity.

4. Although there may be some broadly held norms in any given society, these tend to be specified and elaborated by different groups within the society. Hence normative standards against which health and sickness are judged vary with medical training, social class, and ethnicity.

5. The situations in which these norms for assessing health identity are applied are also variable. Different situations require different capacities and alter the rewards and costs of alternative health identities.

6. Health identities consist of a number of labels applied to an individual by himself and by others with whom he interacts. As with other social labeling processes, health identity consists of those labels agreed on by an individual and various others.

7. The process of assigning health identities consists of interaction between an individual and various others in which normative standards of adequacy are applied to the individual in the context of a specific situation to assess his capacities for present or future role and task performance.

8. The critical parameters for the measurement of health identity must include the criteria employed for assessing health, disease, and illness; the situations in which these criteria are applied; the characteristics of the people who do the defining and whose identity is at issue; and the consequences of alternative definitions relative to behavioral expectations.

Measurement: state of the art

Current attempts to measure health identities with objective quantitative techniques almost uniformly ignore all the parameters just specified. Instead, measurement is likely to be of parameters constructed from more or less arbitrary definitions constructed of data selected because of their easy availability. Although many of these efforts are mathematically sophisticated and some are reliable in the sense that they can reproduce the same results from one application to another, they tend to be of questionable validity in that they fail to relate measures to the events that are most relevant. Consequently, most health status indices are sophisticated tools for measuring something that is not health status.

To illustrate, a recent state-of-the-art book (Berg, 1973) contains the following reports:

1. A factor analysis of 114 variables taken from census reports and health surveys, none of which relate to disease, illness, or sickness
2. A G index consisting of mortality, hospital days, and outpatient visits
3. A functional limitation scale ranging from asymptomatic to death
4. A debility index based on activities of daily living
5. A health status rating system based on physicians' evaluations of clinical descriptions of hyperthyroid patients
6. Several other reports dealing with a range of concerns from health utility measurement to the quantitative evaluation of preferences

Although many of these measures may be useful for program planning or for studying factors related to health status, none makes the issue of health identity really problematic or takes account of the variation in criteria for making health identity judgments. Criteria are almost uniformly selected by the researchers on some a priori grounds or on the basis of data availability. What is produced are indices of debility, functional capacity, disease, and longevity. None is a measure of health identity as defined in this chapter.

Toward measurement

In our opinion, a quantitative index of health identities, or health status, has not yet been developed and a satisfactory index would have to be so complicated that its utility for planning purposes may not be great. Presently several indices measure parts of components that would go into a good index. What has been done may be useful for a variety of special purposes, but the uses to which such measures are put should be carefully circumscribed. The idea that health planning is to proceed on the basis of what has been developed on the false assumption that health status has been measured seems both appalling and likely.

An adequate health identity index would have to deal with many factors and many variables in many combinations, keeping different combinations of variables separate and flexible enough to not miss important ramifications. At a minimum such an index should include the following:

1. The range of criteria employed to define health and sickness as well as measures of the various forms such criteria can take
2. Characteristics of the people to whom the criteria might be applied
3. A full list of signs and symptoms regarded as important by different groups of people
4. Descriptions of the situations within which judgments are to be made
5. Characteristics of the people who are to do the defining
6. The organizational contexts within which decisions are made

All this must take into account available options for placement in one health category or another and most important the range of specific disorders recognized by the culture keeping abreast of the changes over time.

These parameters were identified in a small number of studies, most of which deal with specialized populations such as the aged (Apple, 1960), college students (Mechanic, 1965), symptomatic married men in a specific urban setting (Twaddle, 1969), or patients in highly selective medical care settings (Zborowski, 1952, 1969; Zola, 1966). Although these studies have served to identify some factors that must be taken into account, there is no assurance that all the important dimensions have been discovered. In our opinion, exploratory studies dealing with a larger number of special population groups selected to maximize diversity will be needed before one can generate a definitive listing of what has to be measured to construct a health status index.

Once such a list is generated, we have reservations as to whether it can be measured on quantitative scales without having the mathematical measures depart significantly from the events with which we are concerned. Fundamentally, the question of who is healthy and who is sick is a problem of meaning, the values held by groups and individuals, and the ways in which they conceptualize changes in their physical and psychological feelings and behaviors. The processes are variable and are subject to rapid change over time.

NOTES

1. Kittrie (1971) notes a complementary process in the legal system. He argues with compelling evidence that the criminal law is divesting itself of jurisdiction over a wide variety of deviant behavior.

2. This is assuming that the individual is the unit of analysis. As Parsons (1975) has indicated, sickness is a problem of integration from the standpoint of the social system.

3. Salloway and Dillon (1973) have shown that relatives are less efficient as referral agents than are friends.

CHAPTER 5

The sickness career

Once someone is defined as "sick," which is a complex social process that is only partly understood (Chapter 4), there are a variety of ways in which he can behave. Some persons may change nothing and simply "grit their teeth" and carry on with normal activities. This sometimes requires heroic effort and under some circumstances is much admired. Others may withdraw from almost all activities and become extremely passive and dependent, seemingly "giving up." Some persons concoct home remedies and take them. Others seek out faith healers or other nonmedical practitioners; other individuals immediately make an appointment with a physician or go to a hospital emergency room. Some who see physicians will follow their instructions to the letter; others ignore treatment advice. In short, the question of what happens to people defined as sick has many answers. In this chapter some of these answers will be explored and common dimensions will be sought either in the outcomes or in the processes by which different outcomes are reached. In general, we are asking, "What are the consequences of having the social identity of one who is sick?"

An identity as sick is consequential. Not only is a sick person likely to behave differently from one defined as "well," but also this difference in behavior is permitted and expected. It has been contended that sickness constitutes a distinctive social role de-fined by a cluster of interrelated expectations. This contention will be explored first.

Sickness, however, is not simply a set of expectations. It is also an event that requires that decisions be made either actively or by default. It is also a socially institutionalized process for coping with difficulty. These themes will also be taken into account, after which they will be illustrated with some actual case histories. Finally, we will raise some questions regarding the adequacy of our culture to cope with sickness.

THE SICK ROLE

As noted in Chapter 1, Parsons (1951, 1958, 1964) proposed a concept of sickness that focused on sociological properties rather than medical ones. This was a significant development because it was the first time in which the dependent variable (sickness) had been presented in a way so as to make it relevant to sociological analysis. Parsons' formulation, called the "sick role," has been highly controversial, and it is important to separate what he said from the critical commentaries. After presenting Parsons' proposal and major criticisms of it, we will argue that both sides are right.

Parsons' formulation

Parsons is primarily concerned with the construction of a broad, general sociologi-

116

cal theory that will describe the structure of societies as total entities. His proposal of a sick role was part of this broader concern and cannot be understood apart from it. (Parsons, 1951, 1958, 1964). Specifically he was concerned with two major problems: the modernization of societies and the social control of deviant behavior.

With respect to modernization, Parsons contended that the professions were emerging as a distinctive occupational group at the same time the businessman was becoming dominant. Businessmen and professionals were seen as being distinctive from one another in their orientations and as having different kinds of relationships with the public. One context in which the sick role is to be viewed is as an attempt to describe the expectations brought to bear on people defined as sick, treating these people as a prototype of the professional client. The most important feature is the vulnerability of the client to exploitation and the necessity of some institutionalized system of protection. Discussion of this aspect is deferred to Chapter 10.

With respect to social control, Parsons argued that sickness is a special form of deviant behavior that needs to be differentiated from other forms such as crime, sin, and disloyalty. The primary focus was in differentiating the sick from the criminal. Accordingly, in reading each of the following expectations posited as characteristically held for the behavior of sick people, the meaning will be clearer if the phrase "Relative to the criminal, the sick person is expected to" is used as a preface.

Keeping this background in mind, we can discuss the specifics of the formulation. Parsons contended that when people became defined as sick, the following four institutionalized expectations would be upheld by others for their behavior:

1. *The sick person would be entitled to some exemption from normal social activities and under some circumstances would be required to give up or curtail certain activities.* The degree to which this is the case for any individual is variable, depend-

ing on the specifics of health status, notably the kind of disease or illness involved, the degree of incapacity imputed, and the degree to which the person is a danger to others. In Parsons' terms, exemptions are dependent on the "nature and severity" of the illness.

2. *The sick person would be defined as unable to "pull himself together" and "get well" by an act of decision or will.* In this sense, he is defined as "not responsible" for his condition. He cannot help it and needs to be taken care of.

3. *The sick person would be expected to define the state of being sick as undesirable.* The sick person should want to get well. He should not resign himself to being sick, nor should he take advantage of such secondary gains as being the center of attention and concern of others.

4. *The sick person would be obligated to seek technically competent help and to cooperate in the process of trying to get well.* This may mean seeing someone defined as competent by his community, taking medications, altering life-style, and taking other necessary measures.

Thus the sick role consists of norms defining two rights and two obligations that are attached to being defined as sick. As presented by Parsons, these constitute a unit. The rights are limited in that they are conditional on performance of the obligations. One would not long continue to be granted exemptions from normal activities nor would one continue to be defined as deserving help if he did not communicate a desire to get well and seek appropriate treatment.

Major criticisms

The sick role is not only an analytical concept, but it is also a description of expectations applied to those defined as sick in "modern, western, urban, industrialized societies" (Parsons, 1958). This specification is because medicine is seen as part of an emergent scientific orientation that is part of the modern social structure and that differentiates it from more "primitive" structures. The thought is that a shift in values produces a shift in expectations surrounding sickness.

As a descriptive concept, the sick role has been criticized heavily. Specific criticisms are too numerous to list in detail but are of the following types:

1. *The theoretical domain* (Chapter 2) *of the sick role is too limited.* Because of the focus on Western societies, the concept says little about non-Western experience. In addition, much about the experience of illness cannot be explained by the sick role. Many behaviors surrounding sickness are complex and seem unrelated to the sick role (Freidson, 1962, 1970), and the sick role does not seem to apply to other conditions that come to medical attention such as pregnancy (McKinlay, 1972).

2. *The sick role applies to a limited range of sickness.* Specifically it provides a useful description of the expectations attached to relatively serious acute conditions. It is less useful for understanding trivial conditions that do not result in exemption from normal activities or contact with a physician. Nor is the sick role as useful for incurable or stigmatized conditions or for various legitimate nonhealth roles. In the case of incurable disease, the patient must adjust to the condition rather than expect recovery. Stigmatized conditions such as venereal disease or mental illness do not get treated with emotionally neutral disease orientations and frequently carry an assumption of responsibility for onset. Some legitimate roles such as the handicapped may not involve the attention of a physician, exemption from normal activities, or a recovery motivation (Freidson, 1962). From another perspective, it has been argued that roles of any kind can only arise in stable interaction situations, requiring time and repetition to take form. For this reason, the sick role must be limited to the case of chronic disease (Kosa and Robertson, 1969).

3. *The formulation of the sick role suffers from a management bias that gives undue weight to professional definitions.*

Much of the behavior of sick people consists of self-treatment or consultation with nonprofessionals, and the expectation of consultation with professionals is not applicable. The sick role would be most useful for people who share the values of the professional. It would be less relevant to working class, peasant, and non-Western populations than to middle-class Europeans and Americans (Freidson, 1962).

4. *Although it may be a reasonable description for the society taken as a whole, the sick role reveals little about known variability within societies.* Even if the nature of the society, the type of disease or illness, and contact with a physician were held constant, there is variability in the extent to which recovery is possible, the stigma attached to different conditions, the seeking of help, and the degree of exemption from normal activities (Freidson, 1962). Taking each of Parsons' expectations and looking at the behavior of sick people from the standpoint of conformity or nonconformity, it has been shown that at least seven different patterns exist (Twaddle, 1969).

An assessment

There have been many studies of the behaviors of people with diseases or illnesses or who are otherwise defined as "sick." These studies underline the fact that human behavior is as variable in the face of sickness as in any other aspect of life. The criticisms of the sick role formulation therefore are backed up with considerable evidence. However, most of the research and critical commentary have been from investigators whose major concerns have been with differences within societies, whereas the sick role formulation is part of a theory dealing with the society as a whole. This presents a problem in that the sick role formulation and the major criticisms relate to different theoretical domains. An assessment must take both into account.

With reference to the societal approach, the sick role seems to be a useful concept. The treatment of sickness as a form of deviant behavior has considerable heuristic value in that it serves to order observations and to call attention to needed research into the relationships between medical care and such social control systems as the legal system (Twaddle, 1973b). There is also some evidence that such a relationship exists. Prisoners in a maximum security prison, for example, are less likely to have disciplinary reports written for infractions of rules when they have a history of medical care prior to imprisonment, and medical histories can discriminate between those who get disciplinary reports and those who appear at sick call (Twaddle, 1976).

Aside from the treatment of sickness as deviance, there is evidence that the sick role describes central tendencies in people's attitudes toward sickness. Gordon (1966), in the study discussed in Chapter 4, sampled New York City residents and provided them with a list describing different diseases and illnesses. When asked how each should be treated, the responses were consistent with the sick role, although there was significant variability.

Although there are many unanswered questions, the conclusion must be that at present the sick role is applicable both analytically and descriptively when the society is the unit of analysis. The major questions relate to the fact that there have been no international comparative research efforts to see to what extent the formulation is limited to the industrialized society.

When the focus is on differences within societies, the sick role is less useful, but the usefulness of the concept is difficult to assess. There is considerable variability in the behavior of the sick. Research to date has not adequately distinguished questions of social identity, expectations, and behavior. Although behavior is variable, it is not clear to what extent the same can be said for expectations. The variability of expectations may be a function of variability in health identities as discussed in Chapter 4. Gordon, for example, distinguished an "impaired role," in which people were expected to perform their normal activities within the limits of their handicaps, from

the sick role, in which they were exempted. It is doubtful, however, that those in the impaired role were regarded as sick. In Parsons' formulation, only those regarded as sick would be candidates for the sick role.

It is clear, however, that understanding sickness behavior requires more than the sick role. It requires understanding decision-making processes, socially structured opportunities, and the place of health in personal value systems as these affect social interaction. At the present time, the sick role must be regarded as a useful starting place for the analysis of sickness behavior (Mechanic, 1962; Freidson, 1970).

NORMS AND OPPORTUNITIES

The assumption that the sick role describes a set of general norms for the society must be resolved with the observation that sickness behavior is varied. Either there must be some variation in specific norms at the level of subsocietal populations and interactions, or there must be some features of social situations and personalities that block the implementation of the norms. In fact, both occur.

Normative variation

The specificity of norms generally increases with the specificity of the focal unit (Chapter 2) under consideration. In general, as discussed in Chapter 4, it may be important to know that someone is or is not sick. For casual, everyday discourse, such a designation may be sufficient for most purposes. In a hospital, from the perspective of the administration, it also would be important to know whether the person is a medical or a surgical case. At the level of the ward, it may be important to know the specific diagnosis. In each instance, the expectations (norms) upheld for behavior would be more specific. Knowing that someone is sick indicates that some exemption from normal activity is expected. For example, knowing that a person has diabetes mellitus or acute glomerulonephritis (an acute kidney infection) would lead to different expectations as to the kinds of activities from which he will be exempted and the degree of exemption. For a person suffering from the first condition, there may be some restriction on diet and violent exercise, but otherwise it is expected that the patient will pursue normal activities. The patients suffering from the second condition may be hospitalized with complete bedrest, a total disruption of normal activities.

Another source of variation is ethnicity, the cultural orientations of different groups, generally measured by nationality and religion. As indicated in Chapter 4 different cultures are defined by differences in orientations toward life. When people of one culture live among those from another, many traits of the dominant group are assimilated. At the same time, other traits persist over long periods of time. The differences among Italian Catholics, Protestants, and Jews in their orientations toward symptoms (Chapter 4) seem to persist for several generations after most other "old country" traits have disappeared. In general, the distinctive use of materials disappears first and religious differences last. What is "using good sense and taking care of oneself" in the face of symptoms in one culture may be "acting like a baby and being self-indulgent" in another. This would affect the response to symptoms, including the likelihood of seeking care and the degree of cooperation with treatment agents (Zola, 1966; Twaddle, 1969).

Variations in opportunities

Human action requires resources. These may be internal in the form of capacities, and from this perspective the presence of

Table 5-1. Use of health care services by socioeconomic status, United States*

	Physician visits†	Chiropractor visits	Hospital discharges
Occupation			
Professional	—‡	—	75.6
Farmers and farm managers	—	—	71.4
Managers	—	—	79.1
Clerical	—	—	93.0
Sales	—	—	85.1
Craftsmen	—	—	77.6
Operatives	—	—	90.5
Private household	—	—	66.8
Service	—	—	109.5
Farm laborers	—	—	54.4
Laborers	—	—	65.7
Income			
Less than $3,000	12.4	20.6	31.5
$3,000-$4,999	15.6	31.3	43.3
$5,000-$6,999	17.0	31.7	45.0
$7,000-$9,999	17.7	36.3	44.8
$10,000+	19.2	33.1	42.6
Education			
Less than 9 years	12.3	30.5	37.4
9-12 years	14.5	32.2	43.4
13 or more years	16.7	21.5	38.4

*From USPHS, publication 1000, series 10, nos. 21, 55.
†Physician visits are calculated as number per family in 1963-1964. Hospital discharges by occupation are per 1,000 persons in the labor force, 1961-1963; otherwise, per 100 families, 1963-1964.
‡No data available.

disease is often a resource loss. Or they may be external in the form of the availability of services, money, and other similar resources. All disease, illness, and treatment alter the resources available for behavior. Behavior in response to symptoms to some extent depends on resources available.

The major index of resources as distributed in societies is socioeconomic status measured by income, education, and occupation. Education reflects the level of knowledge about alternative courses of action available, as well as skills in utilizing social facilities. Income reflects economic competence, that is, the ability to purchase goods and services. Occupation reflects available flexibility in the use of time, as well as being a primary source of income.

In general, the lower the socioeconomic status of a population the less their use of medical services approximates the ideal of the medical profession. Persons of lower socioeconomic status are less likely to see physicians for any reason. Physician visits, chiropractor visits, and hospital discharges increase with increasing income (Table 5-1).

Table 5-2. Percent distribution of physician visits by place of visit according to selected characteristics: United States, 1969*

| | Place of visit | | | | | |
Characteristics	Office	Home	Hospital	Industrial unit	Telephone	Other and unknown
Sex						
Male	69.1	2.0	11.7	1.8	10.8	4.6
Female	70.8	2.6	9.4	0.5	12.8	4.0
Age						
Under 5 years	58.9	1.5	11.0	—	23.4	5.1
5-14 years	62.2	1.7	12.9	—	17.5	5.4
15-24 years	71.1	1.0	11.2	1.1	8.7	6.9
25-34 years	71.5	—	11.0	2.1	11.1	3.7
35-44 years	70.0	1.6	13.0	2.0	9.8	3.6
45-54 years	75.6	1.4	10.1	1.4	8.1	3.5
55-64 years	78.3	2.5	7.4	1.3	7.5	2.9
65-74 years	77.6	4.7	5.9	—	9.0	2.4
75 years and over	69.2	13.6	6.3	—	8.5	—
Color						
White	71.1	2.4	8.9	1.0	12.6	3.9
All other	60.6	1.3	22.5	1.7	6.5	7.3
Family income						
Less than $3,000	67.8	4.3	14.4	—	7.3	5.6
$3,000-$4,999	68.7	2.6	13.5	1.1	9.3	4.7
$5,000-$6,999	71.7	2.7	11.2	1.2	9.1	4.2
$7,000-$9,999	71.2	1.6	8.6	1.3	13.5	3.8
$10,000-$14,999	70.1	1.4	8.5	0.9	15.3	3.7
$15,000 or more	69.5	2.0	7.9	—	15.4	4.3
Education of head of family						
Less than 5 years	69.3	4.4	14.3	—	5.2	4.6
5-8 years	74.7	3.5	10.5	1.1	7.0	3.3
9-11 years	70.4	2.7	11.4	1.4	9.6	4.4
12 years	70.5	1.5	9.5	1.0	13.4	4.2
13 years or more	66.5	1.7	9.5	0.7	16.8	4.7

*From USPHS, publication 1000, series 10, no. 75.

Whereas physician visits increase with increasing education, chiropractor visits decrease. Hospital discharges are highest among those with between nine and twelve years of schooling.

The location of physician visits varies with socioeconomic status. People with low incomes are less likely to make office visits or to consult by telephone, and they are more likely to be seen in clinics (Table 5-2).

Several studies have shown that persons with lower incomes know less about their bodies and consequently think of illness as caused by such factors as "tired blood." They are consequently more prone to use patent medicines advertised in the mass media or folk remedies. For these reasons, they are less likely to define their problems in ways that result in consultation with professionals (Koos, 1954, Gurin et al., 1960; Feldman, 1966; Freidson, 1970).

Although some of these patterns are associated with class culture, a set of norms and values arising from position in the class structure, most are directly attributable to opportunities. People with high education, high income, and occupations providing flexibility in the use of time and space have more options available to them. Taking time off from work does not mean reduced income. A given expenditure of money is less catastrophic.

SICKNESS AS A SEQUENCE OF DECISIONS

Sickness does imply changes in social identity and in expectations for behavior. Although some broad general parameters of changes in expectations can be identified, the specifics are highly variable. To understand the richness and complexity of human behavior in response to symptoms requires that one look at the social processes that influence behavior. These include an active process of decision making that leads to a series of discrete identities and expectations constituting a career. At each decision juncture, a variety of influences can alter career patterns. Since each individual

must travel each sickness episode separately, it is little wonder that the variety must be impressive.

The concept of career

Central to the notion of career is the concept of "status passage" in which one passes from one social identity to another. The total sequence of status passages constitutes a career. The growth and development sequences in children provide one example. In this case, the individual moves from infant to child to adolescent to adult. As one passes from one status to another, expectations change relative to intellectual capacity, physical development, athletic skill, and other qualities.

One typically thinks of careers in conjunction with occupations in part because occupation is a key source of social identity and a central mode of participation in the social system. Occupational careers sometimes have clear-cut demarcations, notably in the military. One can obtain a commission as a second lieutenant in the army, for example, and depending on seniority and evaluations of senior officers move to first lieutenant, captain, major, lieutenant colonel, colonel, brigadier general, and higher

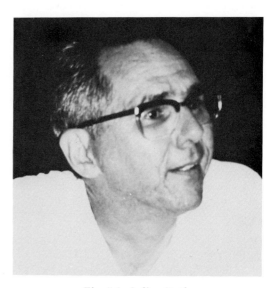

Fig. 5-1. *Julius Roth.*

ranks. With each change there are differences in pay, responsibilities, and ritual prerogatives. Other careers provide moves that, although no less important to the participants, are much less clearly major demarcation points, as in an academic career. One can begin as an instructor and advance to assistant professor, associate professor, and professor with little change in responsibilities or prerogatives but some increase in pay. The benchmarks by which careers are measured may vary therefore in their clarity and significance. That is, careers may be more or less structured.

The concept of career is not limited to the case of occupations. According to Roth (1963:94-95), any life event may be considered as a career if it meets the following criteria:

1. . . . It is something which a person goes through over a period of time and which has
2. definable stages or signposts along the way and
3. A more or less definite and recognizable end-point or goal.

This means that there must be a group definition of success or attainment of the goal. Such definitions may be provided by movement through an institutional hierarchy (such as academic careers), through a series of contingencies moving in a given direction (like the private practice physician getting a better clientele, better office location, better hospital appointments; the school teacher getting better school assignments or more desirable courses to teach), escape from an undesirable situation (the patient getting out of a hospital, the prisoner getting out of jail, the draftee getting out of the army), or development in a given direction (such as children developing toward independent adulthood).

Leisure activities, aging, dying, and sickness are aspects of life that can be seen as careers. In fact, people normally have several careers simultaneously, and a recurrent problem of living is the allocation of energies among them and dealing with career conflicts (Goode, 1960a).

Sickness careers focus on the changes in identity that are attendent on disease or illness. Conceptualizations vary according to the goals of the person formulating the career model. Suchman (1966), for example, was concerned with the place of rehabilitation in the experience of physical handicaps. He focused on a time dimension constructed around antecedent and consequent relationships. He thought in terms of preconditioning variables (the preexisting conditions), independent variables (disability), the intervening variables (rehabilitation), and the dependent variables (consequences). Rehabilitation then was an event that intervened between a disability and its consequences.

Bank et al. (1973) were concerned with the series of identities a patient has during the experience of an illness. They proposed the following model of the transition from health to patienthood:

Health $\longrightarrow$ illness $\longrightarrow$ sick role $\longrightarrow$ patient

The transition has three steps as follows:

1. The healthy person notices some symptom "which interferes with his adequate and painless activity."
2. He adopts the sick role by cutting down or eliminating some activities and/or by initiating treatment.
3. He may seek the help of a professional and become a patient.

Davis (1963) studied polio victims and their families. He analyzed the onset of polio as a disaster that had in common with other disasters certain sequential stages: a predisaster or quiescent stage, a warning or threat stage, an impact stage, a postimpact or inventory stage, and a long-term recovery stage. The identification of these stages allowed him to analyze the response of victims and their families to symptoms, incapacity, and residual disability as a process of coping with what was at that time a catastrophic disease.

The particular formulation of any career is a creative act of an observer. The particular benchmarks or stages identified are more or less useful for understanding an event, depending on the purpose of the investigation.

Decision steps in the sickness career

One useful approach to the sickness career is to employ as benchmarks the decisions made by the sick person or others acting on his behalf. There is a set of logically necessary decisions that must be made for the sick person. Against a background of capacities, feeling states, and biological states that define being well to any given individual, the following decisions seem necessary: that some change from normal health has occurred, that the change is significant, that help is needed, that a particular type of help is preferable, that a particular treatment agent or setting is most appropriate, and that certain types and degrees of cooperation with a treatment agent are optimal. The outcome of these decisions will be either that the person is again well, the person dies, or the changes are reinterpreted as a new state of normality. These decisions are diagramed in Fig. 5-2.

Using this model, much of the literature dealing with "illness" behavior can be tied together. As defined by Mechanic (1962), "Illness behavior falls logically and chronologically between two major traditional concerns of medical science: etiology and therapy." It consists of "the ways in which given symptoms may be differentially perceived, evaluated, and acted (or not acted) upon by different kinds of persons . . . whether by reason of earlier experience with illness, differential training in respect to symptoms, or whatever." Sickness behavior (which we prefer to "illness behavior") encompasses a wide range of activities, some of which have been discussed in Chapter 4.

As we discuss each of the decision steps, it will be helpful to refer to Fig. 5-2.

The baseline state of being well. Being healthy has different meanings to different people. As indicated in Chapter 4, the general culture, ethnic identity, opportunities, influence patterns, and situational factors affect the likelihood of any symptom being noticed or taken seriously. Several studies have tried to identify the common general parameters of good health.

Baumann (1961) studied hospital outpatients and classified their conceptions of being healthy as (1) a feeling of well-being, (2) an absence of symptoms, and (3) the capacity to engage in whatever activities they regarded as normal. Freidson (1970) reported that Herzlich (1964) studied a group of Frenchmen and found "an emphasis on the importance of the capacity to carry on daily activities rather than on 'organic reality which is itself ambiguous.' " Twaddle (1968b, 1969) studied older married men in Providence, Rhode Island, and found that they defined themselves as healthy when (1) they had no identifiable medical conditions, (2) they had had experience with a disease they defined as serious but had recovered, (3) they were told by a physician that their health was good, or (4) they did not expect to become sick. None of those who reported their health as "good" in that sample referred to capacities as the reason for their judgment.

What it means to be normal seems not to

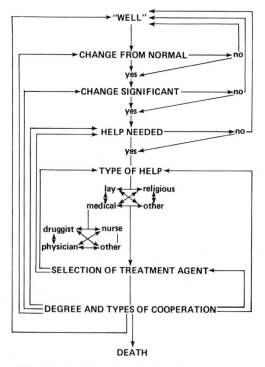

Fig. 5-2. *Decision steps in the sickness career.*

be uniform from one person to another, but whatever it means for any given individual will be the baseline against which changes are measured.

Decision that some change from normal has occurred. Any change in a person's life may produce a situation in which health identities may come into question. Again several studies have attempted to identify the kinds of changes that seem to define health problems. Apple (1960) studied older residents of a city in the United States and found that symptoms were more likely to be attributed to illness when they were of recent onset and were hence regarded as novel or they interfered with normal activities. Baumann (1961) found that the symptoms or signs of illness could be classified as (1) capacity changes, or inability to perform some task regarded as normal; (2) changes in feeling states; or (3) other symptoms regarded as important. Twaddle (1968b, 1969) found that older married men thought of themselves as ill when Baumann's criteria were present. Feelings state changes were most important, "other" changes were least frequently reported. Another study of hospital patients found that most people experienced some combination of the symptom types identified by Baumann (Sweet and Twaddle, 1969b).

Signs and symptoms; as noted in Chapter 4, do not serve to define people as sick; rather they are triggers that raise questions which need exploration. A first step in many diseases is for the symptoms to be interpreted as "normal." Many changes that may be due to disease may also be characteristic of normal life changes such as aging (Mechanic, 1968).

Freidson (1970) has suggested that "laymen everywhere are likely to report spontaneously about the same number of symptoms, irrespective of the number of illnesses discernible to medical men." People become accustomed to symptoms and begin to treat their presence as normal. The fact that comparisons of self-reported symptoms and medical findings consistently conclude that disease is underreported is consistent

with this interpretation (Commission on Chronic Illness, 1957; Freidson, 1970).

Decision that the change is significant. It is not enough to recognize the existence of symptoms. As just noted, frequently, the first step in the recognition of disease is to view the symptoms as normal. That is, they are interpreted as being caused by something other than disease. Fatigue may be treated as resulting from overwork. Muscle pain as the result of unusual exercise. The treatment of symptoms as significant is related to several of their features.

Both Mechanic (1968) and Twaddle (1968b) have listed aspects of symptoms and their interpretation that influence judgments of severity. Combining these lists to eliminate duplications, the following items seem important.

1. *The extent to which symptoms interfere with normal activities or characteristics.* In a sense, the more a symptom inconveniences the individual in question or others who relate to that individual the more likely it will be interpreted as significant. Apple (1960) found that interference with normal activities was a characteristic of symptoms that led to their interpretation as illness. Angrist et al. (1963) found that people were more likely to be defined as mentally ill when they became unable to control bowel and urinary habits, since these symptoms were less tolerable to other people, than were other symptoms that might have been more clinically significant. Barker et al. (1953) found that adjustment to physical handicap was reduced when valued activities or aspects of appearance were destroyed. Suchman (1965) found that the interpretation of symptoms depended on the degree of incapacitation involved. Baumann (1961) found that capacity changes were a major sign of sickness as did Gordon (1966) and Twaddle (1969, 1974). It will be recalled that an inability to perform normal activities is central to the sociological definition of sickness (Chapter 4).

2. *The clarity of symptoms.* The more obvious symptoms are to others and to the individual involved the more likely they

will be interpreted as significant. When a person deviates from social expectations, he becomes more socially visible (Lemert, 1946, 1951). As observed by Mechanic (1968: 143):

Many symptoms present themselves in a striking fashion, such as in the case of a sharp abdominal pain, an intense headache, and a high fever. Other symptoms have such little visibility (as in the early stages of cancer and tuberculosis) that they require special checkups to be detected in their early stages.

Among older men in Providence, Rhode Island, Twaddle (1968b, 1969) found that some people became defined as sick as a result of a routine physical examination or while having a consultation for another complaint. One man, for example, was hit by a car and while being checked by a physician was told he had high blood pressure. Another went for a routine checkup and was told he had a hernia. In both instances medical care was initiated by the physician. Others experienced symptoms that were so dramatic that there was no question that something was wrong. In the majority of cases, however, symptoms were ambiguous as to their meaning, resulting in considerable consultation with family and friends before their meaning was interpreted.

3. *The tolerance threshold and impression management of the symptomatic person.* People differ in their ability to tolerate symptoms and in the ways in which they express their symptomatic states. How a person controls or displays his symptoms makes them more or less visible to others. With similar levels of pain, for example, some people maintain a stoic silence, whereas others cry, complain, and grimace.

To a significant degree, the willingness to tolerate symptoms is a function of the expectations of other people. Zborowski (1952) and Zola (1966) have shown that ethnic groups differ in their responses to pain (Chapter 4). Lambert et al. (1960) have shown that Christians and Jews tolerated more pain when they were told that the study was testing the hypothesis that their particular group could not tolerate as much

as the other group. Several studies have shown that tolerance of the performance of mental patients is higher among parents, the working class, and the unattached as compared with spouses, the middle class, and the married (Brown, 1958; Lefton, 1962; Freeman and Simmons, 1963; Fischer, 1965).

A little reflection indicates the importance of tolerance and impression management (Goffman, 1959). Most people have some symptoms most of the time. Aches, pains, momentary weaknesses, and other such problems are part of normal living. The issue is seldom related to the presence or absence of symptoms but the degree of symptoms that is needed to define one as sick. A study in London at the close of World War II found that only 9% of individuals were free of medically important symptoms (Perse and Crocker, 1944), and a recent study of 10,709 apparently healthy people found that more than 9 out of 10 had some medical disorder. Relative to what these figures would suggest, few people are defined as sick.

4. *The familiarity and seriousness of the symptoms.* The more unfamiliar the symptoms are and the more threatening they seem the more likely they will be defined as serious (Mechanic, 1962). Familiarity refers both to the personal experience of the symptomatic person and that of his group. Common diseases that people have and recover from without treatment are seen as less serious than a symptom that has not been observed in one's social group or one that has been observed to cause incapacity or death. It has also been found that the longer the duration of a symptom and/or the more frequently it recurs the more it will be considered as serious (Mechanic, 1968).

5. *Assumptions about cause.* Symptoms are viewed in Western cultures as being caused, and the cause of almost any symptom can range from something relatively insignificant to life threatening. An episode of chest pain, for example, may be caused by a muscle spasm, indigestion, or coro-

nary heart disease to name a few possibilities. If the episode is thought to be a muscle spasm, it will be considered less serious than if it is thought to be a heart attack. Mechanic (1968) pointed out that most symptoms are ambiguous and may or may not be taken seriously, depending on the people involved. He illustrated this with a study of psychiatric patients and controls (Dinitz et al., 1961a, 1961b, 1962; Lefton et al., 1962, 1966; Angrist et al., 1963) in which the two groups were compared on such symptoms as "moving around restlessly," "always seems tired or worn out," "gets grouchy or ill tempered," "acts tense or nervous," and others. The interesting finding is that the psychiatric patients and controls did not differ on any of the symptoms investigated. It was suggested, although not investigated, that the groups differed in the degree to which they could explain the symptoms in other than an illness framework.

6. *Assumptions about prognosis.* The longer the symptom is expected to last the more the incapacity thought to be associated with it, and the more death is thought to be a likely outcome the more serious the symptom is thought to be. In a study of 1,000 residents of New York City, Gordon (1966) presented a list of disease descriptions. Each respondent was asked to state whether the case described constituted sickness. The more uncertain the prognosis was or the more the disease was thought to be progressively incapacitating, the higher the proportion reporting that the person was sick. Prognosis was relatively more important to middle-class than to working-class respondents.

7. *Interpersonal influence.* Symptomatic people generally confer with other people, and the advice they receive influences the kinds of decisions they make. Freidson (1961) conceptualized the symptomatic person as engaging a "lay referral system," consisting of family and friends who were consulted and who guided the individual toward or away from medical care. Twaddle (1969) studied older married males who had reported an illness and found that at the first appearance of a symptom, they usually consulted their wives. If the husband and wife disagreed or if her opinion was not valued, children, co-workers, and neighbors were consulted.

8. *Other crises in the life of the symptomatic person.* Symptoms are crisis events in themselves, at least potentially. They are also available to be used to solve other problems. Stoeckle et al. (1964) studied patients coming to the outpatient department of the Massachusetts General Hospital in Boston, with a focus on psychological distress symptoms. They found that 8 out of 10 patients had depression, hypochondriacal, obsessional, anxiety, delusional, or conversion symptoms and that these symptoms were often linked to the decision to seek medical aid. In the majority of cases, patients reported symptoms that had been long standing but that had become important because of some social stress. Studies that show increased reporting of chronic diseases immediately after retirement are consistent with the notion that individuals focus on symptoms as a means of coping with other stresses.

Decision that help is needed. If one recognizes that significant symptoms are present, it is necessary to decide whether the help of other people is needed or whether self-treatment will suffice. The phenomenal sales of over-the-counter patent medicines attest to the fact that self-treatment is common (Brecher, 1972). Many observers contend that self-treatment is the norm and that most disease and illness never reach the attention of health professionals (Freidson, 1962; Mechanic, 1968; Coe, 1970).

Several attempts may be made at self-treatment. The patient first may rest to see if the symptoms go away. Failing that, he may try patent medicines, special exercises, and similar measures. For many people, it is only when all efforts at self-treatment fail that the help of others is sought.

Decision as to the type of help needed. When an individual decides to seek help, he becomes immersed in a lay referral system (Freidson, 1961). Friends, family, neighbors, co-workers, and others are consulted and asked their opinions. Their judgments of "what is wrong" are solicited, treatments may be suggested or tried, and referrals are made to people who are presumed to be capable of helping. Such a referral system may or may not lead to consultation with a professional.

According to Freidson (1961, 1970), the likelihood that a person will see a professional depends on two factors: the degree of correspondence between the lay and professional cultures and the number of people consulted. Contact with a professional is most likely when the culture of the individual seeking help is similar to that of the professional and when the referral structure is extended (contains large numbers of people). From data gathered in the Bronx, Freidson (1961:198) reconstructed the typical pattern of seeking help as follows:

The process of seeking help began with purely personal, tentative self-diagnosis that implied their self-administered treatments. Upon failure of those first prescriptions, members of the household were consulted. Aid in self-diagnosis was sometimes sought from laymen outside the household—friends, neighbors, relatives, fellow-workers, a former nurse, or someone with the same trouble. Indeed, when exploration of the diagnosis was drawn out and not stopped early by cessation of symptoms or immediate recourse to a physician, the prospective patient referred himself, or was referred, through a hierarchy of consultant positions. The hierarchy ran from the intimate and informal confines of the nuclear family through successively less intimate lay consultants until the professional was finally reached.

In a study of older married males in Providence, Rhode Island, Twaddle (1968b, 1969) found that symptoms regarded as trivial were generally self-treated while a few were sufficiently dramatic to be taken directly to a physician.

In the majority of cases, however, there were important ambiguities surrounding the meaning of the relevant signs to the individual involved. Under these circumstances, there was a

process of "bargaining" over the definition of his current health status. Generally, for these married men, this bargaining seems to have begun with an exchange of information between the respondent and his wife, and in most cases, there was immediate agreement that the sign required the attention of a physician. . . . In those instances where disagreement occurred between the husband and wife, or where the wife's opinion was regarded as unimportant, other people, such as co-workers, children and friends were consulted. If one of these others were regarded as authoritative, because of professional training or personal experience with illness, and suggested seeing a physician, the physician was usually consulted (Twaddle, 1969:109).

In the absence of an authoritative layman, long delays resulted before a physician was seen, and in some cases the illness went untreated.

Other studies have shown a correspondence between the kind of treatment agent sought and the culture of an area. Members of the farm populations in the midwestern United States make more visits to chiropractors than members of urban populations in the same region. It has been argued that the chiropractic theory fits the mechanistic culture of the area by providing an understandable explanation of disease and a therapy that objectively works well for the most frequent kinds of complaints (e.g., muscle strain and skeletal misfunction) (Wardwell, 1952; McCorkle, 1961). Rural populations in India make selective use of Western medicine and native healing according to the nature of symptoms. Those symptoms that can be treated with Western techniques (i.e., acute infectious disease) are taken to physicians, whereas those that medicine can do little about (i.e., chronic debilitating disease) are taken to shamans (Carstairs, 1955; Marriott, 1955). Paul (1955) has collected impressive documentation on the failures of Western public health programs in traditional areas that have resulted from a lack of cultural fit.

Another body of literature has demonstrated effects of social class on the type of treatment agent sought. In general, persons of lower socioeconomic status are less likely to seek consultation with medical professionals in the presence of symptoms. Koos (1954) in his classical study of Regionville found that individuals of the lower strata made greater use of chiropractors, believing them to have a better explanation of illness and a better relationship with them as people. Lower rates of utilization of medical practitioners among members of the lower strata have also been reported by Graham (1958) and Anderson (1963), although Ross (1962) has argued persuasively that social class differentials in this regard are diminishing over time. With reference to mental illness, Redlich et al. (1955) have shown that positive attitudes toward psychiatry are greater the higher the social class level. These differences are partly the result of differences in opportunities. They also reflect, however, differences in norms. Whether the experience of the National Health Service in the United Kingdom (Stevens, 1966) or studies of public welfare recipients in the United States (Brightman et al., 1958), it has been shown that even in the absence of financial barriers, class differences in medical care utilization persist (Stoeckle and Zola, 1964).

In any given instance, the type of treatment agent to be sought is generally not a major issue. Different groups have traditional sources of help for disease and illness, and the influence patterns brought to bear on individuals will generally lead to that particular source. More at issue is the number of steps before seeking the ultimate source. People who see physicians are most often those who would not consider chiropractors, faith healers, or Christian Science readers. The question of whether the conditions necessary to make a consultation are present is major. In over 200 interviews with medical patients, one of us (A. C. T.) has yet to encounter a single case in which the decision to see a physician was not discussed with others and a recommendation to see a physician was not made.

Decision to see a particular treatment agent. The specific treatment agent sought (physician, chiropractor, nurse, faith healer) may be problematic in situations in which more than one is available. For people who have had prior treatment, it might generally be expected that they would return to the same one. The process of making a selection, however, has not been systematically studied. The only study found bearing on this topic was one investigating the use of National Health Service physicians in the United Kingdom. Gray and Cartwright (1953) found that most people used National Health Services physicians, and about half chose their physician without any prior knowledge or even hearsay. Presumably selection was based on geographical convenience. Whether these findings would apply to a country with a less evenly dispersed physician population or one in which the services were provided under different financial arrangements is not known.

Research has provided some suggestive leads. In studies of medical practice in Toronto, Ontario, and Providence, Rhode Island, Hall (1946, 1947, 1949) found that patients tended to be ethnically matched with their physicians. Jewish patients tended to go to Jewish physicians, Irish patients to Irish physicians, and so on. This suggests that the sharing of a common culture, which includes assumptions about disease and treatment, is one factor taken into account when particular physicians are selected.

Freidson's (1961, 1970) account of the "lay referral system" suggests that particular treatment agents are selected as the result of a referral from a medical layman who has had prior contact or knowledge. It also suggests that the problem of selection on the part of the patient may be limited to "client dependent practices," which get new patients from the recommendations of old ones. In specialized practices, referrals are made by other professionals, and after first contact the patient is immersed in a "professional referral system." Both of these are discussed more fully in Chapter 10.

Decision as to the degree and types of cooperation offered to the treatment agent. It is often thought to be axiomatic that treatment agents will prescribe a course of treatment to be followed by the patient and that the patient will follow the treatment prescribed. Among professionals, it is often assumed that the "uncooperative" patient is the exception to the rule and that failure to cooperate is to be explained as a negative character trait of the patient who "doesn't care about his own health" or "lacks a will to live." For the most part, this is shown to be a defensive posture by the consistent finding of sociological investigations that most patients do not cooperate with all the treatment prescribed (Twaddle, 1969; Vincent, 1971). People differ in the degree of cooperation they will offer. Total cooperation with all measures prescribed is a rarity.

Several factors influence the degree and kinds of cooperation offered with treatment programs, including the following: the kind of treatment involved, changes in symptoms in response to treatment, the fit between the treatment and expectations of the patient, and the support of the patient's family and friends. Every treatment has a cost not only in monetary terms but also in terms of discomfort, degradation, and the sacrifice of alternative pursuits. If this cost is higher than corresponding benefits, at least as perceived by the patient, the likelihood of cooperation is reduced.

In his Providence study, Twaddle (1969) found that it made a difference whether the treatment was active (i.e., required the patient to do something such as take medications, exercise, or modify diet) or passive (i.e., required that the patient allow something to be done to him such as an injection or surgery). The rate of noncooperation was high among those involved in active treatment and low among those involved in passive treatment. In a comprehensive literature review of the process of recovery from heart disease, Croog et al. (1968) reported that the Purdue Farm Cardiac Project found that patients reported high degrees of compliance with dietary restrictions and low compliance with changes in "personal habits." Johnson (1966) found compliance with taking medications high but lower cooperation with avoiding "stress and strain."

In a pilot study of factors leading to preventable hospital admissions, Sweet and Twaddle (1969a) found that some patients' admissions were "preventable" because they had discontinued treatment sooner than their physicians had desired. Generally, these patients took their medications until their symptoms disappeared but discontinued treatment before the infection had been eliminated. A similar pattern was found by Twaddle (1969) particularly among the Protestants. Italian and Jewish respondents were more likely to take medications but less likely to adhere to dietary changes.

Davis and Eichhorn (1963) found that rural Indiana men were more apt to comply with treatment for heart disease when they had a relatively low work orientation, were less educated, and had a more formal as opposed to friendly relationship with their physicians. Compliance increased with increasing duration of symptoms.

In a study of hospitalized patients, Davis and von der Lippe (1967) found that discharge from the hospital against the advice of the physician resulted from a lack of fit between the expectations of the patient and his treatment in the hospital. Especially important were the diagnostic tests, which convinced many patients that they were the subject of experiments. Those who expected events similar to those that actually occurred were less likely to leave treatment.

New et al. (1968) studied patients discharged from a rehabilitation center in Boston to discover the extent to which they followed the prescribed rehabilitation program. They found that most patients did not because others in their household discouraged them from doing so. The program often involved the collaboration of other household members, and treatment was inconvenient for many people other than the patient.

The nature of the communications between the physician and patient has been identified as critical by Croog et al. (1968), including what the physician and patient tell each other and the adequacy of the communication, that is, how much each understands of what the other tells him. Szasz and Hollender (1956) described three "doctor-patient relationship models" that apply here: the activity-passivity model, in which the treatment agent is active and the patient passive; the guidance-cooperation model, in which the patient cooperates with the guidance of the treatment agent; and the mutual participation model in which the physician helps the patient to help himself. Thus the range is from complete dominance-submission to complete negotiation. It is presumed that the mutual participation model minimizes miscommunications and leads to greater cooperation on the part of both the therapist and patient.

Career contingencies

The seven steps just discussed are points at which some decision gets made, which takes into account a set of norms regarded as appropriate to a given situation as negotiated with a set of other people whose opinions are significant. As shown in Fig. 5-2, alternative decisions at any step can either lead to further decisions or to a reconsideration of earlier ones. Hence several pathways are possible for the sickness career.

Assuming that someone makes the necessary decisions to be under the treatment of an agent regarded as appropriate and to some extent cooperates with that agent, three outcomes seem possible: the patient can recover and again be defined as well, the patient can partially recover but in a way that necessitates a redefinition of what it means to be well, or the patient can die.

Getting well. In most cases of acute disease, it is expected that the patient will get well. Motivation and cooperation toward this goal are explicitly part of the sick role formulation. At some point in the treatment process a decision is made, usually by the treatment agent and sometimes by the patient or those with whom he interacts, that (1) the symptoms that initiated the redefinition of health identity have disappeared and (2) they are not likely to return. At this point, sometimes abruptly and sometimes gradually, the patient withdraws from treatment and resumes normal activities at the level preceding the onset of symptoms. That is, the well role is resumed.

Becoming impaired. Alternatively, resulting from most chronic conditions and some acute ones (e.g., polio), the sick person may not get well. Instead the disease process may be arrested in such a manner that although no longer sick the patient is still not normal. Either continuous treatment is needed to forestall death (e.g., diabetes) or permanent residual damage may be done by the disease process (e.g., paralysis from polio). Such persons are not generally considered to be sick, but neither are they considered to be well. From the perspective of societal standards, such persons are incapacitated (deviant) to some degree, and at the same time they must define the new capacity level as normal for them. Both the normal expectation for well people and the special expectations for sick people would be considered inappropriate.

In exploring the sick role as applied to a variety of case descriptions, Gordon (1966) found that the expectations held for people of this type could be described in terms of an "impaired role." The impaired role parallels the sick role with the exception that people are not exempted from normal activities but rather are expected to engage in them as much as possible within the limits of their impairment.

The handicapped person shares with many other people the problem of being stigmatized (Goffman, 1963). That is, they have some characteristic that is deeply discrediting to their personal identities. This characteristic leads to a "spoiled identity, and renders the individual suspect in moral character." Mental illness, imprisonment, drug addiction, alcoholism, homosexuality, and unemployment are characteristics that, in addition to physical defects (what Goff-man calls "abominations of the body"), re-sult in the same generic outcome:

An individual who might have been re-ceived easily in ordinary social intercourse pos-sesses a trait that can obtrude itself upon atten-tion and turn those of us whom he meets away from him, breaking the claim that his other at-tributes have on us. He possesses a stigma, an undesired differentness from what we had an-ticipated (Goffman, 1963: 4-5).

To be impaired is to be "different"; val-ued attributes have been stripped away. Frequently, one believes that it is no longer possible to expect to be treated as a person. Those confined to wheelchairs often report that "people only see the chair, never me." The point is that an impairment to varying degrees imposes a social as well as a physi-cal handicap, complicating all aspects of liv-ing (MacGregor et al., 1953).

Dying. The third possible outcome, that the patient may die, deserves special atten-tion. As noted in Chapter 3 death has been a taboo topic until recently (Farberow, 1963). Not until the mid-1960s was there any sociological literature on death. Most of this literature has focused on the manage-ment of death in hospital settings, which will be discussed later. Some findings should be noted here, however.

There may come a point at which it seems impossible to arrest the disease pro-cess. From the standpoint of the health pro-fessional, who is trained to cure, there is "nothing left to be done." Typically the staff abandons the patient. They drop in occasionally to "see how things are going" but spend as little time as possible. To be defined as dying is to disrupt social interac-tion patterns (Glaser and Strauss, 1967, 1968).

When the patient discovers that he is dying, he begins a psychological career con-sisting of five stages: *denial,* manifested by assertions that it is not happening and that there must have been a mistake; *anger,* dominated by the question "why me?"; *bar-gaining* with family, professionals, and God for more time; *depression,* a period of griev-ing for the impending loss of contact with other people; and *acceptance,* a readiness to face the inevitable (Kubler-Ross, 1970). Each of these stages presents special prob-lems for people interacting with the pa-tient, especially if they are unaware of the causes for the behavioral changes.

Patients differ in the social worth they have to the professional staff. Those who are defined as having more value receive more attention from the staff, and fre-quently, more effort is expended to prolong their lives and to ensure their comfort (Glaser and Strauss, 1967; Twaddle, 1973a; Crane, 1974).

SICKNESS AS A COPING PROCESS

With the kind of analytical approach taken here, it is easy to lose sight of the human problems of sickness. The response to symptoms is seldom if ever as dispassion-ate or rational as we have suggested. The benefit of a model, such as the decision steps listed previously, is its usefulness in imposing order on our observations. It is a way of dealing with reality and should not be confused with the reality itself.

Many events in life are sources of stress, events that interfere with the capability of people to deal effectively with their lives (Levine and Scotch, 1970). One response to stress is to develop symptoms (Wolff, 1953). As indicated in Chapter 3, stress in social relationships is one factor implicated as a major cause of disease.

There is also reason to believe that the appearance of symptoms is always stressful. In some instances, such as the case of pain, the stress may be physiological; in others, such as depression, it may be psychological; and in others, such as inability to carry on one's job, it may be social. Increasingly it is being recognized that these dimen-sions interpenetrate and that social stress can cause biological symptoms and vice versa (Mauksch, 1973).

In addition to physical discomfort, the emergence of symptoms is generally accom-panied by fear or anxiety. Symptoms may mean death, personal degradation, and lost chances. They require efforts to cope: to come to terms with the event, to make sense of it, and, if possible, to overcome it (Mechanic, 1968). This is often accomplished to the tune of much personal anguish both for the individual involved and for others with whom he is in contact. In addition, symptoms can disrupt organized activities and relationships in the family, at work, and among recreational groups. In short, the implications of any individual getting sick are not confined to that individual but ramify throughout all the social networks in which he is engaged. The introduction of a symptom presents a confrontation with the unknown for all involved, an element of uncertainty and unpredictability that is itself stressful. It may be necessary to contend with incapacity and dependency and call for mobilization of all the resources of the group to protect its integrity and to restore predictability to life, if not the status quo ante.

Unfortunately, although there has been much polemical literature in social work and community psychiatry that reports case studies of people coping with the stress induced by symptoms, there has been little systematic research beyond noting that people often seek medical attention in direct response to stress (Kadushin, 1964; Rosenstock, 1960; Mechanic, 1962; Stoeckle et al., 1963; Zola, 1964; Twaddle, 1969; Mauksch, 1973). It has also been found that the failure of one kind of treatment sometimes leads to search for another type. When cancer patients are not successfully treated by medical practitioners, they often detour to other types of healers (Cobb, 1954).

The process of coping with symptoms is a fruitful area for research that needs work in the development of hypotheses and methods. Although it can safely be presumed that illness in an individual disrupts the whole network of family relationships, for example, little is known about this phenomenon. Following models proposed by Bott (1957), Wheaton (1970) analyzed the experience of families with a member hospitalized in a rehabilitation center. She found two "crisis points." The first occurred at the time of injury (most of the patients had strokes) when the family had to reorganize to reallocate the tasks performed by the sick member. The second occurred with recovery when family members were asked to return to the patient the tasks he previously performed. In the interim it was presumed that other family members developed "vested interests" in performing the tasks, making recovery a threat.

Stahl (1971) has suggested that families have a "health estate" consisting of the ways in which they view illness and respond to symptoms. This estate includes levels of health and disease and tends to be passed on from one generation to the next.

The family is only one area that needs investigation. Perhaps some idea of the complexity of the problems can be gained from considering a few case histories. What follows is a series of statements by patients at the Massachusetts General Hospital, Boston, Massachusetts, during the summer of 1968 (Sweet and Twaddle, 1969). They are not representative of hospitalized patients much less sick people, nor do their reports take them beyond the point of entering the hospital.

CASE 1. Mr. O'Donnell* was a 67-year-old divorced, retired salesman who was hospitalized with a severe respiratory disease. He had a long history of heavy cigarette smoking and obesity and had been hospitalized several times for bronchitis, obesity, shortness of breath, and unnatural drowsiness. He related the following story:

I put on weight in the last couple of years. I was in the C ———— Hospital in 1965. I lost 60 or so pounds and got down very well. Of course, when you get out, you start to get a little careless. If you eat out, you can't get diet meals. You go into a restaurant, you wind up having a sandwich or meat and potatoes, and maybe you get tempted and have some ice cream. First thing you know, you built up your weight again. I've been through this thing three times.

I haven't been feeling well since Christmas, maybe back further. Different friends of mine would say, "Donney, you got to watch that belly." I also noticed that I had shortness of breath.

—————

*All names are fictitious.

When this first happened, I didn't think it was important. All of a sudden, I got pains in my side with coughing. I had pleurisy. I felt on the sick side, called my doctor. I went down to see him. He gave me penicillin (this was in the second week of June). I went back the next day. Two days later, I looked at my abdomen and there was a big purple mark. I couldn't wait to see him that afternoon. I told him about it and showed it to him. The doctor said, "That must have happened from coughing, I'm pretty sure you broke blood vessels." He asked if I fell, if I had blood in my throat, or if I had passed blood. He said it was just small blood vessels that wouldn't matter. He said, "I think I want a blood test." I got the test Saturday morning and saw him Saturday afternoon. He felt I had passed a crisis.

When I went home that Saturday, I went across the street to a restaurant for lunch. It took me a long time to get back across. I couldn't get my breath. I didn't feel right that afternoon.

Sunday, Father's Day, I had no pep. My grandchildren came to see me. Monday, I was really going. I got up and then got back in bed and stayed there until now. I called the restaurant across the street and asked the waiter, who I know pretty well, to bring me over an eggnog. That's all I felt like. I didn't feel like anything too solid.

Tuesday morning I was still lingering around. Each night I perspired, so I was weak in the morning. My landlady said, in severe talk, "You're going to get out, eat, and go to the doctor." I felt sick. I called the doctor. He came to see me. I just got to the point where I was just all in. I threw up my hands. I said, "Doctor, what hospital are you connected with?" He said, "Mass. General, Don. You grab a cab and go down."

Mr. O'Donnell had different decision careers for different symptoms. He apparently attributed his shortness of breath to obesity. Although both he and his friends noticed the symptom, it was seen as not significant. The same was true of his not "feeling well" until, after a lapse of some 6 months, he developed pain connected with his coughing. The pain was new and regarded as abnormal, significant, and something he could not treat himself, so he called his physician. Even though he was under the care of a physician, he did not seek help for his loss of energy in late June. Instead he defined the symptom as something significant that he could handle alone. He went to bed for several days. It was not until his landlady insisted that he get treatment that he called the physician.

CASE 2. Mrs. Dolliver was a 72-year-old woman who had been widowed seventeen years earlier.

Before her marriage, she had worked as a school teacher. When her children were grown, she returned to teaching and later secretarial work, from which she retired at the age of 69 years. At the time of her admission, she was a housemother in a dormitory serving several small art colleges. Her story follows:

They tell me I had a heart attack. I had been getting the feeling of being terribly tired for 2 weeks. That's not usual for me. I'm an active woman. I noticed I was short of breath.

Last Friday, I woke up with a terrible pain that I thought was indigestion. It got worse, but I never thought it was my heart. My mother lived until 87½ years of age, and I thought I was following in her footsteps. I thought I was just like my mother; that I wouldn't have a heart attack until I went. I didn't do anything. I just felt it was an effort to be alive. I walked up two flights of stairs. The pain got worse all day. About 2:00 PM, I thought I'd forget about it. I walked to the store. Thinking back, I remember I would go into a dead sleep for a few minutes at times during the last few weeks. Between 5:00 and 5:30 PM I went for supper to the cafeteria around the corner. A retired nurse, a housemother, said to me at the table, "What's the matter, Mrs. Dolliver?" I guess she could tell by the way I looked that something was wrong. I said, "Something's going to happen to me." She took my pulse and said, "As soon as you get back to your room, call your doctor."

As I was walking back, the pains were shooting in back. I went to my room. It's funny, I left the door to my room open, and I never do that. The pain was so terrible, I was having to struggle to breathe. I still didn't think it was heart. I thought of calling my sister-in-law, telling her that something may happen to me and that she'd better call me later. But I didn't call.

I can't remember what happened next. I told two of my girls, "I don't know what happened to me, girls." They said that another girl had gone by my room at 7:00 PM, and my door was open. She looked in and I was bent over. She went downstairs and then came back with another girl. They found me unconscious on the floor. I remember seeing a girl call someone. Then I remember a policeman say, "Oxygen." Then he said, "Mass. General or St. E———'s," and I remember thinking "Mass." The policeman said, "can't wait for St. E———'s, take her to Mass." I'm glad they took me here. I came into the Emergency Room.

I didn't think it was important until Friday. I knew it was wearing me out. I thought, "I wonder if it was my heart." But it got me before I could decide.

I was going to call Dr. W——— that Friday. I was very confused. I dialed the wrong number a couple of times. Then I decided not to bother him.

If I had it to do over, I'd never walk up five flights of stairs again. For a couple of weeks, I had had spells of indigestion. Now, thinking about it, I guess it wasn't indigestion. For the past 2 weeks, I've had to hold my head. It thumped so hard. I'd be dizzy. I thought my blood pressure was up. I was worn out. Maybe if I had stopped then and gotten a vacation, I might have warded this off.

Mrs. Dolliver had spent 2 weeks noticing "something wrong" but apparently attaching little significance to her symptoms. Even with substantial pain, she was uncertain as to whether anything needed to be done. After talking with her friend at dinner, she became convinced that the symptoms were important and the she needed help. At that time, she tried to call her physician but was too confused to complete the call. When she lost consciousness, others defined the situation as important and took the steps that led to her being admitted to the hospital.

CASE 3. Mr. Trano was a 47-year-old, married truck driver who was admitted to the hospital with a major heart attack.

I first thought I might not be well Thursday morning. I woke up and was getting all sorts of funny feelings in my chest. I had a breathless feeling. Also my heart was missing beats and had extra beats. I worked all day. I'm a truck driver; I handle heavy stuff, light stuff, anything I can wrestle around. I figure if I outweigh it, I can handle it.

At 2:00 in the afternoon, I developed pain in my chest and arms. Those feelings had been getting worse all day. I came to the hospital between 10:00 and 10:30 at night.

Thursday morning, when it first started to happen, I didn't know what to think. I thought I had a cramp in the muscle, or something. I didn't think much of it until it got progressively worse, until I got pain in my chest and arm. I told a couple of fellows at work before noon. They didn't give me any advice. When a fellow of my size and strength complains, people ignore it.

I first thought it might be important when I got the pain in the afternoon. My heart started skipping beats and there were extra heart beats. I had to slow down. Actually, I worked at practically nothing all afternoon. On the way home from work, I decided I had better go and have it looked at.

If the dog wasn't so sick, I could have come in sooner. I thought there was something wrong. When I got home, my wife said that my son had a fever and the dog had diarrhea and vomiting. She said, "the dog had to go to A———— (a veterinary hospital) now!" I didn't have a chance to tell her

about myself until we were in the car. She very definitely thought I should have it looked at. I very seldom complain of something wrong. When I did, she knew something was wrong.

Mr. Trano first noticed some "funny feelings" but apparently interpreted them as either normal or as insignificant. The symptoms gained salience during the day when they became defined as chest and arm pain. He attempted to get confirmation from his co-workers but failed to get a response. Even so, he began to treat himself by "slowing down" and resting. After meeting the medical needs of his dog, he was able to get confirmation from his wife that he needed medical attention.

A NOTE ON HUMAN RESPONSE

Although in Western societies and perhaps in others we have come to think of resources for coping with disease and illness as technological, the previous analysis suggests that they are at least equally human. It is a hallmark of Western civilization that life has become depersonalized or in the language of Max Weber (Gerth and Mills, 1946), rationalized and disenchanted. Although producing enormous economic benefits, at least in the short run, this process has taken place at a high cost, which is just now coming to be recognized.

The response to disease and illness has been to seek better technology. The volume of food production per acre has been improved. Storage facilities and transportation systems have been created that have almost eliminated endemic famine. Much has been learned about the structure and function of the human body. A formidable armamentarium of drugs, surgical technique, and sophisticated equipment has been created. In short, the biblical injunction to subdue and dominate the earth has been followed (Deloria, 1969, 1970, 1972, 1973).

One mechanism for subjugation has been the development of an ideology, which came to dominate Europe by the eighteenth century, that emphasized individualism and competition. The ideal was for each person to be on his own and prepared to deal sharply with his fellow man. This ideology was quickly recognized at the time of colonization of the New World by the Native-American populations, who believed that man is an integral part of nature and cannot subjugate it without ultimately destroying himself and who had an ideology of cooperation (Council on Interracial Books for Children, 1971; McLuhan, 1971; Vogel, 1972). The alternative they proposed was to emphasize human rather than technological resources (Deloria, 1972, 1973).

The Native-American argument has merit when applied to illness behavior. As we have seen, human resources are of enormous importance. To recognize and respond to symptoms, people need to interact with others. They need to have help to understand and interpret what is happening to them and to decide a proper response. There is evidence that in the absence of this human resource base, people fail to link up with appropriate sources of help (Sweet and Twaddle, 1969a).

We raise the question as to whether our culture is adequate to cope with sickness. Might it not be better had we followed the Native-American approach, emphasizing communion rather than competition? Then the isolated of Western cultures would have a home among people who care. They would not be denied the human resources necessary to the solution of their problems. This question is a serious one, since our individualistic, property-oriented, technological approach to problems may be leading to ecocide and our ultimate destruction.

PART THREE

THE HEALING OCCUPATIONS

As noted in Chapter 1, the response to sickness is not random. Every society makes some provision for the treatment of the sick. Every society has some people who are to some degree specialized in taking care of sick people. In this section, we will look at some of the occupations that are so specialized.

Most individuals who have been exposed to Western medical ideology develop a kind of medicentrism. In this state, they tend to think of healing occupations as synonymous with Western medical professions. They miss the extensive diversity of traditional healing occupations that do not derive from the established Western medical profession. Not only are non-Western medical practitioners extensively used, but non-Western healing systems serve the important societal functions of promoting ethnic solidarity and providing needed medical services. Chapter 6 explores faith healing, Chinese-American medicine, Native-American medicine, and the Mexican-American practice of *curanderismo* as a few examples of widely used and important traditional healing practices in the United States.

Chapter 7 deals with the most central occupation in health care, both from the standpoint of public opinion and political power, the physician. Some historical background on the modern physician sets the stage for an analysis of major trends in medical training, the organization of medical practice into specialties, and the nature of the medical career. The discussion encompasses the osteopath and chiropractor, as well as the more dominant medical physician. We anticipate that some may object to the inclusion of chiropractic, and in fact we have already heard such objections. Nevertheless, whatever differences there may be on other grounds, these fields are sociologically equivalent and should be dealt with together, hence our decision to do exactly that.

In Chapter 8 we examine another occupation that has a history that antedates the twentieth century, nursing. As with the physician, the process of becoming a nurse and the organization of nursing practice are briefly reviewed. Nursing, however, is in a special kind of ferment, trying to define and redefine its mandate vis-à-vis medicine. We give considerable attention therefore to the changing role of the nurse and the currently enacted conflicts with the medical profession.

During the present century, there has been a rapid proliferation of new occupations in the health field. Medical care is now dependent on armies of technicians and specialized therapists. In Chapter 9 some of these new occupations are described: the physician's assistant, community health worker, and nurse practitioner. We also identify some of the issues that these new health workers raise for the nature of health care occupations and for the organization of health care systems.

The student will note some important "holes" in our discussion of health occupations. We do not present any information, for example, about dentists, veterinarians, physical therapists, occupational therapists, learning disability specialists, laboratory technicians, medical social workers, or any number of occupations that are increasingly important for the delivery of health services. The reason for this is simple. There is little sociological literature on any of these. For some reason, sociologists have focused almost all their attention on a limited range of occupations. We hope that by the next edition of this text, this situation will be remedied.

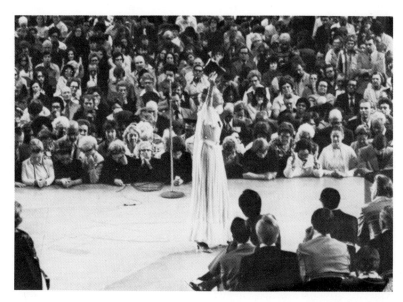

Courtesy Doug Grandstaff Photography, Tulsa, Okla.,
and Kathryn Kuhlman Foundation, Pittsburgh, Pa.

CHAPTER 6

Types of healers

For those individuals who have been educated in the Western Judeo-Christian tradition, this chapter will create some anxiety and difficulty. They will be made anxious, possibly even angry, because concepts about healing and medicine that comprise part of their fundamental epistemology will be challenged. The difficulty will arise because of their trained incapacity to recognize the diversity of healing roles in all societies the world over, North America included.

We have come to accept the dogma, on faith alone, that healing and medicine are the exclusive domain of physicians, nurses, and other Western-trained health professionals. Furthermore, we are convinced that medicine as practiced by Western-trained health professionals is primarily a logical discipline based on methods derived from the natural sciences. The ethos has it that Western medicine has been with us from

time immemorial, and other healing systems are viewed as third-rate attempts at emulation. Legitimation for these beliefs occurs through licensure procedures and civil laws that effectively control and determine who practices medicine legally in our society.

This chapter shall attempt to examine or, at least, classify these points. To do this, our medicocentric concept of healing will have to be put aside long enough to permit the discovery of great diversity in the types of healers and systems of medicine extant in our society. This process in no way diminishes the vitality and importance of the dominant form of medical practice that is called "Western medicine." Instead, by carefully looking at alternative types of healers and their respective systems of medical beliefs, one can better appreciate the rich heritage and contribution

139

which they have made to Western medicine and to our lives.

Specifically in this chapter, we present a frame of reference and then discuss the following types of healers and healing systems: (1) *curanderismo,* (2) spiritual (faith) healing, (3) Native-American healing, and (4) Chinese-American healing.

A FRAME OF REFERENCE

Every society, if it is to survive at all, must see to it that diseases and illnesses are contained at least to the extent that the majority of its members are able to function adequately. For this reason, healing is one of the most important roles in a society, and great prestige is accorded those who occupy the status "healer." Society's confidence in healing and healers goes far back historically. Ancient Mayan or Greek writings illustrate how the patient's confidence in healers was based on the religious belief that the gods taught the art of medicine (Greek, *technai*) to mortals, thereby lending great social prestige to those who took up the role of healer and practiced medicine.

In the practice of healing, four elements are constantly at work: (1) the symbolic, (2) the technical, (3) theories of disease and/or illness, and (4) the social organization of the healing role. These elements are value added in the sense that if the healer has a theory of disease causation, he will also have technical and symbolic facets to his healing. Conversely, possession of symbols or techniques does not imply necessarily that the healer subscribes to a particular theory about disease etiology. Western use of Chinese acupuncture is a good example of how some healers utilize techniques with little or no knowledge of the theory behind them.

The symbolic

Healing has its origins in religious beliefs of which symbolic representations of good and evil constitute an important component. It is not surprising therefore to find a significant use of symbols by all heal-ers, Western and non-Western. Symbols include the healer's particular style of dress, the kinds of tools or instruments used by the healer, and a particular language as well. For example, Western physicians have symbols that include a white coat, high technology, and the use of Latin words such as "edema" and "hematoma" to describe swelling and bruises. Symbols are important to the healer primarily because they signify in a graphic way to all interested parties that the society or some group within the society considers the bearer uniquely qualified to practice some form of medicine. Symbols communicate to others the identifying characteristics of healers and help to maintain the professional dominance of healers relative to their patients and other healing occupations.

The technical

The technical side of healing includes the use of remedies, therapeutic procedures, and hygienic practices for preventive and primary medical care. For the treatment of medical problems, techniques can be divided into those which do or do not utilize drugs or herbs that can be applied to internal disorders versus external conditions and injuries (Fig. 6-1).

As shown in Fig. 6-1, different types of healers can be placed within one or more of the four cells, depending on the techniques they use to treat patients. For example, Swanton (1928) described how the Chickasaw Indians used herbs to treat internal infection. For one disease called the "burning ghost disease," in which large sores appear on swollen feet, the Indian healer took soil from the top of a grave, baked it in a pan, and applied it to the sores. Vogel (1970) has suggested that antibiotics may have been used unknowingly through this technique long before Western medicine "discovered" them in the midtwentieth century.

As another example, herbs are applied to external injuries for therapeutic purposes. A traditional Chinese healer will not use a Western-type cast for the repair of a

DIAGNOSIS

	Internal disorder	External disorder
Drugs/herbs	Medicine man	*Curanderismo: sobador* (bone manipulator)
No drugs/herbs	Spiritual healer	*Curanderismo: bruja* (witch)

TREATMENT MODE

Fig. 6-1. *Types of healers according to diagnosis and treatment mode.*

broken bone. Instead the injured part is wrapped with herbs, and a soft bandage is wound around the affected area. At no time is the injured part immobilized in the fashion of Western orthopedic practices.

With regard to prevention of disease, techniques exist for preserving or improving health. These can be classified according to whether the specific technique is applied or taken internally (e.g., dietary practices) as opposed to measures applied to the body externally. This would include practices such as sweat baths or the placing of hot herbal compresses against the body.

Theories of disease

This is the ideational component of healing and medical practice. Generally, symbols and techniques of healers are derived from theories about causes of disease held by the healers. Of course, these theories are influenced by the discovery of new techniques, beliefs of the members of the larger society, and, at a level closer to home, beliefs of the consumers.

Theories about disease and illness can be thought of as containing two major dimensions: an explanation of the cause of specific diseases or illnesses and a classification of diseases based in part on knowledge of the causes and effects of diseases.

For example, Rivers (1924) and later Clements (1939) argued that primitive societies worldwide have evolved theories about disease and illness that are predicated on the notion that disease is an ab-

normal phenomenon. Furthermore, they pointed out that there are three general categories or classes of disease: (1) disease due to natural causes; (2) disease related to human actions, usually defined as evil; and (3) disease resulting from supernatural forces. More specifically, five causes of disease and illness were defined as follows:

1. *Sorcery.* Disease due to the manipulation of persons either skilled in magic or with control of supernatural forces. Two types of sorcery exist: imitative sorcery (e.g., voodoo dolls) and contagious sorcery, in which the sorcerer induces illness through a personal item of the subject.

2. *Breach of taboo.* Disease resulting from the punishment of the gods for violating religious or social norms.

3. *Disease-object intrusion.* Disease due to the presence of a noxious foreign substance in the body.

4. *Spirit intrusion.* Disease that is the result of the presence within the body of demons or evil spirits.

5. *Soul loss.* Illness due to the loss of one's soul leaving the body.

Although this classification scheme is not inclusive of all theories about disease causality, it gives one a sense of how disease theories penetrate many aspects of one's life, exerting control over the sick and the well alike. Theories about disease causation are primarily logical and are deeply embedded in societies' attempts to define the purpose of man and his relationship to the environment (Ackerknecht, 1942). As such, the religious, philosophical, magical, and scientific collective representations by society are used by healers to devise theories that can explain the mysteries of why people get sick, why they recover, or, perhaps, why they die.

The social organization of the healing role

The healer may have symbols, techniques, and even some theories about the cause of diseases, but unless some form of social organization exists for the healer to operate within, there will be no delivery of medical services.

Perhaps the most fundamental aspect of the organization of the healing role is the matter of the healer-patient relationship. Before any healing can be performed, norms must be established that govern the nature of the healer-patient relationship. Three important aspects of this relationship must be considered. First, the question of patient pathways to the healer must be understood. That is, why did the patient decide to use this healer, and what were the decision paths that led to the healer? Second, one must understand the expectations of the healer and patient as they meet in the medical encounter. These expectations will determine to a large extent what type of communication transpires between the patient and the healer and what goes on in the healing process. Often if barriers to communication exist, they can be traced to differences in expectations.

For example, at the simplest level, a healer or patient may approach the relationship with either instrumental (discipline, punishment) or expressive (conciliation, solicitousness, warmth, affection) expectations. Problems in the relationship can occur when expectations of the patient and healer do not match, for example, cells b and c in the diagram below. What goes on in the healing act depends on these two dimensions of the organization of the healing role.

Finally, the status of the healer within the larger community or society is an important aspect of the social organization of healing. Depending on the prestige of the healer vis-à-vis the patient, the nature of the relationship will be determined to a large extent in terms of how the patient approaches the healer, how much control the patient has over his body during healing, whether the patient feels free to confront the healer about problems, how much the healer and patient can discuss, and how close the healer and patient can get to each other socially. If the healer and patient share similar cultural experiences and come from similar socioeconomic backgrounds, their relationship will be much closer and open than in cases in which healer and patient diverge culturally or economically.

A brief comment is necessary concerning the issue of why patients utilize healers who are not Western-trained physicians. Research has opened our minds to the fact that many patients "veer off the orthodox path" and seek advice or health services from healers who are not trained in the Western scientific schools of medicine and related fields such as nursing, pharmacy, and physical therapy. Traditional healers (non-Western–trained practitioners) are seen

HEALER EXPECTATIONS

		Instrumental	Expressive
PATIENT EXPECTATIONS	Instrumental	a	b
	Expressive	c	d

by the medical profession as unscientific or magical, and studies tend to juxtapose science and magic (Hsu, 1952; Stekert, 1970) by assuming that patients who utilize Western medicine are scientific and are forsaking traditional healers. This could not be farther from the truth. Instead of falling into the trap of assuming that only the Western-trained physician is the right and legitimate healer to go to for help, we take the position that patients take many different paths, some orthodox, others unorthodox, to reach the goal of obtaining relief from their physical, social, or emotional problems. This is the norm rather than the exception, and studies support this (Maclean, 1969; Press, 1969; Schwartz, 1969).

We suggest that pathways to care be viewed as completely open in which beliefs based on magic and science can and do coexist in a person's mind and their health-seeking behavior may take the individual down one or more of several paths. Some of these pathways may never enter the orbit of the Western-trained professional, as seen in the following discussion of some types of healers.

SPIRITUAL HEALING

The longest recorded history of healing going back to the Old Testament can be found in the voluminous accounts of healings performed in the name of religion through the power of God (Dawson, 1935; Frost, 1940; Scherzer, 1950). Out of this historical context, modern-day spiritual healers have emerged to "lay hands" on countless thousands of persons seeking help for ills of every conceivable type.

"Spiritual healers" refers to individuals who are recognized by others for having the unique ability to cure physical and emotional illnesses. The healer most often works out of one of the organized churches, but there are spiritual healers who are not attached to any specific denomination. A distinguishing common characteristic, however, is that spiritual healers, for the most part, do not attribute their healing powers to personal abilities but rather view them-selves as a conduit or conveyor of the power of a transcendent, superior force identified as "God."

Insight about spiritual healers can be gained by considering the motivations for becoming a healer. Data on this subject were gathered through personal interviews with six nationally known spiritual healers and by attending a number of healing ministries to observe the healers at work (New et al., 1971).

Persons became spiritual healers suddenly. A conversion process occurred precipitated by a certain event that made a drastic change in their lives. The healers were engaged in careers or work unrelated to spiritual healing when suddenly something happened to them, and they rededicated their lives to spiritual healing. In many instances, they were floundering, not knowing what to do next, when they "found the light." According to one healer, when he was in the Navy, he met a sailor:

God put a Christian sailor on our ship. He knew where he was going. I watched his life for 9 months and I became very impressed. I was basically a playboy.

The Christian sailor became a model for the healer and gradually he learned to pray. He said:

One night I read 51st Psalms, David's Repentance. I prayed, "If you are really God and if Jesus Christ was really your Son—there were lots of ifs—then you renew in me the right heart and give me the right spirit." I was already in bed when I prayed and I fell asleep. The next day I woke up and I had a tremendous change of attitude.

However, this change of attitude was minor compared with a dramatic event that occurred a little later:

One night I was praying in a radio shack. I was concerned about a few things. I was going to stay in the Navy as a Christian sailor, but something was nagging me. I felt that God had something else for my life. I prayed, "Lord, I don't know what the trouble is. But you've got to let me know what I should do. My enlistment is coming up again." Suddenly there was this tremendous experience. The whole room seemed like it was just flooded with light. There was a presence of God that I had never experienced in my life and I was rendered speechless. I wanted to pray, but I couldn't talk.

Another man, already a minister, was invited by another minister to a prayer session in the latter's home. The former was skeptical of what the healing ministry could do. At this gathering, he heard a singer, dying of cancer, render a song:

She had at one time of her life been a great singer of this land. And she got up (after she had been invited to sing), put her hand on her forehead and straightened up her body. Now I have been following operas ever since the days when I was a child—back in the days of Tetrazini, Lotte Lehman—I've heard them all, but I have never heard anyone sing the way she sang that night. Her voice production—it was the most beautiful thing that I had listened to.

However, he was not yet willing to be saved. After some time, he became more convinced, until one day he decided to review his life:

I fell down on my knees and took another look at myself. I didn't like what I saw. I saw the skepticism, agnosticism, and nihilism that I had preached through the years. I saw hundreds of people coming and getting nothing. I belonged to the Shriners and all the ranks of Masonry. And I was at the bottom of a dirty pit. I was ashamed of myself. I had no defense. I had no excuse. I had this plain self-righteousness and self-conceitedness that I had to get out of me. Well, I began to cry and I cried so hard that it was almost hysterical. I finally turned to S——— and said, "Well, I give up. I've gone too far away. I'll never find Him. God couldn't save a rotten sinner like me." And this is where the transformation came.

This was a miracle. I'm going to describe to you the new birth that took place with me. He (S———) just put his arms around me and said, "Ray, Jesus said, 'Behold, I stand at the door and knock. If any man hears my voice and opens the door, I will come into him and suffer him with me.'"

It was just that quick—this is the psychology of it. You can call it subjective, but it doesn't make any difference. It was a reality to me. I

was surrounded by a world of peace, most beautiful peace. It was like a plateau. I could put my hands on it. I've never felt anything like it before or ever since. I don't expect to feel it again until I cross over. God gave me a little sight of it that night. It was like I was transformed into a different room. It was paneled on all the sides. And think what you will, this is what I have to tell you because this is what happened.

The fact is that it opened up and Jesus came in. I saw it. I looked at Him. I looked at Him from head to foot. I could tell you what He was dressed like, I could tell you the color of His hair, I could tell you about His hands, I could tell you. I looked at Him just like I am looking at you. He walked right up to me. He didn't say a word. His lips didn't move. His face was radiant with love, just filled me with it. I was born again in Christ.

Of course, not all conversion processes are as dramatic as the ones just described. Another healer, who was also a skeptic, mentioned that as a free-lance writer, she was assigned to do a story on a famous spiritual healer. In the process of writing the story, she became converted:

Now, as a free-lance writer I was constantly searching around for new ideas and my original idea had been to write an expose of this fraudulent thing of faith healing. So, I began to investigate and I myself was converted in this process. There were too many cases and I know they weren't all coincidences. I was trained as a reporter to be objective about things and I had to report the truth as I saw it.

Symbols

The major symbols used by spiritual healers are religious. Aside from crucifixes and long flowing robes or sequined suits, prayers constitute the major symbolic domain of spiritual healers. Prayers are offered prior to and during the actual healing, and this is symbolic of the link between the spiritual realm and the earthly needs of the patient. Prayer establishes for the patient the fact that his problems are in the hands of a great force, more powerful than he and the healer together, and the healer thereby identifies himself as a tool of this force. In fact, some healers claim that the patient does not need to have faith to be healed. As one spiritual healer told a skeptical patient who had stated boldly that he had no faith in the power of prayer, "Don't worry about it, brother. I have enough faith for the two of us."

The most famous and well-known healers have established international foundations, foreign missions, and various media programs, all of which symbolize their respectability and legitimacy in the eyes of the larger society.

Techniques

Touching or the laying of hands on the patient is the core technique of spiritual healing. One healer described in minute detail how he lays on hands:

Laying on hand is a focusing on a particular person with a particular need. Some persons use oil. I've never done that. It's a physical contact. There is no particular power in the hand. Many times, there is a prayer. You just want to make sure that everyone realizes there is no particular power in these hands. It is just a method. It is a physical movement that is used to focus.

I use the particular method of placing both my hands on the sides of the head with my thumbs immediately on the forehead. Then at the end of the individual prayer, the sign of the cross is made on the forehead. I do this for two reasons. There is a remaining sensation. If you do this on the forehead, you'll notice that the remaining sensation some time after the sign is made. You can still feel this. And this is a significant sign for the Christian faith. The Christian faith is very materialistic. The New Testament places a great deal of emphasis on the body, not only the spirit. Jesus was very concerned with the sick.

Some healers lay on hands gently (Fig. 6-2), whereas others either shake the patient violently or deliver a sharp blow to the patient's head. At one healing service, one of us (R. M. H.) observed the healer delivering sharp blows to the carotid sinuses of patients who had come forth to be healed. This invariably knocked the patient unconscious, which added to the dramatic effect of the laying on of hands not to mention the severe headaches that some of the faithful patients seemed to experience on arising from the floor.

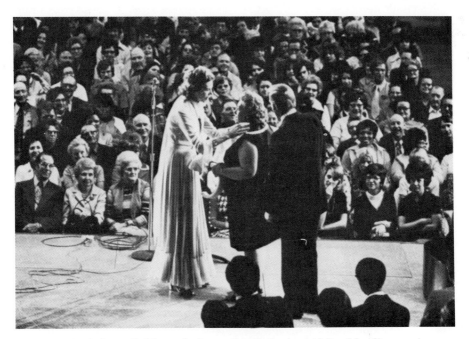

Fig. 6-2. *Kathryn Kuhlman laying on hands during spiritual healing service.*

(Courtesy Doug Grandstaff Photography, Tulsa, Okla., and Kathryn Kuhlman Foundation, Pittsburgh, Pa.)

Some healers work on a one-to-one basis, but most heal in front of large audiences. However, even in mass audience situations, the healer will make an effort to single out individuals from the audience for healing. The following description of this technique comes from a case in which the father-in-law of a healer attended a healing service. The father-in-law, who was a physician, was extremely skeptical of spiritual healing at the outset of the services.

In the middle of the service, Kathryn Kuhlman points in his (father-in-law's) direction. She has never met them (the mother-in-law was also present), and she doesn't know they're there. She said, "There is a man here who is receiving a healing. There is a burning in his ear and I see a lump the size of the walnut beginning to dissolve" and something about his head passage being cleared—I don't remember the exact words. She said this a couple of times, My mother who was sitting close to him said, "That's you." He said, "It's not." He wasn't going to make a fool of himself and go up there so he didn't.

Kathryn Kuhlman said, "I don't want him to miss his healing. Won't he please come forward?" But he wasn't going to go up. So, he noticed this warmth in his ear, but he thought it was just a hysteria kind of thing so he passed it off that way. They drove home and it was a damp, rainy time and it was a several-hour drive and it wasn't the kind of condition to improve your sinus any. . . . They got home and he decided to blow his nose and all the bloody business came out, and that was the end of his sinus trouble.

They were talking and they went up to the bathroom. I should mention that a couple of weeks ago we had been in their home, and I had noticed that when he took a cup of coffee in his right hand—his right shoulder was haywire—it shook so that it went all over everywhere. So, they went up to the bathroom and without thinking he put his right hand up to the shower curtain behind him. And she said, "Do you realize what you are doing?" Well, he moves his arm around, and there is no pain there. He had the freedom of motion. His lump had gone down a little bit. Within a few weeks, it was gone. We came down for Thanksgiving— it was a Thursday after this had happened. He was all excited about it. He's touching his toes,

showing us how he can do everything. He wrote a letter to Kathryn Kuhlman, and I wrote a note and said that I saw it. That captured my imagination and it also touched me. An x-ray taken for another purpose on June 20 showed no difference between the right and left clavicle. The healing of this fracture was permanent and complete. He said that it was beyond his medical knowledge.

Theories of disease

Spiritual healers use four theories singly or in combination to explain the presence of disease or other medical problems: the spiritual, the psychological, the germ-mechanical, and the parapsychological.

The spiritual explanation attributes disease and illness to original sin and the disenchantment of heavenly spirits with the afflicted mortal. Similarly, the human soul, viewed as a vital principle, is believed to be activated in an extraordinary manner so that physiological processes are altered in ways never observed in normal biology (Leuret and Bon, 1957). Few spiritual healers subscribe to this theory in their healing practice, but few, if any, would deny the probability of its existence.

Psychological theories are much more commonly utilized by the healers. Most of these theories define illness and disease as something that occurs when psychological processes such as needs, drives, and dispositions of the individual are countervailing and at odds with each other. This psychological stress leads to physical, social, and emotional breakdowns, according to this perspective. An example would be an individual who has a strong need to succeed at business and an equally strong desire to spend more time with his family. These two needs are in conflict, according to the theory, and this conflict can lead to mental, physical, or social breakdowns.

Resolution occurs when the psyche is ordered once again, that is, when the needs and dispositions are working together in the same direction. This ordering can be accomplished by means of spiritual healing whereby the healer helps the patient to accept God's divine plan. This plan includes the patient, and according to the theory, the patient's psyche will order itself once the patient has given himself over to the larger plan of God.

Spiritual healers who accept and use this theory for the most part reject the more mechanistic approach, which places the burden of discovering the patient's disorder and treating it actively squarely in the hands of the healer and patient. The psychologically oriented healers, similar to psychoanalytical schools of thought, accept the hypothesis that intrapsychic conflict is related to manifest illness. However, the spiritual healer counsels patients to open their hearts and minds to God the Spirit rather than to a psychiatrist actively seeking to understand the root of the problem. As far as the spiritual healer is concerned, knowledge of the origins and causes of one's problem is neither necessary nor desirable for healing to take place. What is critically important is to achieve psychic peace and harmony through the process of giving oneself over to God's master plan.

The germ-mechanical theories of disease are not held by any one group of spiritual healers as such, but there is a strong tendency among them to accept the concept of germs and the deterioration of physical systems as causes of disease. However, we did not interview any healers who utilized drugs, surgery, or other forms of treatment associated with the germ-mechanical theories. Instead the healers seemed to recognize not only the validity of this perspective but also their own ability to treat patients in the fashion dictated by this point of view.

Along this line, healers believe that Western scientific medical care should not be ignored. Most go as far as to state that patients would be foolish to ignore the healing capabilities of Western scientific medicine, and in fact they advise people to see a Western-trained physician when they think it would be appropriate. Some healers who are more oriented to the Western scientific perspective believe that the severe germ and mechanical problems of patients must be resolved first before spiritual healing can succeed. As one healer said:

If people are very sick, emotionally or really psychotic, they are not able to receive the healing power of God. They are so filled with obsessive fear, they are not able to receive it. Very often, it'll take a psychiatrist to remove this barrier; then this person can receive the healing power. If a person is going to blow his brain out or jump out of the window, I am not trained to deal with this.

Another healer acknowledged the validity of modern medicine as part of his obligation to his clients. He stressed the need for modern medical practitioners and spiritual healers to work together as follows:

Spiritual healing and medical healing are complementary. You must see doctors. Ours is no substitute for medical care. Everyone who is in the healing ministry should make this very clear to the people. In fact, I go out much more than most others. I tell people, if they do not consult with doctors, they are committing a sin because God is knowledge and medicine is knowledge and that is given to us by God. What you see in more and more places is a cooperation between doctors and the healing ministry.

I think if someone has a broken leg, he should go to a doctor and have the leg set and come to the healing services, pray that God will hasten the healing process. If someone has cancer, he should be under the care of a doctor, utilizing all that medicine has to offer, as well as come to the healing services and use the spiritual power—use everything that is available to us.

This healer gave an example of a close working relationship with a Western-trained physician:

A young woman had been coming to my service three or four times. I didn't know who she was. A few weeks ago she came to me and told me that she had told her doctor that she was going to a healing service. She expected him to go, "tsk, tsk" but he said that he hoped she was going to the C——— Church (where the respondent holds her services). He had some of my books and he pulled down some of these books to show her. It turned out that this doctor was my doctor. Since then, she has had a test of her blood and now it is negative.

Several healers told us of the existence of the Order of St. Luke in Philadelphia, Pennsylvania, which attempts to bring together professionals of different disciplines in the common cause of healing. This Order has even formalized some aspects of the laying on of the hands (Ousler, 1957).

A third healer agreed with the proposed convergence of healing professions, adding:

The majority of illnesses are psychiatric. Psychiatry can do so much and I can only do so much. We need to work hand in hand. If we think we can exclude the other, then we're first-class idiots, because we are denying reality. The spiritual pride, professional pride, and intellectual pride are our worst enemy. So, I acknowledge the validity of modern science and medical science. I acknowledge their conclusions insofar as the evidence supports them. We do have diseases, we have bacteria, that's a reality. But I have seen what might be called miraculous healings—cancer healings in their last stages.

Leuret and Bon (1957) have defined parapsychological action, the basic concept of parapsychological theories, as including "instantaneous replacement of tissue" and "disappearance of substance." Many of the case histories of cures presented to validate the claims of spiritual healing describe incredibly rapid restoration of severely damaged tissue. Such a case follows:

Sister Marie Marguerite, born on April 13th, 1872, a religious in the Poor Clare Convent of Rennes, as a result of troubles of a cardiac and renal nature, spread over the years 1924 to 1934, was suffering from suppurating nephritis which, coupled with complications due to cardiac failure, in 1936 developed generalized edema, particularly in the legs where bullae formed, burst and began to discharge serum constantly. Cardiac dyspnea made it impossible for her to stay in bed, and the patient had to remain seated in an armchair day and night.

On January 20th, 1937, the community began a novena to Our Lady of Lourdes to beg for a cure. "On January 22nd, 1937," writes Dr. Philouze, the doctor in charge of the case, "at eight o'clock in the morning, the patient dragged herself painfully to the chapel adjoining her sickroom in order to assist at Mass. At the moment of the Elevation she suddenly had a feeling of compression all over her body, es-

pecially in her legs, where the swellings seemed to subside instantaneously; the bandages round them fell to the floor of their own accord. As soon as Mass was over the patient returned to her room without any difficulty and found that the edema had completely vanished. She put on her slippers, which she had been unable to wear for more than a year, went downstairs and walked about the house all day without feeling any fatigue and without any sign of a heart attack."*

Gross (1971) has developed possibly the most advanced parapsychological perspective. He uses the hypothesis developed by Roll (1957-1964) that links the physical and psychological so that when the psyche interacts with physical or organic elements in the environment, energy is exchanged between the two in such a fashion that "total energy" is conserved. Gross goes on to link psi energy with Jungian "psychoid" energy. In this sense, there is no reason for treating the relationship between the psychological and physical in cause-effect terms.

Gross analyzes spiritual healing sessions and argues that there may be an extraordinary investment of individual and collective energy among the participants, both healer and patients. At most healing services, intense prayer sessions are offered prior to and during the actual laying on of hands, and according to Gross, this produces large-scale collective exchanges of energy among the participants. This emotionally charged atmosphere was observed by one of us (R. M. H.) at several different spiritual healing services.

Services are designed in such a manner as to excite the emotions of all present with songs and prayers. When the audience is at an emotional peak, one can observe many instances of individuals going into trances. More interestingly, the charged emotional atmosphere can be felt physically in the form of intense body heat that radiates from many individuals in the audience. At first, we doubted this and assumed that the perception of heat was an artifact of our

*Reprinted with permission of Farrar, Straus & Giroux, Inc., from *Modern Miraculous Cures* by Dr. Francois Leuret and Dr. Henri Bon © 1957 by Farrar, Straus & Cudahy, Inc.

own doing. However, more recent research has demonstrated through the use of infrared measurement techniques that an abnormally large amount of heat is generated within the bodies of persons attending the services. Most intriguing of all is the finding that heat is produced between the healer's hands and the head of the patient at the precise moment of contact.

Thus the parapsychological theory argues that there is a radical interchange of energy between body, mind, and the psychoid or Jungian collective unconscious. No longer is one dealing with the body-mind duality per se but instead must consider three factors as energy transfers occur between the physical, psychological, and psychoid levels. These transfers of energy occur, according to Gross, in concert with laws that exist in and govern the psychoid realm. Gross argues that these laws are not visible to direct measurement or observation. For this reason, cause-effect, and space-time explanations cannot be used to analyze what occurs during spiritual healing sessions. According to Gross' analysis, spiritual healing sessions produce intense exchanges of energy, whereby matter and energy become interchangeable at the physical, psychological, and psychoid levels. In this fashion, extremely rapid and highly unusual healing can take place.

We should not be misled into thinking that all or even most spiritual healers are as sophisticated as Gross about their theories of why and how healing occurs. On the contrary, most healers stress the mysterious and miraculous nature of their work, viewing their role as an instrument of God's vast and unknowable power. In the words of one healer, "I am not a spiritual healer. We hate to be called a healer. It's only God who heals. We are an instrument." Another echoed her views: "I've not healed anyone. I am not what you call a faith healer. Most of the faith healers would say that too—they do not do the healing." Yet another healer attributes healing to God:

God is and does operate supernaturally. He bypasses the natural medical process. How is this accomplished? It is accomplished primarily by the belief in communion. Just simply trusting that God will work. Jesus said he didn't do any miracles in his hometown because of the hardness of their hearts. There is an aspect here where disbelief will not allow these things to occur. So, there is an element of faith involved here. The burning question is this: Why are some healed and some not? At this juncture, I can't answer this. I don't know other than ultimately we do have to put it in the hands of God and ask Him for the wisdom and knowledge to understand these specific cases.

Organization

Spiritual healers work as solo practitioners. Seldom does one find more than one healer in any healing setting. Nevertheless, a distinguishing organizational feature is that some healers work exclusively on a one-to-one basis with their patients, others work only with mass audiences, and still other healers do a little of both. For example, some healers will lay on hands only when the patient and healer are alone together, similar to the typical physician-patient relationship. In these practices, the spiritual healer deems it desirable to know as much as possible about the problems and personal history of the patient.

The mass-audience approach is a much more common form of organization among spiritual healing practices. In these settings, the healer may know nothing about the patients, or they may learn only the barest of facts concerning the patients' health problems moments prior to laying on hands. Generally, with this type of organization, the healer must rely on countless ushers to provide contact with the patients. Healing is performed through the laying on of hands, which the healer alone does to patients who elect to step up to the front of the church or auditorium. Frequently, patients line up, and the healer lays hands on one person after the other, almost in assembly-line fashion.

Financially, healers depend primarily on contributions for their income rather than a fee-for-service structure. Investment, publications, and audiovisual materials constitute other important sources of funds. In the mass-audience setting, collections are taken up formally once the audience has been primed sufficiently. The priming usually involves group singing and reminders that God has called on specific individuals to give, the implication being that to refuse to give may preclude healing. Group recitations of prayer are important aspects of the services as well. The group or mass-healers are knowledgeable when it comes to audience control, and this knowledge is used maximally to create the appropriate atmosphere for healings to occur.

Spiritual healers make heavy use of electronic media, especially radio, to reach patients who cannot attend the services. Occasionally patients call the healer on the telephone, and healing is conducted over the telephone lines. Frequently, persons will attend healing sessions on behalf of a friend or relative who is too sick or who lives too far to attend in person. The healer in these cases will lay on hands and heal by proxy. These outreach efforts by spiritual healers greatly increase the range of their influence, and they are able to reach many more thousands of persons than they could if their work was organized similarly to the private practitioner or group practice model so common to modern western medicine.

CURANDERISMO

Modern *curanderismo* is the medical care system utilized by many Mexicans, Latinos, and Mexican-Americans. *Curanderismo* is an extremely popular and well-used form of medical care, and as a folk system of medicine, it owes much of its current popularity to its cultural richness and sensitivity to the norms and values of its users. Modern *curanderismo* represents the blending of ancient Mexican folk medicine, Native-American medicine, European medieval medicine, and African folk medical practices into one system of care independent of what is known as the "Western scientific system." Willard, a Native-American anthropologist who is noted for his work on Mexican folk medicine (1972), has concluded that the practice of *curanderismo* or *los remedios Mexicanos* is a matter of cultural pride and constitutes a declaration of cultural identity over and above the practical consideration of obtaining relief from illness and suffering. In this sense, the practice of *curanderismo* is closely bound to the values, norms, and life-styles that give meaning to the Mexican, Mexican-American, and Latino cultures.

Symbols

The use of religious or magical symbols and objects takes many forms. For the most part, this facet of *curanderismo* is used to place a hex on an enemy, remove a hex, or ward off illness caused by dysfunctional environmental conditions, actual or potential. Regarding the third point, for example, a Mexican-American woman who believes in *curanderismo* would be concerned, especially during pregnancies, about the effect that a lunar eclipse might have on her unborn child. To prevent possible disfigurement of the child due to viewing an eclipse, the woman will tie a *hila* (a string or cloth line) and a small wooden or leather half-moon around her abdomen, which theoretically will prevent or ward off the disfiguring effects. *Curanderos* can place curses or hexes on individuals, generally at the request of someone who wants to destroy another. A common form that the curse takes is to place a small wax figurine, representing the intended victim, on or near the victim, in a pillow, for example. The figurine will have pinpricks in areas representing vital organs scheduled for breakdown. The only remedy, should one be fortunate enough to discover the fact that he is cursed, is to employ a *curandero* who is willing to attack the hex, a risky job from the perspective of the *curandero*, given the belief that the curse can be dissipated only by taking the full power of the curse into one's own body first. Hence it is possible, according to *curanderismo*, for the *curandero* to succumb to the curse should his power fail to prevail.

Techniques

Three major types of healing techniques are used in *curanderismo:* the use of foods and/or herbs to be taken internally or applied topically, massages and manipulation of the body similar to chiropractic, and the use of religious or magical objects and symbols.

Foods and herbs are given orally to counteract the illness, defined as either "hot" *(caliente)* or "cold" *(frío).* For example, cold foods defined in *curanderismo* as lamb, corn tortillas, peas, cow milk, and oatmeal are prescribed by a *curandero* for hot illnesses such as bleeding or certain types of skin disorders. Hot foods, such as rice, pork, beans, onions, beer, and goat's milk are prescribed for cold illnesses such as measles, ear infections, and others.

Body manipulations are performed by the *sobador* to set bones or to realign organs with nerves. These manipulations are similar to the range-of-motion exercises and massages performed by chiropractors, with the exception that the *sobador* will occasionally place poultices of herbs onto the affected area.

Theories of disease

The most prevalent conception of disease causation within *curanderismo* is that which identifies imbalances of heat and cold within the organism as the major cause of illness. According to this theoretical construct, certain diseases are hot diseases and others are cold. A hot disease will become manifest when the delicate balance within one's body between hot and cold forces breaks down and hot forces take over. The converse is true for cold illnesses. This theory not only identifies the cause but also the cure, which lies in the judicious use of foods and herbs to restore the balance among the two forces. Foods and herbs are classified as hot or cold not according to their actual temperature but rather on their relationship to the hot and cold forces within the body. Hot foods are used for cold illnesses, and cold foods are used to cure hot illnesses. A diet consisting of bal-anced proportions of hot and cold food is viewed as a major preventive medical practice to ensure the proper bodily balance necessary to maintain health.

In addition to the hot-cold concept of disease, *curanderismo* contains other distinct categories of disease that constitute theories about their causes and cures as follows: (1) diseases of magic or witchcraft, (2) diseases of organ and body dislocation, (3) diseases of the emotions, and (4) Anglo diseases originating in Anglo-cultural practices and other facets of Anglo life-styles.

To better understand the *curanderismo* concepts of disease, one must study its concepts of health. For example, Mexican-Americans who accept *curanderismo* view health as something that they have little control over, since it is believed that health comes from God in the form of a gift. Furthermore, health is considered as that state which allows one to maintain a high level of physical activity and to perform activities of daily life independently and without pain. Clark (1970) has pointed out that Mexican-American members of *el barrio* are reluctant to assume the sick role because they believe that family and friends will lose respect for them. This is especially true for males for whom the important cultural norm "macho" (strong, durable, brave, independent) is threatened by the image of one who is sick, weak, or infirm. The ethos is one of "I shall endure," and there is little room for the sick role (Chapter 5). A man who gives in to illness, especially if he lets others know of his problem, is not a macho but is treated as weak and dependent. In this culture, even though health is one way of maintaining one's independence and dignity, medical care is far down on the list of priorities.

Organization

Curanderos practice as soloists within the private, entrepreneurial framework of organization. They are respected and valued by their patients because the social organization reflects and reinforces the culture of the barrio. The practitioners live and work in the barrio, speak Spanish, and share with their patients the values, norms, and experiences unique to the ethnic group. If their patients are working class, the *curandero* is also working class. Rural Mexican-Americans can go to a rural Mexican-American healer; the same holds for the urban scene. In short, *curanderismo* fits the life-styles and cultural needs of its patients through a complex process of the social organization of the healing practices.

One of the most important concessions to culture is the amount and quality of time the *curandero* spends with patients. For the most part, Mexican-American patients expect the healer to take time for a thorough physical examination. If the examination is hurried or if the healer does not cover the entire body during the examination, he will be suspected of incompetence or, worse yet, of trying to make a profit from the misery of others by neglecting to do one's best to cure the illness.

Since most patients of *curanderismo* have relatively low incomes, the fees charged by the *curandero* are much lower than those incurred for Western scientific medical care. If a patient has no money, then payment can be in the form of food and goods. The fee structure is informal and is worked out between the healer and the patient according to the patient's ability and willingness to pay.

In summary, the social organization of *curanderismo* reflects a high degree of cultural congruence between healers and patients. This mutual sharing of values, norms, and symbol systems such as conceptions of illness produces a close healer-patient relationship infrequently found in the Western scientific counterpart.

NATIVE-AMERICAN HEALING

Native-American healing systems have opened more frontiers in Western scientific medicine than any other non-Western healing system, past or present. Native-American tribes are responsible for the discovery of the cure for scurvy, oral contraception, the use of antibiotics, and more than two hundred drugs that have been listed officially in *The United States Pharmacopeia* since the first edition in 1820 or in *The National Formulary* since it began in 1888 (Vogel, 1970).

Our Western ethnocentric views on medicine have severely limited our understanding of the role that Native-American healing arts have played in the development of modern scientific medicine. This is a great shame, since by our collective ignorance, we have misplaced an important part of our medical culture and subsequently lost some of the ability to assess where we have been and where our medical care system is taking us. Certainly it is common to believe that knowledge and other benefits flowed exclusively from scientific Western culture to the so-called lower cultures of Native-American civilizations. What escapes most historical treatises about the contact between Native-American healers and white physicians is the rather sobering fact that Native-American healers benefitted white society more than their white counterparts did during the eighteenth and nineteenth centuries. During this period, Native-American healing arts were well in advance scientifically of their European counterpart. Thomas Jefferson in a letter to Dr. Caspar Wistar, professor of surgery at the University of Pennsylvania, scorned the Western-trained medical practitioners of the day:

I believe we may safely affirm that the inexperienced and presumptuous band of medical tyros let loose upon the world, destroys more of human life in one year, than all the Robinhoods, Cartouches, and Macheaths do in a century. It is in this part of medicine that I wish to see reform, an abandonment of hypothesis for sober facts, the first degree of value set on clinical observation, and the lowest on missionary theories (Koch and Peden, 1944:584-585).

With Western medicine in this state of disrepute, people were reluctant to entrust themselves to physicians who endangered lives with majestic determination. It is small wonder that Native-American healers were much sought after for advice by white patients and physicians alike. The Native-

American healer frequently assumed the superordinate role of teacher and doctor to whites, an almost quixotic notion according to modern conceptions that define Native-American healing as primitive and folksy with little or nothing to teach Western medical practitioners. Alas our memories are short and we forget that modern medicine emerged from ancient medicine. Thus Native-American medicine made a lasting but unappreciated mark on modern medicine.

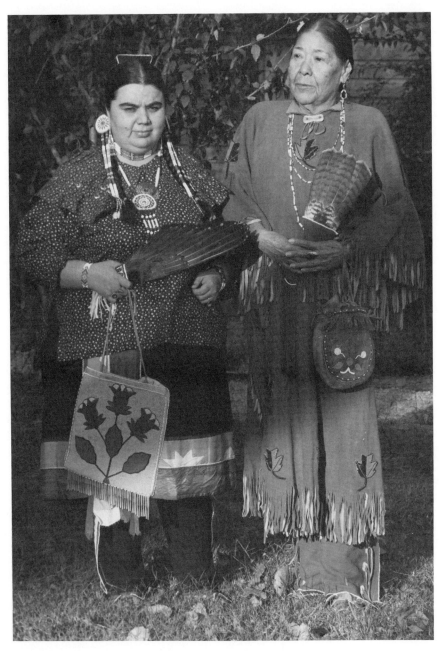

Fig. 6-3. *Nora Thompson Dean ("Touching Leaves") (right), a Delaware Indian traditionalist and medicine woman, pictured with her daughter, Louise. Both are in traditional dress and carry fans used in purification ceremonies.*

Symbols

The Native-American healing symbols portray Indian conceptions of the sacred relationship between man and nature. Unlike Western scientific medicine, symbols used by Native-American healers have deep spiritual as well as medicinal meaning. This is because Native-American healing is both pragmatic and spiritual. It encompasses disorders such as broken bones, skin rashes, and wounds in which the causes are defined as mechanical in nature. Similarly, other health problems, for example, certain internal diseases such as cancer, are considered supernatural in their etiology. Therefore Native-American healing symbols represent both the empirical and the supernatural, the profane and the sacred. Humans are considered intimately bound to nature with its physical and spiritual laws and processes.

The healing symbols represent the physical and spiritual aspects of the Native-American culture and its surrounding natural environment. The symbols are tremendously stimulating to the people and carry great meaning and significance for both healer and patient. Although most adult Native Americans heal others occasionally, only a specially recognized healer, a medicine man, can legitimately manipulate or otherwise use the symbols of healing (Fig. 6-3). This is decreed by the members of the society.[1]

The symbols, although different for various tribal groups, commonly include the pipe and tobacco (Kemnitzer, 1971), sacred masks, effigies, rattles, medicine bowls, sucking cups and tubes, drums, and medicine lodges. These are just a few examples of the many symbols used in Native-American healing.

Techniques

Native-American healing systems contain three basic techniques for achieving the desired state of health: (1) the use of drugs, (2) mechanical intervention, and (3) religious or spiritual actions.

Historical accounts of Native-American healing tend to emphasize the spiritual aspects to the exclusion of the less magical and pragmatic. Perhaps this accounts in part for almost automatic labeling of Native-American medicine as primitive and ineffectual. On the contrary, stimulant and anesthetic drugs, astringents, cathartics, emetics, antibiotics, and even effective herbal contraceptives were developed and used by Native-American practitioners (Humbolt, 1877; Hrdlicka, 1908).

Mechanical interventions include the use of sweat baths, soaking in mineral springs (Lawson, 1937), isolation of ill persons, surgery, and the application of herbal poultices, especially to broken limbs.

Spiritual techniques include prayer, group singing and incantation, and the manipulation of physical objects considered sacred. Much of what is called "shamanistic healing" falls under these sets of spiritual techniques. Perhaps the best modern example of the application of spiritual techniques in healing is found among the Lakota Sioux at their Yuwipi medicine meetings. Supplicants and participants bring to the medicine man problems that have been made more confusing or indeterminate by previous attempts to resolve them or when there is no other means for dealing with them. Thus only the most difficult to resolve medical and social welfare problems are presented to the Yuwipi healer. The central concept of Yuwipi is the concept of spirits or *managi,* defined as immaterial gods who can communicate with mankind directly or through the medium of the Yuwipi healer. The spirits can be associated with any natural object or living thing and are used by the medicine man to affect cures either by direct intervention of spiritual power or through the spirit telling the healer which herbs and other techniques to use.

The most important symbol of Yuwipi medicine is the peace pipe. Similar to the Christian belief that Mary brought Christ to the people, so Lakota people believe that the White Buffalo Calf Woman brought the pipe to the people to be used as an intermediary between man and God. The bowl of the pipe must be of stone, representing the earthly permanence, and the stem must be of wood, representing all growing things and the shortness of life. The pipe symbolizes the world in its entirety (Kemnitzer, 1971).

Theories of disease

Rivers (1924), and later Clements (1932) (who never formally recognized the intellectual debt owed to Rivers' work) categorized Native-American theories of disease etiology into the following general causes: (1) human agency, (2) supernatural agency, and (3) natural causes. Clements delineated sorcery, taboo violation, disease-object intrusion, spirit intrusion, and soul loss as specific types of supernatural causes of disease. Certain tribes may stress one or more of these theoretical orientations, and there is considerable variation among tribes concerning the central theory of disease causation.

Sorcery or witchcraft is cited by some tribes such as the Zuni (Hrdlicka, 1908), and Yaqui (Spicer, 1940) as the cause of economic or health problems. Taboo violation occurs when one behaves imperiously before the spirits, either neglecting to thank them properly or deliberately wasting natural resources. Disease-object intrusion is a concept whereby disease is deemed caused by an animal or inanimate object that enters and resides in the body. Spirit intrusion is a familiar concept to white society, especially within religions that believe in possession by the devil. The Native-American concept is similar. Disease is thought to be caused by spirits, symbolic of animals or even humans, that enter the body or home and wreak havoc. Some tribes define the intruding spirit as the soul of the dead returning to reside in the bodies of the living. Soul loss occurs during dreams when the soul is thought to leave the body. The soul could do this voluntarily or be coaxed out by evil shamans or spirits. Without the soul the victim is believed doomed to die. Some tribes have no mechanism for recovering the soul, whereas others place the burden on the medicine man, whose function it is to come up with effective techniques to ensure recovery.

Organization

Native-American healers work in solo practitioner settings for the most part. "Calling," a divine vocation to be a healer, usually occurs at a young age and singles out the healer as someone with special qualities whom the spirits have designated as their choice for the role of intermediary.

Patients seek out the healer and go to him much as one goes to the Western-trained physician. However, the healing rituals generally include the kin of the patient and even the larger community as participants. Thus healing has an integrative function not found in the Western scientific model. Native-American healing serves to reaffirm the social and cultural bonds among the participants as they unite in petitioning the spirits or seeking harmony with the laws of nature.

Payment may be made with money. More often than not, however, the healer is paid with goods and services instead of cash. This is particularly true on reservations where goods and services have much greater utility than cash per se.

Native-American healing rituals have distinct phases or stages that correspond to the process of natural entropy, human intervention, the mobilization by spiritual forces, and the renewal of nature. Kemnitzer (1971) summarizes the relationship between the modern Oglala Dakota healing ritual and the decline and renewal of natural resources at the Pine Ridge Reservation. Kemnitzer distinguishes four major phases of the Sioux healing ritual: (1) the light phase in which men build the altar, which is an offering representing the corporeal world, (2) the dark phase in which the spirits come into the room, communicate with and heal troubles through the medium of the shaman or medicine man, destroy the altar, and take up other offerings; (3) the marginal phase in which the congregation asserts the power of the pipe, the most important Dakota healing symbol of tribal unity and identity, and the dependence of the people on it; (4) and the feast,[2] which is a proper component of all sacred and secular gatherings among Dakota people.

Native-American medicine, together with Indian social life, quests for visions, personal power, and practically every other aspect of their lives, is affected by religion. Historically Native Americans have been intensely religious, although not in the same ways of the white society. Their religion may be incomprehensible to "Sunday Christians" who find it difficult to fathom that reverence for all forms of natural processes is the core characteristic of Native-American religious beliefs. From the Native-American perspective, medicine is a system designed to preserve or reestablish the integration of man and nature. The goal of medicine in this context is harmony or balance between all living things, inanimate objects, and man. For Native Americans this is the true meaning of health.

CHINESE-AMERICAN HEALING

Before one studies modern Chinese-American healing, it is important to look at the origins of this unique system of medical practice. Chinese medicine in the United States has its origins in the People's Republic of China and the development of Chinese medicine in that society. As such, it is important to once again shed Western perspectives to examine the social and cultural underpinnings of Chinese medicine. Chinese theories of disease, conceptions of health, techniques of healing, and the organization of medicine are grounded in the social and cultural order of Chinese society. The Chinese views of man and his responsibilities to society are radically different from Western concepts of social order. This is especially true of modern mainland China where the individual is expected to place the common good and good of the state above any personal or familial needs. In China one is expected to remain healthy for the good of the state (New, 1974), where

people help each other and actively seek self-criticism. According to New (1974) who visited China in 1973:

As you can see, every time I try to solve the puzzle of applying the lessons I learned in China to the western world, I remain in the web that is China. . . . I see the people going at their task with a unity of purpose that is lacking in the western world. They start with self-criticism in the context of how best to serve the people and the country. Through this mechanism, they are able to weed out the old and adopt the new and constantly accept change.

This adaptability is characteristic of Chinese institutions, including medicine. Born of this social order, the Chinese-American healing system retains this central characteristic. It has adjusted to United States society well, so well in fact that most of us never encounter a Chinese physician in spite of the growing interest by Westerners in acupuncture.

Similar to the other healing systems discussed in this chapter, frameworks that delineate healers and health care systems into primitive, folk, and scientific categories are not applicable to Chinese-American medicine. For example, Coe (1970) defined primitive medicine as "basically non-scientific medicine where it's causal roots are located in beliefs and practices which are founded in traditions and magic, lending a moral imperative to its credence." Chinatown medicine is not primitive according to this definition, since it is not founded on magic. Rather it harks back to a long tradition of scientific medical practices on mainland China and in Hong Kong.

Furthermore, Coe defines folk medicine as "medicine of the people—a set of beliefs and behaviors shared and practiced by everyone—which may be based on theories either nonscientific or quasi scientific in nature. It is to be sharply distinguished from the specialized and more or less codified medicine practiced by specialized healers." He goes on to argue that folk medicine persists alongside Western scientific medicine, for example, in an urban setting, when the consumers of folk medicine do not come into contact with scientific medicine. Again Chinese-American medicine does not fit this description exclusively, since not all Chinese-Americans adhere to its beliefs and norms. Furthermore, one cannot distinguish Chinese-American medicine from specialized or "more or less codified medicine practiced by specialized healers." Chinese medicine exists alongside the Western medical care system, and there is considerable contact between Chinese-Americans and Western medical care.

Symbols

The basic symbol of Chinese-American medicine is the concept of vital force, that element which represents life itself. The essence or primary matter of individuals is the vital force, without which one ceases to be. It is a symbol of life, of intrinsic and essential unity of being, and everyone who is living has a vital force.

Techniques

Minor illnesses are treated through the use of Chinese medicine. Two aspects of Chinese medicine are involved: the use of Chinese doctors and the use of Chinese medicine for illnesses.

Within the Chinese system of *yin yang*, preventive care is viewed from a hot and cold perspective by both the Chinese herb doctor or specialist and the Chinese consumer. The body must be balanced, which means avoiding conditions in which the body is excessively hot or excessively cold. Certain Chinese foods and herbs have hot and cold value, and these are used to keep the body balanced or to correct an imbalance.

If one's body is too cold, one takes hot foods, herbs, or both and vice versa. Most minor problems of the body such as minor colds or sore throat are considered to be due to too much heat in the system, and hence one would use cold foods, herbs, or both to counteract this situation. One of the most common types of herbs taken is *dong Kuei (Angelica sinesis Diels)*, which is

a root used to make a soup with chicken fruit flesh *(longan)*. Also there is *gay tse*, which women usually take because it reportedly builds blood lost during menstruation. In addition, this herb is commonly taken after a woman has given birth.

The equivalent of *dong Kuei* for men is *look mai ba* (deers tail), but men take this herb less frequently than women take the *dong Kuei*.

Another herb is *buck kay fong dong suin*. This is a stimulant of sorts that helps one gain energy. It is a combination of two herbs, *buck kay* and *fong dong suin*, and it is usually made in a soup with pork or other meats.

Also *wak san, lin tze*, and *bak hap* are three herbs used for cleaning the lungs and keeping the lungs clear. They are usually made with chicken in a soup.

Foods like winter melon soup, beef broth, and certain fruits and vegetables are also used as folk medicine to prevent illness. When taken alone or out of the context of soup, herbs are bitter to the taste. However, when they are made with soup, the bitterness vanishes and the taste is pleasant.

Another much publicized healing technique is acupuncture. This is used primarily to combat pain but may also be used to cure and even to prevent disease. Needles are inserted subcutaneously into highly specific points along theoretical meridia through which pass vital forces. The needles when manipulated in precise ways cause changes to take place within the meridia, and if done correctly, the desired balance of heat and cold will be reestablished or the pain will be anesthetized.

Theories of disease

In Chinese-American medicine, the vital forces are believed to be part of a dynamic process within each human organism. The dynamic is grounded in the ancient principle of hot and cold forces *(yin yang)* in which a balance of heat and cold must be maintained within an organism to ensure good health. Foods and herbs are characterized as hot or cold as are specific bodily disorders, and a counterbalance of food and body is sought to prevent or cure illness. This dialectic, when translated into forces of hot and cold, represents the traditional Chinese system of palliative and preventive medical care (Basil and Lewis, 1940).

Organization

Specialized Chinese medical practitioners serve as healers or physicians for the Chinese-American medical care system. There are basically two categories of Chinese physicians. The physician treats illnesses like colds, flu, diarrhea, and other similar conditions by prescribing Chinese medicine. He is analagous to the Western medical physician who treats problems in a clinic setting. Also there is the "chiropractic" physician who treats bone fractures, dislocations, sprains, and other muscular problems. His treatment typically includes use of his hands to feel and massage and straighten the affliction by manipulation. This technique is held in high esteem by Chinese-Americans primarily because confining casts are not used by Chinese physicians, a distinct advantage from their perspective.

Chinese physicians work on a solo practice, fee-for-service basis. They are primarily located in Chinatowns in the cities of the United States and practice medicine in the back rooms of gift stores. They are extremely difficult to locate if one is not Chinese, and consequently most, if not all, of their patients are Chinese-Americans.

Chinese physicians learn their profession through a lengthy apprenticeship with a practicing Chinese physician. Unlike the other healers discussed in this chapter, the Chinese physician does receive a diploma of sorts after successful completion of the training.

Most patients who use Chinese healers are working-class individuals with low or fixed incomes. Thus fees for services are low compared to Western medicine. However, herbs are costly, with some of them running as high as $80 for a fourth of an ounce.

As mentioned earlier, it is unlikely that any Westerner seeking Chinese medicine would find a Chinese physician. Chinatown society is closed to outsiders, and community affairs are considered confidential and private by Chinatowners (Hessler et al., 1975). Outsiders to the community are viewed with suspicion and are barred access to all Chinese institutions, including medicine.

CONCLUSION

The dominance of Western medicine is intimately bound up with the process of secularization in United States society. This growth of secularization is characterized by a shifting of man's attention to this world, to the here-and-now. Inevitably tradition is deemphasized and ultimately forgotten. Secular man is preoccupied with pragmatic tasks at hand and is highly mobile both physically and mentally. Therefore in secular society deep roots are not grown in any place or tradition.

Prior to urbanization and secularization, when the largest social unit was the tribe and the resources to master nature were primitive, people had little faith in themselves and their meager knowledge. They had to rest their faith in nature and gods who were considered omniscient and omnipotent. As man proceeded from the tribe to the megalopolis, they have moved to a religion of faith in mankind and its own powers. This has led to an inevitable acceleration of the acquisiton of knowledge and skills, increasing specialization of occupations, and the vertical integration of societal institutions. Western scientific medicine is caught up in this process as well.

In spite of the odds against such an occurrence, modern scientific medicine is showing a growing respect for the theories and techniques of healing systems developed outside of the Western tradition. The ancient and contemporary traditional healers would find this new attention flattering, especially in light of the angry denouncements in the recent past by Western-trained physicians. The development and incorporation of aspects of traditional healing systems into modern Western systems would be a healthy antidote to the specialization, mechanization, and high technologizing in modern medicine.

Perhaps the most intriguing aspect of the healing systems discussed in this chapter is their holistic approach to medical practice, in which the patient is considered a total human entity—a unit of physical, mental, and emotional processes subject to natural, social, and personal influences.

NOTES

1. It should be noted that although we speak of the "medicine man" as a unitary role, many tribes recognize a multiplicity of healing roles. The Navajo, for example, have three types of healers: the singer, who "alone has the ability to cure illness, that is, to restore the individual to a state of harmony"; the diagnostician, who ascertains the etiology of disease but does not treat; and the herbalist, who uses medicines to relieve symptoms but cannot cure. The Western physician practices in a manner analogous to the herbalist from the tribal perspective (Kane and Kane, 1972).

The Delaware traditions recognize two types of healers: the *maternu,* or healer, who has spiritual powers and can cure by restoring harmony between the symptomatic and individual and the *manituik,* the spirit forces of the world; and the *nantpikes,* or herbalist, who can treat symptoms. Again Western medicine corresponds to the lowest order of Native-American healing traditions (Dean, 1975; Westlager, 1973; Vogel, 1970).

2. The term "feast" is used by the Dakota. It should be noted that other tribes, including the Delaware, reserve the term "feast" for those dinners that are part of funeral rites or are held in commemoration of the dead.

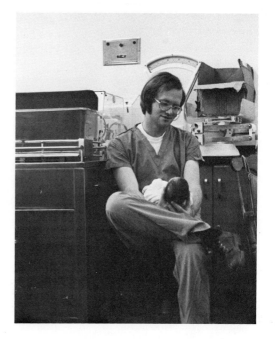

CHAPTER 7

The physician

. . . what profession is there equal in true nobleness to medicine? He that can abolish pain and relieve his fellow mortal from sickness, he is indisputably the usefullest of men. Him savage and civilized will honor; he is in the right, be in the wrong who may.

Carlyle

Our body is a watch, intended to go for a given time. The Watchmaker cannot open it, and must work at random. For once that he relieves or assists it by his crooked instruments, he injures it ten times, and at last destroys it.

Napoleon Bonaparte

All professions are conspiracies against the laity.

George Bernard Shaw

The physician as an occupational type is of special sociological interest. The relatively early emergence of medicine as a distinctly professional type of activity has made the physician a prototype of the professional. The understanding of the work roles of physicians is important for the understanding of professional roles in general. The physician is also of special practical interest for understanding the nature of the health care systems of at least the relatively modernized societies. More than any other occupational group, physicians have come to dominate the activities of health and sickness care in recent years. They are thus a key occupation in the health care system.

In this chapter we will explore the nature of the beast, *homo medicus*. Our attention will turn first to the nature of professions and then to the historical origins of the physician and chiropractor in the controversies between osteopathy, allopathy, and homeopathy during the last century. Then the processes by which some people

160

are recruited, socialized, and certified to engage in medical practice will be examined, with particular attention to selective processes at each step. Following that, our attention will be directed to the variety of types of physicians that have emerged through a complex process of specialization. Finally, the organization of medical practice at both the informal and formal levels will be outlined.

CONCEPTS OF PROFESSION

The term "profession" refers to a class of occupations that is distinct from other kinds of work. On this much, there is agreement. The term, however, is not simply descriptive; it is evaluative. To call an occupation a "profession" is to call forth images of high prestige and to suggest a high moral character for those who ply that particular trade. To be a professional is "good." A profession is better than other occupations. The values associated with the term "profession" are such that many, if not most, occupations aspire to being called "professions." Many occupational groups have embarked on a self-conscious program to gain public acceptance of their claim to professional status, sometimes at the expense of their social usefulness to others. At times these claims are serious, and real benefits to the public are associated with changes in occupational behavior, as may be the case with nursing. In other cases, the efforts border on farce. One of us (A. C. T.) attended a graduate school where wearing a white shirt and tie was enforced on the grounds that it would make the students more "professional."

The evaluative connotations must make us cautious in using the term descriptively. Because everyone wants to be considered professional, many efforts to describe the characteristics of a profession are bent to assure that the writer's occupation is included. Also there are many ways in which occupations can be classified; with prestige, content of work, general goals, internal organization, reward systems, career patterns, and educational requirements

being only a few. No system of classification is exhaustive.

Keeping these reservations in mind, we will review some efforts to define professions and then look briefly at the process of professionalization by which occupations assert their claims. This background is important because medicine is the most successful occupation in establishing such a claim and tends to be a model for aspiring occupations.

Definitions of profession

In an early work dealing with the concept of profession, Carr-Saunders and Wilson (1933) identified five characteristics that they thought to be distinctive of professional occupations: (1) specialized skill and training, (2) minimum fees and salaries, (3) professional associations, (4) a code of ethics, and (5) work consisting of the provision of a skilled service or advice. Many of these characteristics were restated in later attempts at definition.

Greenwood (1957) distinguished professions as those occupations (1) that had a basis of systematic theory, (2) whose authority was recognized by a client population, (3) that had community sanction and approval, (4) that had a code of ethics, and (5) the members of which had a professional culture built on their occupational identity and formalized in a professional association.

Gross (1958) characterized professions as those occupations that had (1) an unstandardized product, (2) personality involvement in the occupation on the part of those who practiced it, (3) a base of specialized knowledge and techniques, (4) a sense of obligation to the occupation, (5) group identity, and (6) a product or service which was significant to the society.

Goode (1960b, 1961), in one of the most elaborate attempts at defining profession, identified two "key" characteristics and ten "derived" characteristics. Central was the presence of prolonged, specialized training in a body of abstract knowledge and a collectivity or service orientation. The ten derived traits were as follows:

1. The profession determines its own standards of education and training.
2. The student professional goes through a more far-reaching adult socialization experience than the learner in other occupations.
3. Professional practice is often legally recognized by some form of licensure.
4. Licensing and admission boards are manned by members of the profession.
5. Most legislation concerned with the profession is shaped by that profession.
6. The occupation gains in income, power, and prestige ranking, and can demand higher caliber students.
7. The practitioner is relatively free of lay evaluation and control.
8. The norms of practice enforced by the profession are more stringent than legal controls.
9. Members are more strongly identified and affiliated with the profession than are members of other occupations with theirs.
10. The profession is more likely to be a terminal occupation. Members do not care to leave it, and a higher proportion assert that if they had it to do over again, they would again choose that type of work (Goode, 1960b:903).

Examining Goode's definitions, Freidson (1970) noted that five of the ten derived traits (the first, third, fourth, fifth, and seventh) referred to the profession controlling its own work, standards, and membership. He concluded that "the core characteristics are critical criteria for professions insofar as they are said to be causal in producing professional autonomy." A professional occupation is one that controls the process by which its members are recruited, the content and duration of training, and the licensing of practice; defines the scope of its work; and sets and polices its own standards of practice.

Reviewing these criteria, the greatest consensus is found in the assertion that a profession is an occupation with specialized skills based in a body of abstract knowledge and that it provides a service to others. Although there is less consensus on the following point, most define professions as

having some formal occupational organization, community recognition (usually in the form of licensing), and autonomy in the definition and organization of work. A minority hold that professions have codes of ethics, a special degree of commitment of members to the occupation, special social significance, unstandardized products, and minimum fees. In comparing occupations, we will focus on skills, service orientation, formal organization, community sanction, and autonomy as especially important characteristics.

Professionalization

Although it is clear that law and medicine are uniformly considered professions in the twentieth century, the classification of many occupations is ambiguous. It is equally clear that many occupational groups aspire to be considered professions, generating much self-conscious literature among educators, librarians, nurses, social workers, engineers, and business managers (Volmer and Mills, 1966). Such occupations are making a claim that they are worthy of special recognition, high prestige, and high moral worth and should be granted the right to autonomy and official community sanction. Characteristic of these occupations is their attempt to define an area of special expertise, create occupational organizations, establish codes of ethics, and enforce standards of dress and decorum (Caplow, 1954; Hughes, 1958; Wilensky, 1964).

In many instances, changes are taking place, and occupations are moving toward professional characteristics over time. Such occupations are becoming professionalized, and some of them will be dealt with in later chapters. For the present, we focus on one that is clearly defined as a profession, explore how it became one, and look at some of its salient characteristics.

THE EMERGENCE OF MEDICINE AND CHIROPRACTIC

Although medicine has a long and fascinating history (Bullough and Bullough, 1972), it has only recently emerged as a profession with a distinct body of scientific knowledge, standards of performance, and occupational autonomy (Freidson, 1970). The immediate roots of modern medicine are found in the nineteenth century. At that time, allopathy, homeopathy, and osteopathy were distinct schools of thought that in the absence of good information warred with each other on ideological grounds much as described in George Bernard Shaw's *The Doctor's Dilemma.*

In the late eighteenth century, several medical colleges were established in the United States, the first in 1765 in the College of Philadelphia. No standards existed, and more than 400 schools were established by the middle of the nineteenth century, since "anyone could claim to be a doctor and even establish a medical school" (Bullough and Bullough, 1972). The typical medical schools were:

. . . proprietory institutions, run on students' fees, and designed to show a profit; the more students, the more profit. Few of them required a high school degree, let alone any college work, for admission; and the student, regardless of qualification, usually graduated at the end of two or three years without any real practical experience. . . . All awarded the title of doctor, so that all kinds of practitioners from natural healers to graduates of Edinburgh claimed the title of doctor (Freidson and Lorber, 1972: 97).[1]

Given the lack of an objective empirical base for the discussion of disease and any effective mechanism for transmitting the information available to those who were to practice the healing arts, it is not surprising that various cults emerged, each with a simplistic explanation of disease processes and a distinctive preference for mode of intervention. Although none of these proved to be satisfactory for long, each provided a stance that led to the emergence of modern empirical medicine.

Nineteenth century developments

The mainstream of establishment medicine of the early nineteenth century was in a "heroic" period. The prestige of a physi-

cian was marked by his courage in applying treatments that by modern standards are known to be dangerous. The favored tool was the lancet, and the favored treatment was bleeding the patient. Often huge quantities of blood would be drawn in the treatment of fevers and other disorders. A leading figure of the day, Benjamin Rush, asserted, "Tis a very hard Matter to bleed a Patient to Death, provided the Blood be not drawn from a Vital Part." He advocated bleeding patients "till they were as pale as Jersey Veal," often to the point of unconsciousness. His commitment to this practice is indicated in his exhortation to medical students at the University of Pennsylvania to "do homage to the Lancet . . . I say venerate the Lancet, Gentlemen" (Kaufman, 1971).

In addition to bloodletting, the establishment physicians, or *allopaths,* engaged in cupping, blistering, purging, and sweating along with large doses of calomel (mercurous chloride). Cupping was a procedure in which blood was drawn to a local area where small amounts could be drained; blistering was the creation of second-degree burns in which the formation of pus was interpreted as the drawing out of infection; purging consisted of the adminstration of emetics and cathartics, which induced vomiting and bowel evacuation to "cleanse the system"; and sweating was induced by means of diaphoretics. Calomel was administered in large doses, sufficient to produce symptoms that now would be recognized as mercury poisoning (salivation, loosening of teeth, falling out of the hair, lethargy).

Needless to say, such practices did much more damage than good, and the commitment to their massive (heroic) use caused many deaths, including that of George Washington, who died of treatment for a sore throat (Kaufman, 1971). The public in its infinite wisdom entertained a healthy fear of allopathic treatment. The physicians also recognized the dangers, but it was an important part of their professional self-image to have the courage to proceed in spite of the odds.

It was largely because of such abusive treatment that many alternative schools of medicine were able to take root and have an impact on the development of medicine. Each of these was thought a heresy by the establishment.

Samuel Thomson, a New Hampshire farmer, became locally noted for his ability to effect cures with herbs and other local plant life. In 1813 he patented a series of proprietary medicines and undertook to teach his system. He held that disease was caused by reduction of body heat. Cure was effected by increasing temperature, cleansing the body, and proper feeding. Thomsonian practitioners administered herb preparations in specific sequences along with steam baths and came to be known as "steam doctors" or "steamers."

Thomsonianism was a short-lived heresy, much opposed by the allopaths but much in tune with the public. Although popular, his efforts to "make every man his own physician" was soon replaced with another and more important school.

In 1825 Hans Gram returned to the United States after spending time studying with a German physician, Samuel Hahnemann. Hahnemann had developed a system of medicine based on two laws: the law of similia, and the law of infinitesimals, which together he called *homeopathy*. The slogan "let likes be cured by likes" summarized a position that diseases could be cured by drugs that produced the symptoms of that disease. It was based on the discovery that a bark which produced fever in healthy people could also control fever in sick ones. It was posited that the drug introduced a mild form of the disease that the body could combat, assisting the "vital powers" of the body in combating the main disease. From this it followed that the smaller the dosage of any drug the more potent its effect. It was asserted that "in illness the body is enormously more sensitive to drugs than in health" (Kaufman, 1971).

As an attractive alternative to allopathic practices, homeopathy was quick to take hold in the United States. Not only was the treatment less fearsome, but it was objectively less harmful. In several instances in which allopathy and homeopathy were compared, mortality was lower for the homeopathic practitioner. This was not because of effective treatment (dosages used by homeopaths were probably much too small to do any good) but rather because the treatment did little or no direct harm to the patient. It was nevertheless derided and opposed by orthodox physicians, who used their control of state licensing laws and publicity organs to attack this "absurd" and "ridiculous quackery" (Holmes, 1842).

Riding the crest of Jacksonian democracy, the Thomsonians succeeded in gaining the repeal of all state licensure laws. Since 1827 only physicians were able to sue to recover payment. Although others could practice healing arts, it was difficult to make one's living doing so. However, by 1849 anyone "male or female, learned or ignorant, and honest man or a knave, can assume the name of physician, and 'practice' upon anyone, to cure or to kill, as either may happen, without accountability. It's a free country!" (Shattuck, 1948).

The situation fell to such a sorry state that a group of physicians met in New York in 1846 to form a national organization designed to protect the interests of the medical community and to further the development of medical skills. They passed resolutions calling for standards for professional training and for a code of ethics. One concern was with the "struggle against homeopathy (Kaufman, 1971). One article in the code passed in 1847 contained a "consultation clause" that forbade physicians from consulting with "irregular" practitioners, including Thomsonians and homeopaths. The growth of the American Medical Association served to polarize the medical community even further. The AMA succeeded to a large extent in preventing homeopaths from access to public facilities such as city hospitals and blocked the military from admitting homeopaths to the medical corps.

In the second half of the nineteenth century, however, cooler heads began to prevail. Both the allopaths and homeopaths had national organizations devoted to upgrading medical practice and improving the efficacy of treatment. Both sides retreated from their extreme doctrinaire positions, and practitioners became more eclectic, incorporating both allopathic and homeopathic treatments and applying them selectively. Over time the objective differences between the schools was reduced. By 1905 the leading physician in the United States, Dr. William Osler, asserted in the *New York Times* that "a difference in drugs should no longer separate men with the same hope . . . the homeopaths should not allow themselves to be separated by a shibboleth that is inconsistent with their practice today" (Kaufman, 1971).

Even though similarities of training and practice were noted, bitter feelings from past conflict might have prevented a merger of allopathy and homeopathy had the two fields not encountered a new common enemy, *osteopathy.* The doctrines of Andrew Still were repugnant to both groups. In joining for the common fight, allopaths and homeopaths abandoned their separate identities and became "medicine."

Still was an army physician in the United States Civil War who became dissatisfied with the treatment of military patients and with the state of knowledge of his time. He founded a reform movement within medicine (allopathy) that focused attention on body mechanics. He viewed disease as primarily resulting from problems with the skeletal and muscular systems and curable through physical manipulation. Finding no success in convincing his colleagues, he founded a new school in Kirksville, Missouri, in 1894, at which he granted the degree of doctor of osteopathy (D.O.) (Still, 1908; Bourdillon, 1973; Crowell, 1974).

The opposition to Still is not surprising if one considers the vast difference between his conception of disease and that of either allopathy and homeopathy, indicated by the following:

I have concluded after twenty-five years of close observation that there is no such disease as fever, flux, diphtheria, typhus, typhoid, lung-fever, or any other fever classed under the common head of fever or rheumatism, sciatica, gout, colic, liver disease, nettlerash or croup, on to the end of the list, they do not exist as diseases. All these separate and combined are only effects. The cause can be found and does exist in the limited or excited action of the nerves which control the fluids of part or the whole of the body (Still, 1908).

If this doctrine and the claim that he was divinely inspired were not enough, established medicine could not take kindly to his hostility toward orthodox practice, born of the loss of his own children and events he witnessesd as a physician.

They met pain with anti-pain medicines and bleeding of the bowels with astringents that closed the issues from which the blood came, following such remedies to death's door, and then lined up for another battle and defeat with the same old failing remedies, and opened fire all along the line on symptoms only (Still, 1908).

Although there was merit in the manipulative therapies developed by Still (Bourdillon, 1973), the claims were extravagant, being seen as a cure for all disease.

Not long after the founding of the first osteopathic college, D. D. Palmer founded a second school of manipulative therapy. Describing himself as a "self-educated erstwhile grocer," Palmer was credited with treating a man for deafness by spinal manipulation and then successfully treating a case of heart disease by adjusting a vertebra. From these experiences, Palmer reasoned that other diseases might have a similar cause, leading him to create a system of therapy called *chiropractic.* Originally intending the system to be a family secret, he was persuaded by his son, B. J. Palmer, to go public with the founding of the Palmer Infirmary and Chiropractic Institute in Davenport, Iowa, in 1897 (Stanford Research Institute, 1960). Harkening to Hippocrates' injunction "Look well to the spine for the cause of diseases," chiropractic began in a manner similar to osteopathy. It was a complete system of healing based on a mechanistic theory and techniques of physical manipulation of the body. Although more exclusively focused on the spine than was osteopathy, the similarities were sufficient to cause speculation that Palmer had experienced osteopathic treatment.

By the end of the nineteenth century, allopathy and homeopathy became more similar in practice and joined in common opposition to osteopathy and chiropractic. Mainstream medicine based its practice on the use of drugs and surgery. Both in terms of numbers and in terms of public acceptance, combined allopathy and homeopathy clearly dominated the healing professions. It had gained control of the licensing of its members and was gaining control over the licensing of other health occupations, in some states succeeding in barring osteopaths and chiropractors from practice. The allopathic practice of the early nineteenth century had disappeared, and only a small group, calling themselves "naturopaths," still adhered to the original doctrines of Hahnemann. By any of the criteria discussed earlier in this chapter, medicine was close to completing a change from a segmented set of healing occupations into a unified profession.

Consolidation of medical dominance in the twentieth century

The consolidation of medicine as a profession is a phenomenon of the twentieth century. It is this recently that medicine gained significant growth in numbers, a base in applied scientific knowledge, and an exclusive legal mandate. This century has also been one of growing prestige and income for medicine, deriving from both the increased technical sophistication and effectiveness of treatment and monopoly position of the profession. Although there are still divisions such as between traditional medicine, osteopathy, chiropractic, and naturopathy, increasingly these seem to be best characterized as internal disputes rather than competition among competing systems.

Numbers of physicians. At the turn of the century, there were approximately 121,000 physicians in the United States of whom 119,749 had doctor of medicine (M.D.) degrees, 1,136 were doctors of osteopathy (D.O.), and almost 100 were chiropractors. Clearly the doctor of medicine was in a dominant position and has remained there to the present. For every 1,000 population, there were almost 160 physicians (American Osteopathic Association, 1901; Stanford Research Institute, 1960; Fein, 1967).

In the first half of the century, the number of doctors of medicine almost doubled, and the doctors of osteopathy increased by a factor of eleven. The population, however, increased faster, and the combined number of physicians per 1,000 population declined to under 150. There was also an increasing tendency for physicians to specialize in nonpatient-related activities, which reduced the ratio to under 140. Between 1950 and 1963 the number of physicians kept pace with population growth, and between 1963 and 1971 they increased at a faster rate than the population, bringing the ratio of physicians per 1,000 population to an estimated 170 (Table 7-1).

In relative terms, chiropractic grew even more rapidly than either traditional medicine or osteopathy. In 1917 there were 19,151 chiropractors in the United States, or eight for every 100,000 population. Although there are more chiropractors than osteopaths, osteopathy is still in a dominant position because of mode of practice. Osteopathy is an unlimited form of practice that is indistinguishable from traditional medicine in the training of its members and the forms of treatment actually given to patients. Although maintaining some important ideological differences from traditional medicine, osteopathy has joined the mainstream and shares in the power of the doctor of medicine. Chiropractic, on the other hand, is a limited practice that does not allow the use of drugs or surgery, and chiropractors are looked on by both tra-

Table 7-1. Physicians in relation to population: selected years, 1900 to 1972*

Year	M.D. degree	D.O. degree	Physicians per 100,000 population
1972	356,534	14,900	174
1970	334,028	14,300	166
1968	317,032	13,700	161
1965	292,088	13,027	153
1960	260,484	14,349	148
1950	219,997	12,700	149
1942	180,496		134
1936	165,163		129
1927	149,521		126
1921	145,404		134
1916	145,241		142
1910	135,000		146
1900	119,749		157

*Data for 1900 to 1942 based on Fein, R. *The doctor shortage: an economic diagnosis.* Washington, D.C.: The Brookings Institute, 1967, p. 66; Data for 1950-1972 based on United States Department of Health, Education, and Welfare. *Health resources statistics.* Publication No. 75-1509, p. 169.

ditional medicine and osteopathy as being a "cult."

There is little information available on naturopathic medicine. It was founded in the 1890s by a group who went to Germany and rediscovered the doctrines of Samuel Hahneman. The first licensing act for naturopaths was passed in the District of Columbia in 1869, and between 1923 and 1935 specific acts were passed in five other states and six provinces of Canada. Little is known about the training of naturopaths other than there was a Central States College of Physiatrics that folded between 1966 and 1968, and there is a National College of Naturopathic Medicine, which is based in Seattle, Washington. The curriculum of the National College is similar to that of most medical schools with the exception of major surgery and the addition of courses in botanical medicine and nutrition. It may be cautiously inferred that there are changes in naturopathy that are bringing it in line with the mainstream of medicine. In 1971 there were 170 members of the National As-

sociation of Naturopathic Physicians, making this a small group with little present impact on physicians as a whole (Rogers, 1949; Mills, 1966; National College of Naturopathic Medicine, 1974).

The convergence of medicine and osteopathy. At the turn of the century, medicine and osteopathy were bitterly opposed. Medicine was based on the treatment of disease with drugs and surgery, whereas osteopathy was based on manipulative therapy. Writing in the *Journal of Osteopathy* in 1904, F. J. Fascett listed fifteen theories that distinguished osteopathy from traditional medicine, including the notions that obstructed nerve centers affected the blood flow of the body, manipulation of bone displacements could alleviate nerve obstructions, and manipulation was safer than the use of drugs (Peterson, 1974). These beliefs were characterized as a "cult" by the AMA, and in 1923 the AMA Judicial Council ruled that consultation with osteopaths was unethical for physicians.

The differences between medicine and osteopathy were probably exaggerated by both sides. Although seen by traditional physicians as a radically different form of practice that rejected medicine and surgery, such practices were never excluded by Still. In 1902 Lewis wrote an article in the *Journal of Osteopathy* that clearly viewed manipulation as an addition to medicine and surgery rather than a replacement and questioned the extent to which manipulation should be used in comparison with alternatives. In 1904 the American Osteopathic Association (AOA) evaluated the colleges and set a standard curriculum for training, which was implemented between 1914 and 1945. That curriculum included medicine, surgery, and manipulation (Cole, 1957).

The battle lines were drawn, however, and each side viewed the other from a position of committed hostility. By the 1940s the differences that had existed between the two fields had diminished considerably, and each perceived that the other had changed. On the side of medicine, increased attention was being given to manipulative therapy under the title of physical medicine, which was interpreted by some osteopaths as medicine adopting osteopathic technique (Evans, 1941). On the side of osteopathy, greater attention was being given to traditional medical subjects such as pharmacology and surgery in school curricula, which was interpreted by the AMA as the modernization of osteopathy and the abandonment of its committment to the cult of manipulation (Cline et al., 1953).

Both traditional medicine and osteopathy seemed to be holding positions on ideological grounds that distorted the facts. Both had changed in a direction toward convergence, and each field had distorted the position of the other on medical issues. Although osteopathy placed greater emphasis on manipulation and medicine placed greater emphasis on drugs and surgery, these were always relative differences, and both fields incorporated the full range of treatment.

Early in the twentieth century, medicine recognized the usefulness of manipulation but called it "physical medicine" and did not acknowledge its similarity to osteopathy. Osteopaths recognized the limits of manipulation at least as early as 1903 in the *Journal of Osteopathy* (Peterson, 1973), and in 1904 osteopaths were being warned of the dangers of "faddism" (Peterson, 1974).

Nevertheless, from the 1890s until the 1950s, osteopaths were outsiders (Becker, 1963). In 1938 the AMA House of Delegates ruled that any relationships between physicians and osteopaths was to be forbidden, and osteopaths were excluded from hospitals and consultations with orthodox physicians. The first breach in this isolation occurred in 1950 when the exclusion of osteopaths from the Audrain County Hospital in Mexico, Missouri, was ruled illegal by a court. In 1952 the president of the AMA suggested that the stigma be removed from osteopathy and appointed a committee (Cline et al., 1953) that approved the training of osteopaths. In 1958 the Kansas Medical Society ruled that consultation with osteopaths was to be considered ethical and opened the Kansas University Medical Center to osteopaths for postgraduate work.[2]

At about the same time, R. C. McCaughan (1949) noted:

Nearly all the drugs and most of the surgical techniques extant in 1874 have been discarded because they did more harm than good, or at best turned out to be useless. . . . About the only safe philosophy has been one of negativism, "medical nihilism" someone has called it. . . . But what of Still's theories? It may be said today that they stand like a rock as the logical basis for a modern school of the practice of the healing art. . . . Everybody knows them to be acceptable biological principles. They are not unique to osteopathy (Peterson, 1974:143).

In the late 1950s, at the initiative of the AMA, negotiations were opened between the California Medical Association and the California Osteopathic Association for a merger of the two organizations. The CMA made the osteopaths "an offer they couldn't refuse," that the osteopathic colleges in California should become medical schools and that osteopaths currently practicing in California should be awarded doctor of medicine degrees in place of their doctor of osteopathy degrees. The hooker was an agreement that the examining board for osteopathy would be dissolved and that no new osteopaths would be licensed in the state. In 1960 the AOA revoked the charter of the California affiliate, and in 1961 the merger was completed. In 1974 the California Supreme Court upheld the contention of the AOA that the law enacted to facilitate the merger was unconstitutional and "removed the one remaining legislative barrier to the practice of osteopathic medicine in all of these United States" ("California Reprise," 1974).

Currently in the United States the training of medical and osteopathic physicians is virtually identical with respect to course content, and each group recognizes the qualification of the other to practice medicine. Although there is some division within osteopathy, it is generally believed that osteopaths do not wish to merge with medicine. Largely this may be because of resentment over past treatment by organized medicine, and to the extent that this is the case, opposition to merger may subside in the future.

There are additional ideological differences, however. Relatively speaking, orthodox medicine has specialized to a far greater degree than has osteopathy, which maintains a commitment to general practice. There is also a belief that medicine has focused too exclusively on diseases and too little on sick people, as reflected in the following statement:

The whole substance of osteopathic medicine is a reformation in our time so that the person not the disease is the central figure in medicine's stage. We must not become that toward which we have sought equality (Northrup, 1966).

As expressed elsewhere by Northrup:

Repair, removal or relief—the three r's of medicine—do not mark the zenith of achievement by physicians. Safeguarding health and preventing disease, which osteopathic medicine stresses, are higher goals. . . . The medicine may be the same, but the hands are different.

These statements would suggest that considerable sentiment on the part of osteopaths to maintain a separate identity will exist for some time to come, although as orthodox medicine turns attention toward family practice and health maintenance, the road to merger will be smoothed. No predictions are offered.

Although osteopathy is an American development, there is a college of osteopathy in the United Kingdom. The situation in that country is much different, however, since the course of study is strictly postgraduate. The British physician first earns his bachelor of medicine degree and then takes a one-year course in osteopathy. There the two groups are fully merged, and osteopathy is a subspecialization of orthodox medicine.

MEDICINE

Knowing something of the broad historical developments that led to the present state of medicine is only part of the sociological problem. The historical background is necessary to appreciate that the present state of medical practice is grounded in prior events and that a history of conflict and realignment partially explains the present. Equally important is the way in which medicine is currently organized. In this section, attention will be directed to the major social processes and structures that characterize modern medicine. That our reference is to the United States for the most part will be quickly evident. This does not reflect a bias that the United States' physician is in any way a prototype for the rest of the world. On the contrary, it is our belief that several European systems are more the tide of the future. Rather the study of occupations and professions first developed at the University of Chicago and the information available is overwhelmingly American.

We will focus on four concerns:

1. How does one become a physician? When and why is the decison made to study medicine? What happens during the course of premedical and medical training that molds the process of professional socialization?

2. What are the processes by which medical practices are differentiated or specialized? What are the dimensions along which specialization occurs? What are some major types of medical practice?

3. What is the nature of the informal organization of medicine? How does the medical profession cope with the quality of its membership? How are practices interrelated through referral? What are the dimensions of a medical career?

4. What is the formal organization of medicine like? What is the organization and role of national medical organizations?

Becoming a physician

Physicians tend to be recruited disproportionately from the higher socioeconomic status levels of the society. Although in this century an increasing proportion have come from the ranks of middle- and working-class families (Adams, 1953; Schumacher, 1961), more than half the medical school graduates in 1960 came from professional or managerial families (Becker et al., 1972). As described by Hall (1949), a large proportion of medical students have fathers or other close relatives who are physicians. Such students have an advantage in growing up in an environment in which people can guide their interests along lines that maximizes the chances of success. At Cornell Medical College in the early 1950s, half the students had relatives who were physicians (Thielens, 1957). This is not simply an United States' or Western phenomenon. In 1970 medical sociologists attending the International Sociological Association meetings in Varna, Bulgaria, were able to compare notes, and the proportion of medical students who were the children of physicians was the same in the United States, the Soviet Union, Poland, East and West Germany, the United Kingdom, Bulgaria, France, and the Netherlands.

International comparisons show great variation, however, in the relationship between sex and entrance into medicine. In the United States medicine is overwhelmingly a male occupation. Data compiled by the AMA show that in 1963, 6.3% of all physicians were women. This increased to 7% in 1967 and 8.1% in 1972 (Theodore and Haig, 1968; Martin, 1973). Limiting the figures to those engaged in active practice of medicine, however, shows that 6.3% of physicians in the United States were female in 1972 (Vahovich, 1973). Compare this to the situation in eastern Europe. More than three out of four physicians are female in Poland, and in 1970 more than 80% of physicians in the Soviet Union were women. It has been argued that in the West, medicine is popularly identified with science and is thought of as masculine; in the East it is identified with nurturance, and thought of as feminine (Sokolowska, 1972).

Thus becoming a physician is something that is more likely to happen to a member of the upper class than to one of the lower class and more likely to happen to a male (in the United States and western Europe) than to a female. The transition from medical layman to physican is a process that focuses on socialization. According to Merton, Reader, and Kendall (1957), "The technical term socialization designates the process by which people selectively acquire the values and attitudes, the interests, skills and knowledge—in short, the culture—current in the group of which they are, or seek to become, a member."

The decision to be a physician. As compared to other professions, persons who enter medical training are noteworthy for the age at which the decision is made. Students at Cornell Medical College in the early fifties were studied by Rogoff (1957). Over half (51%) first considered a medical career before the age of 14 years, and more than one out of five made a final decision before the age of 16 years. Of those studied, 86% decided before the age of 18 years. Medical students make their decision much earlier than do law students (Thielens, 1957).

The decision to enter medicine is strongly influenced by whether the student has a relative in medicine. Students whose fath-

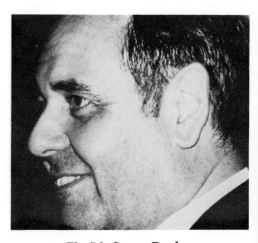

Fig. 7-1. *George Reader.*

ers are physicians are most likely to choose medicine as a career. If his father is not a physician, having another relative in medicine is important for middle-class students, but not for upper-class students (Rogoff, 1957). Also those with relatives in medicine make their decision earlier than did those without.

These data, which come from studies of medical students, have been confirmed by Bourgeois (1975) in a study of premedical students. Of ninety-two freshman students at "Catholic College," eight were the children of physicians and fourteen had relatives who were physicians. Only four had parents who were not in occupations regarded as professions. Almost one fourth had made the final decision to become physicians before the age of 16 years, and more than 90% had made the decision before the age of 18 years.

Premedical training. A student who enters college with the objective of becoming a physician generally takes a premedical course of study that emphasizes biology and chemistry. Although there are some small shifts in undergraduate majors over time toward the social sciences, this most often means that the student majors in biology. In part this is because biology and chemistry courses are required for admission to almost all medical schools, and to major in these areas is the course of least resistance. Also many schools center the premedical advising program in the biology sector of the faculty.

Bourgeois (1975:122) found that the freshman premedical student has a long-range perspective composed of the following elements:

1. A definite interest in, if not always a definite decision to pursue, a medical career
2. A view that medicine is a very good, though not necessarily the best, or only, field to be in.
3. An expectation that the practice of medicine will provide interesting and creative work, financial independence and security, and an opportunity to serve others
4. Idealistic and highly indeterminant con-

cepts of the medical profession and its work
5. A general inability . . . to envision and describe in specific terms their future either in medical school or in actual medical practice

Since only 40% of freshman premedical students will return to the program in their sophomore year, the perspective of the first-year student is dominated by the need to get high grades and to avoid being "weeded out" by the faculty. Isolated from other students and involved in dense interaction with other "premeds," the student tends to know where he stands relative to other students and is in a situation in which each comparison underlines the need for learning to study harder. Also a set of norms develops, ordering the importance of courses (i.e., biology is most important, chemistry next, and the humanities last). Although faculty are regarded as important contacts for recommendations to medical schools, they are not regarded as helpful in mastering the materials to be learned.

By the junior and senior years, premedical students have not become much more sophisticated about the nature of medicine, but they have become significantly more committed to a medical career. As described by Bourgeois (1975:172), long-range perspectives are as follows:

1. A definite interest in a medical career as well as a definite decision to become physicians; both are perceived as having developed at a very early stage in the respondents' lives
2. A view that medicine is not merely one of several excellent occupations, but clearly the best of all fields to be in
3. The expectation that medicine will, above all provide the opportunity to serve others; other rewards are also mentioned, but they are invariably listed after the service aspect
4. A generally idealistic and indeterminant view of the medical profession and its work
5. A general inability . . . to envision and describe in specific terms their actual future in medical practice; this is true in

spite of the fact that these "premeds" demonstrate somewhat more factual knowledge about medical practice than do the freshmen

By the junior year, students must live with the grades they have achieved, since there is little opportunity to greatly improve their averages. The main preoccupation becomes "getting into medical school." Although much more elective time is available in the curriculum, most students continue to concentrate their energies on biology. For most students, living with their grades means living with the realization that they are unlikely to be admitted to a medical school in the United States, a fate generally considered a failure even though they are assured of graduation. Those not accepted generally take one of three courses of action. They apply for graduate study in related fields with the plan of reapplying for medical school at a later time, they apply to a foreign medical school, or they consider alternative careers such as osteopathy and optometry.

Those who drop out of the premedical curriculum are most often led to that decision on the basis of their college grades.

During this century, the proportion of applicants to medical school who were accepted increased from 51.5% in 1929 to 1930 to 60.4% from 1961 to 1963. Since then it has declined in the United States to 42.3% in 1971 to 1972 (Sedlack, 1967, 1973; Dube et al., 1971). Given the emphasis of the premedical-biology curriculum on the part of premedical students, it is of interest that just over 20% of applicants had been accepted as of March 30, 1973, and this figure was not affected by whether the applicant's major was premedical (American Association of Medical Colleges, 1973).

Given the importance of premedical colleges in the selection of physicians, it is unfortunate that more work has not been done. It is not known to what extent these patterns are specific to the school studied by Bourgeois or to what extent they are general. It would be especially valuable to have some international comparisons.

Medical training. Once admitted to medical school, the student enters a world in which emphasis is placed on the acquisition of technical knowledge and skills and their application to the diagnosis and treatment of disease. On the one hand, the student becomes socialized into the medical profession, becoming more and more of a physician as training proceeds. In addition to technical skills, however, the student also learns a set of attitudes toward medicine, sick people, and other health professionals. At the same time, the student must contend with the problems encountered as a medical student. Thus the student is socialized into the medical school, becoming enmeshed in a situation in which student and professional interests may conflict.

During the first two years of medical school, students take courses in basic sciences, including anatomy, physiology, biochemistry, pharmacology, microbiology, pathology, and behavioral sciences. Toward the end of the second year, there is a course that deals with the conduct of a physical examination and one that provides practice in synthesizing information to make a diagnosis and decide on a course of treatment. At the end of the second year, students in the United States take an examination that is administered by the National Board of Medical Examiners and that covers the course work of the preclinical years.

The second two years are devoted to clinical training. Students are rotated for specific blocks of time among the various clinical departments of the medical school and hospital. Time is spent on both medicine and surgery, as well as a selection of medical and surgical specialties. In these clinical years, students serve as junior physicians under the supervision of interns, residents, and medical school faculty. They are given progressive responsibility for the management of patients, generally starting with the collection of samples for laboratory analysis and progressing to having primary responsibility for treatment to the extent of being fully involved in making the diagnosis and suggesting a mode of therapy.

At the end of this period, students take the second section of the National Board Examination and graduate with a professional degree.

During this period, students learn more than scientific and clinical knowledge and skills. They are also being socialized into the values of the profession and the role of the physician. In a study of several medical colleges in the mid-1950s, the following was found:

1. As they advance in medical training, students are more and more likely to express a preference for specialized practice (Kendall and Selvin, 1957).

2. As students are allowed to do activities they thought of as characteristic of doctors, they more and more think of themselves as "doctors" (Huntington, 1957).

3. With increasing experience, students learn to deal objectively with patients' problems, even with uncooperative patients, and those who are most secure relative to their mastery of technical skills are also most secure relative to attitudinal skills (Martin, 1957).

4. As students progress, they learn to live with uncertainty arising from the state of medical knowledge, their own mastery, and the ambiguities of clinical application (Fox, 1957).

In short, students learn norms, values, and attitudes that help them adapt to the real world of medical practice.

At about the time of the publication of the *Student Physician* by Merton et al. (1957), a second major study of medical schools was undertaken at the University of Kansas by Becker et al. (1961). That study, published under the title *Boys in White*, focused attention on the fact that although students acquired skills and attitudes that prepared them for medical practice, they were also faced with a set of problems as students. According to Becker et al. (1961), "How to climb the distant mountain may be a vision in the backs of their heads; how to make their way across the swamp they are floundering now and over the steep hill just ahead engages their immediate attention."

The Kansas study found that in their freshman year, students entered with the perspective that medicine was the "best of all professions," a view that Bourgeois (1975) found developed during the premedical years. They were confronted with a vast amount of material to learn, and early in the year students make an effort to "learn it all." Faced with the limits of their own capacities, they soon discover that "you can't do it all." Their perspective then changes again, and a consensus emerges as to what is essential and what can be left unlearned. At this point, effort is concentrated on "what they (the faculty) want us to learn," and much student interaction is focused on the problem of selecting out the so-called important materials.

In the third and fourth year, students enter clinical training in which they are used to carry out many routine tasks of the hospital, as well as to learn clinical technique. Students learn to differentially value the activities of this period according to two major themes: responsibility and experience. Responsibility "refers to the archetypal feature of medical practice: the physician who holds the patient's fate in his hands and on whom the patient's life or death may depend. . . . The physician is most a physician when he exercises this responsibility." Since a "doctor can only exercise responsibility in a situation in which his action or failure to act can produce some change in the condition of the patient," students learn to place a higher value on those tasks that are the more consequential.

Experience refers to actual practice in dealing with patients. Learning that takes place in this way is seen as opposed to "book" learning and "gives the doctor the knowledge he needs to treat patients successfully, even though that knowledge has not yet been systematized and scientifically verified." Knowledge gained from experience tends to take precedence over research findings. Students notice that if information from a book is not confirmed in the experience of the clinical faculty, the faculty trust their experience. Hence students tend to seek experience, placing a greater value on doing activities that they have not done before. Tasks that are new and exciting become "scut work" after the student has gained all the knowledge that performance of the task is thought to provide.

During the course of medical training, students' attitudes are shaped. Several studies have suggested that one effect of medical schools is to make students less idealistic and more cynical. Eron (1955) and Christie and Merton (1958) in studies using different instruments found that senior students are more cynical than freshmen and that they are more cynical than other occupational groups. Controversy exists, however, on the duration of this cynicism, with the emerging consensus being that cynicism is a veneer of the student that relates to his situation as a student and that after graduation a suppressed idealism reappears (Callahan et al., 1957; Beal and Kreisber, 1959; Becker et al., 1972).

Osteopathic students have an almost identical program with respect to their formal training as medical students. They take the same courses as medical students and in the same sequence. In addition, they have a course in osteopathic theory and technique. According to New (1960), the specifically osteopathic training is more to provide a sense of the history of the discipline, since most students do not think they will make much use of osteopathic techniques.

In addition to similarities, which suggest that osteopathic students face all the problems faced by medical students, there are some important differences, which mean that osteopathic students face important additional problems. One of these is social origins. Whereas medical students come overwhelmingly from upper-class backgrounds, osteopathic students come more often from middle- and working-class backgrounds. As a group, they are more upwardly mobile. In addition, whereas medi-

cal students usually decide on medicine early in their lives and pursue a course of premedical and medical studies, going straight from one to another, osteopathic students make their choice later in life. Frequently, osteopathic school is a second choice, taken after failure to gain admission to a medical school. In many instances, persons who enter osteopathic college have begun on another career, usually in a health-related field such as optometry, pharmacology, or chiropractic. As a consequence, osteopathic students are usually older than corresponding medical students (New, 1960).

One major problem for beginning osteopathic students is the recognition that osteopathy has less prestige than medicine. To deal with this, they develop an ideological stance that their lack of acceptance by medicine is due to prejudice and that osteopathy represents "the ultimate in medical science development." As summed up by one of New's respondents (1960:113):

> There are four methods of treating human ailments: the use of surgery, the use of drugs, psychotherapy, and the use of osteopathic manipulation. The M.D. uses the first three, and the osteopath uses all four. This means to me that the M.D. knows less about treating human disorders than a D.O.

Beginning osteopathic students often have anxieties as to whether they are entering a second-rate field. These anxieties are allayed during the Christmas vacation period when they have a chance to compare notes with friends in medical school. The discovery that the course work is identical allows students to settle into the work and be comfortable with their choice (New. 1960).

In the clinical years, osteopathic students must confront some practical problems regarding the relationship between osteopathy and medicine. New (1960) described these in terms of three "dilemmas." First, although the student will graduate well qualified in medicine, the opportunities for osteopaths are fewer than for the medical student. There are fewer specialties in osteopathy, fewer hospitals available for continued training, and a tendency for doctors of medicine to look down on doctors of osteopathy. The student "wishes to be on an equal footing with the orthodox physician, yet his public treats him as a 'specialist' at best, or a 'quack' at worst." The second dilemma, is the potential merger between osteopathy and medicine. At the time of New's study, the AMA was beginning overtures to absorb osteopathy, a move that later resulted in the merger of the California Medical Society and the California Osteopathic Association. A few students were opposed to this step. A majority were either in favor with qualifications or resigned to its inevitability, and a sizable minority favored merger on grounds that it would provide them with greater opportunities. Third is the dilemma of what to call themselves: osteopathic physician and surgeon, or just physician and surgeon. Here opinion was divided.

The fact that osteopaths have merged with orthodox medicine in California has probably reduced the first and third of these dilemmas. Many orthodox hospitals are now open to osteopaths for graduate specialty training. There is agreement between the AMA and AOA that osteopathy is not second-rate or cultist medicine. The question of the meaning of the label "osteopath," however, has probably intensified. By entering the same work settings as orthodox physicians and because there are ten orthodox physicians for each osteopath, a problem exists of osteopathy being totally absorbed by medicine. This is especially acute with reference to medical politics, since many, if not most, osteopaths are opposed to the AMA's conservative stance regarding health programs and financing. At present the AOA and most osteopathic physicians are opposed to merger.

Specialization of practice

One major trend in medicine over the past fifty years has been the increasing specialization of medical practice. A physician can become licensed to practice after a year of internship, a period of supervised practice in a hospital setting after graduation from medical school. To be recognized as a specialist, however, requires two or more years of residency training beyond the internship and passing examinations in a subarea of medicine. Although there are these commonalities, vast differences can be found among specialties and among countries relative to specific requirements, the process of becoming a specialist, types of specialties, dimensions of different specializations, and implications of specialization for the organization of medical practice.

The importance of this problem area is indicated by the recent trends in specialization. In the United States, for example, only 20% of physicians were specialists in 1940 and eight out of ten were in general practice. By 1962, 57% were full-time specialists; eight out of ten were specialists, and only 18.7% were in general practice (Stewart and Pennell, 1960; Peterson and Pennell, 1962; Martin, 1973).

Processes. The decision to specialize is made early in some instances. About 35% of first-year students studied by Kendall and Selvin (1957) were planning on a specialized practice. For most, however, the decision is made during the course of medical training, with the biggest shift taking place between the third and fourth years of medical school. Among fourth-year students, 74% planned to specialize, and only 16% planned to enter general practice. Two major influences seem to be important in the decision: first, the mass of medical knowledge and second, sponsorship.

It has become commonplace that the expansion of medical knowledge has made it impossible to learn everything about medicine (Becker et al., 1961; Millis, 1966). Students have a choice of knowing a little about a wide variety of medical concerns but knowing nothing in depth or becoming expert in one segment of medicine. Although students may be trained to tolerate uncertainty (Fox, 1957), they generally try to minimize that uncertainty by electing to specialize.

In medical school the student is taught by specialists, and clinical training consists of rotation through a variety of specialty services of the hospital. The role models with whom the students identify and take as referents for their own development are in most schools exclusively specialized. Few schools provide any opportunities for generalists to teach or for students to see a general practice. General medicine becomes second-rate medicine.

Which specialty a student selects is influenced by background characteristics, sponsorship, performance in medical school, and values. Comparing students in six medical schools, grouped according to an expressed interest in general practice, surgery, internal medicine, psychiatry, and undecided, Pavia and Haley (1971) found that those electing general practice were more likely to be Protestant, had less exposure to medicine, were higher in religious interest, had a greater belief in inner values, and were lower in aesthetic interests than others. Those students electing general medicine and surgery were higher in economic interests and lowest in social values, whereas students interested in psychiatry were more verbal and less religious.

The decision to study surgery was more stable throughout the years of training than was a decision to study pediatrics (Geertsma and Grinoils, 1972). Three classes at the University of Rochester were studied. Of these students, 26% were stable in the selection of specific specialties. When the specialties were grouped as person oriented, technique oriented, and mixed, 42% had stable choices. Students with fathers who were physicians were the most stable in their choices. Those electing pediatrics had more science training than those who had elected psychiatry.

Fishman and Zimel (1972) found that the image of each specialty was important in selection. Each student from two consecutive classes at the University of Colorado attributed higher status, more social attractiveness, and greater similarity to self to the specialty he had selected. Overall, surgery was seen as having the highest status but the lowest social attractiveness, an assessment with which the surgery students agreed, although thinking of themselves as exceptions. General practice was seen as the opposite of surgery.

The importance of sponsorship has been known since the pioneering studies of medical careers by Hall (1946, 1947, 1949), in which he demonstrated that career lines were largely influenced by the student coming to the attention of a senior physician who then sponsored the student. Sponsorship took the form of writing letters of recommendation, interceding to gain good appointments, and otherwise boosting the student's career. That this sponsorship affects choice of specialty is indicated in Lorne's study (1949) in which it was found that anesthesiologists were often individuals who had initially wanted to go into surgery but had not succeeded in finding adequate sponsorship from a surgeon.

Dimensions of specialization. There has been a tendency to think of specialization as unidimensional. Such an approach is not only inaccurate, since there is much segmentation among physicians that cannot be simply summarized by dividing generalists and specialists, but also it leads to the misrepresentation of some trends. For example, much has been made of the disappearance of the general practitioner on the assumption that general practice is synonymous with primary care. It has been argued that with an increasing proportion of physicians as specialists, the patient has fewer places to turn for initial diagnosis and for the treatment of routine problems (Millis, 1966).

In fact a decline has occurred in both the proportion and number of physicians who identify themselves as general practitioners. In the United States in 1945, 75,000 physicians reported themselves as general practitioners, representing 80% of all physicians. By 1967 general practitioners had declined by almost 10% to just over 67,500, representing only 20% of all physicians.

This must be offset by the fact that some specialties are also engaged in primary care, and the specialization is based on the elimination of surgery from practice and on the limitation of practice to certain age groups. Both pediatric and internal medicine specialists fit this category. Over the same period, pediatricians increased from 3,496 to 16,898 or from 3% to 5% of all physicians. By 1972, 54,558 (18.6%) of United States physicians were general practitioners, 43,118 were specialists in internal medicine (14.7%), 17,726 (6.1%) were pediatricians, and 4,542 (1.6%) had specialized in family practice. In short, 41% were practicing a form of general medicine, more than twice the proportion the original figure would have indicated (American Academy of Pediatrics, 1971; Martin, 1973).

Even this tends to understate the differ-

Table 7-2. Classification of medical specialties

Dimension of specialization	Medicine	Surgery	Other
Age	Internal medicine Pediatrics		
Organ	Cardiology Dermatology Gastroenterology Pulmonary medicine		Neurology
Technique		General surgery Plastic surgery	Anesthesiology Diagnostic radiology Radiology Therapeutic radiology Pathology Forensic pathology
Setting			Aerospace medicine Occupational medicine
Etiology	Allergy		Psychiatry
Age and organ	Pediatric cardiology		
Age and etiology	Pediatric allergy		Child psychiatry
Organ and technique		Neurosurgery Ophthalmology Otolaryngology Colon surgery Thoracic surgery Urology Orthopedic surgery	
Setting and etiology			Public health Preventive medicine

ence, since we have not considered those specialties that are specialized according to the settings in which they are practiced (e.g., aerospace medicine, occupational medicine), nor have we considered the patterns of osteopathic medicine, which is overwhelmingly general practice oriented.

The major line of specialization has been between medicine and surgery. Medical specialties that have not been oriented toward primary care tend to be limited to specific organ systems, whereas surgical specialties tend to be limited by both technique and organ system (Table 7-2). Physicians tend to specialize along one or more dimensions such as age groups (pediatrics), organ systems (cardiology), techniques (surgery, radiology), or setting (occupational medicine), or some combination (pediatric cardiology, thoracic surgery).

Specialties tend to differ in prestige within medicine such that high involvement with technique is given high prestige as in the case of neurosurgery, and specialties not easily classified as either medical or surgical that occur in particular settings and have no direct use of either drugs or surgery as a major component of practice (e.g., physical medicine and rehabilitation, public health) are accorded low prestige. The selection of specialties is a process that is sensitive to these prestige dimensions.

As discussed in Chapter 10, which deals with the organization of medical services, degree and type of specialization is associated with the location of medical practice and with the settings in which it takes place.

Informal organization

Relationships among physicians, and career contingencies, are regulated through a system of informal organization in which friendship patterns and sponsorship influence the referral of patients from one physician to another, hospital appointments, and other selection processes. Incorporation into the "right" network spells success for the young physician; exclusion relegates him to a lower order of practice. Exclusion

is also the major form of discipline within the profession.

The earliest studies of the informal organization of the medical profession were done by Hall in Toronto, Ontario, Canada and in Providence, Rhode Island (1946, 1947, 1949, 1954). His findings, many of which were confirmed in later studies by von der Lippe (1968) and Coleman et al. (1966), related to the selection of a specialty, hospital appointments, the referring of patients, and the delineation of types of careers as defined by relationships between physicians and the inner fraternity that controls medical practice.

Basic to Hall's analysis is that there is a small group of physicians in any community who have become established in a position of power within the medical profession. This group commands great prestige and controls access to those appointments that lead to prestige. Sponsorship by this inner fraternity is essential to gain the professional recognition that spells success in medicine. One can be a financial success without such sponsorship, but one cannot be a medical success.

To be accepted by the inner fraternity it is necessary to be defined as "promising," which means that the young physician has the requisite skills and "has the makings of a good physician." In addition, however, it means that he is the "right type" of person, that is, has a "good personality" and is of the "right" ethnic and religious backgrounds (usually white and Protestant). One with these characteristics can enter a colleague career beginning with appointment as an intern, with successive promotions to extern, hospital staff positions, office practice with an established physician, and incorporation into a pattern of referrals. At each step, the physician is expected to carry a defined load of charity work and to extend uncompensated services to the medical community. Success comes with loyalty to the institution and "sticking to one's knitting."

Those who are not accepted by the inner fraternity may enter an individualistic career pattern characterized by intense competition for patients and fees with a goal of high income and a large number of patients. Such physicians, unlike those in colleague careers, seldom specialize because they are outside the networks that refer patients. Alternatively the physician excluded by the inner fraternity may enter a friendly career pattern, which is less oriented toward financial success. Primary goals are to maintain friendly relationships with other physicians. This career is less competitive and abides more by the etiquette of colleague relationships than does the individualistic pattern.

A specialized practice, which we have seen to be the pattern for a majority of physicians in the United States, requires that one have the kind of relationships with other physicians in which those who deliver primary care will refer patients. It also increasingly requires hospital admitting privileges. Whereas primary physicians must maintain a good reputation among patients who refer other patients to them, specialists must have good relationships with other physicians who are the major source of referral. To be part of a professional referral system (Freidson, 1961, 1970) means to have a colleague career pattern as described by Hall.

The informal organization of medical practice is not only a facilitator of careers but also a system of social control. As described by Freidson (1970), formal mechanisms of control over physicians who practice substandard medicine are seldom used. Hence, although every county medical society in the United States provides for disciplinary hearings, expulsion of members, and the initiation of procedures to revoke the license to practice, the exercise of such sanctions is extremely rare. Instead the ultimate sanction is more often exclusion from the colleague group.

When a physician makes mistakes repeatedly, the first step is usually for a colleague to "talk to" the offender to see if the behavior can be altered. If the offending physician is unwilling to make changes or seems unable to bring his practice up to standards, colleagues will stop referring patients. Should this fail, the offender may be excluded from admitting patients to the hospital. Although the offender may become isolated from colleagues and lose admitting privileges, it is unlikely that any further sanctions will be attempted. Frequently, a physician so sanctioned can gain privileges at another hospital and become part of another group of colleagues. Although he enjoys lesser prestige, the right to practice will not be revoked.

Formal organization

Although the informal organization of medicine is the aspect of most immediate relevance to the practicing physician, the formal organization is important primarily as a political arm of medicine. Moreover, the informal and formal structures overlap in a manner that ensures that the large formal structures, for example, the AMA, reflect the most conservative political views within the profession.

The student will recall that the AMA was founded in the middle of the nineteenth century to protect the interests of allopathic physicians who were then facing a threat from various "irregular" practitioners. From that time until the third decade of this century, the organization probably reflected the wishes of a relatively homogeneous profession composed of general practitioners by promoting the scientific base of medicine. The AMA sponsored the influential Flexner Report and organized the political activity that led to the passage of licensing laws and minimal standards for medical training (Harris, 1966).

With increasing specialization, the interests of different types of physicians became more divergent, and the AMA became increasingly less representative of all physicians. With respect to national health insurance, for example, the AMA has consistently taken the most conservative stance, probably representing the views of most general practitioners, surgeons and family practitioners, who tend to be more conservative on both political and medical issues, while failing to reflect the views of the more specialized medical practitioners, who tend to be more liberal. Some specialty groups such as the American Academy of Pediatrics represent people whose views are considerably to the left of medicine in general and have endorsed a number of federal programs opposed by the AMA (Harris, 1966; American Academy of Pediatrics, 1971; Goldman, 1974).

Little work has been done on the organization of the AMA. The major source document in this area is a study by the editors of the *Yale Law Review* (1954). Membership is organized at three levels: county, state, and national. To be eligible for membership in the AMA, a physician must be a member of his county medical society, which automatically carries with it membership in the state society.

Officers of the AMA are selected through a process that makes the organization unrepresentative of its membership. Those physicians that get involved in medical politics tend to have more free time than others. Since a great deal of time and effort are required to build and maintain a practice, the politically active physician tends to be older, often semiretired, or for some reason has a small practice. They tend to run for office in the county medical societies. Slates of officers are drawn up by incumbent officers, serving to create a self-perpetuating body. Election to office in state medical societies is controlled by the county officers, who make nominations to a committee appointed by officers of the state society. National officers, including nomination for the powerful House of Delegates, the official policy organ of the AMA are elected from slates drawn up by state officers and screened by the national organization. As a result, the policy-making organs of the AMA tend to be more conservative ideologically. They are composed of members who are older than the average and who have been successfully screened by an entrenched establishment.

That the AMA has become increasingly unrepresentative of its claimed constituency (i.e., all physicians) is reflected in its dwindling membership. At the end of World War II, almost all physicians in the United States belonged to the AMA, with the exception of black physicians who were excluded from the county societies (Editors of the *Yale Law Review*, 1954). By the early 1970s, only a third were members.[3] Much of the loss of membership occurred during the battle against the Medicare legislation, which reinforced the emerging dissident physicians who had formed alternative organizations such as Physicians for Social Responsibility, designed originally to take a stand on atomic warfare, and the Medical Committee for Human Rights (MCHR), organized to provide a medical presence at civil rights demonstrations. MCHR particularly coalesced around the issues of national health policy, having become an ideological force in opposition to the AMA's policies on health insurance. They also undertook to fight elitism, racism, and sexism in medicine and in some areas have provided tactical support for local communities to organize their own health services.

Although the AMA (and its counterpart in other societies) has often fought changes in the health system, it is also organized to capitalize on changes when they occur. Hence the basic policies and rules for implementing legislation are often worked out by committees dominated by national medical organizations. Such was the case with the National Health Service in the United Kingdom (Mechanic, 1968a) and the Medicare legislation in the United States (Zappel, 1967).

National organization of physicians is also important for other health professions. The licensing boards for many other occupations, including nursing, physical therapy, and most of the other fields discussed in Chapter 9 are controlled by physicians.

Hence the AMA and most other national organizations of physicians serve as a coordinating mechanism to defend the autonomy of the profession and to enlarge the sphere of its dominance. It is a formal structure that reinforces the informal mechanisms of the profession.

CHIROPRACTIC

Chiropractors have been studied much less than physicians representing more mainstream traditions. Virtually all that is known comes from studies by Wardwell in the early 1950s and Lin in 1972. Each of these dealt with different situations: Wardwell's work was with chiropractors practicing in a state where chiropractic was illegal and many of his respondents had served time in prison for practicing medicine without a license, and Lin's work was in a state where chiropractic was not only legal but well established.

Compared with medicine and osteopathy, chiropractic is less professionalized on all the dimensions discussed at the beginning of the chapter. Chiropractors have a shorter period of training, less consensus on the content of their curriculum and work, and less autonomy in defining the scope and conditions of their work.

Becoming a chiropractor

Relative to medicine, chiropractors are drawn from the middle- and lower-status levels of the society. One third of the respondents in Wardwell's sample and one fourth of those in Lin's sample were previously in working-class occupations, and presumably a somewhat higher proportion came from working-class families (Wardwell, 1952; Lin, 1972).

The decision to be a chiropractor. Relative to medicine and osteopathy, the decision to enter chiropractic training comes late in life. Half of the chiropractors make the decision after the age of 25 years (Lin, 1972). Also, unlike medicine, chiropractors are not only likely to have seriously considered other lines of work, but they also are likely to have actually worked in other fields. As compared with almost all medical students, only 6% of chiropractors had not considered anything other than chiropractic, and almost all these were the sons of chiropractors (Lin, 1972).

Motivations of chiropractors are not that different from those of physicians on the surface. Wardwell (1952) found that humanitarian concerns predominated, followed by status aspirations and financial ambitions. Some, however, seemed to have no specific motivation, having drifted into chiropractic because of a relative in a chiropractic college or other coincidences. Some common experiences, however, were found by Lin. Among these were "(1) an early childhood association with a chiropractor which provided a role model; (2) experiences in chiropractic treatments which provided the individual's acceptance of chiropractic culture; and (3) some situational factors which (shifted) the individual's . . . career choice to chiropractic . . .," including dissatisfaction with work and the desire for upward social mobility (Lin, 1972).

Chiropractic training. Originally chiropractic training consisted of only 2 months of apprenticeship training. However, by 1912 it had increased to 18 months. No prechiropractic schooling was required. By 1970 the chiropractic course had increased to four years. Thirty-five states required two years of college as a prerequisite to admission, and two states required one year. As a result of this upgrading, the performance of chiropractors on basic science examinations has improved steadily over this century (Wardwell, 1952; Lin, 1972; National Center for Health Statistics, 1973).

Although chiropractic schools now require at least two years of preprofessional training, there is no evidence that college students who are to become chiropractors have identified themselves, much less become a cohesive group, as college undergraduates. It might be reasonably inferred that there is little or no prechiropractic socialization that can be identified with an educational curriculum.

Course work in chiropractic schools consists of 4,000 hours, 1,840 of which are in the basic sciences of anatomy (640 hours); physiology (320 hours); chemistry, including biochemistry and nutrition (320 hours);

pathology and bacteriology (480 hours); and hygiene, sanitation, and public health (80 hours). Clinical subjects cover 2,080 hours of training and include physical, clinical, laboratory, and differential diagnosis; gynecology, obstetrics, and pediatrics; roentgenology; geriatrics, dermatology, syphilology, taxicology, psychology, and psychiatry; principles of chiropractic; and jurisprudence ethics and economics.

In what has been characterized as the "chiropractic Flexner Report" (Lin, 1972), Haynes (1967) called attention to problems in the quality of instruction in chiropractic colleges. One of these was the poor quality of instruction. According to Dubbs (1970), "Too many instructors are teaching the basic sciences without having any advanced or graduate training in these sciences. Too many instructors are not trained or qualified as teachers nor masters of their fields." In addition, teaching loads were heavy, and little research was done by chiropractic faculties. Partly because of these internal pressures and partly because of federal pressures to qualify for participation in governmental health programs, chiropractors have recently developed a self-conscious literature aimed at upgrading the quality of their training (Kimmel, 1964; Haynes, 1967, 1969; United States Department of Health, Education, and Welfare, 1968; Dubbs, 1970).

It seems possible that chiropractic will follow a pattern taken earlier by osteopathy. That is, chiropractors may become more like mainstream physicians, either becoming an alternative source of medical training or a subspecialty of medicine. In the absence of good sociological studies, however, it is not possible to predict this course with confidence.

Most impressive is the lack of any sociological studies of the chiropractic student. Compared with medical and osteopathic students, nothing is known about the socialization process either into the student culture or the professional culture of chiropractic.

Organization of chiropractic

Other than that chiropractic is almost exclusively a solo, fee-for-service–type of practice, almost nothing is known about its informal organization. There is no literature that deals with the process of becoming established in practice, the effects of sponsorship, and other organizational factors. Referrals among chiropractors are rare, however, as each chiropractor is a general practitioner. To date, there is no evidence for specialization within the occupational group (Lin, 1972).

There is evidence, however, for a split among chiropractors on ideological grounds. One group, called "straights" by the Stanford Research Institute (1960) and "traditionalists" by Lin (1972), have adhered to the original teachings of Palmer. These chiropractors limit their practice to the adjustment of subluxated spinal vertebrae by hand, concentrating on the upper spine. They use no other therapies and consider themselves as the only "pure and unadulterated" chiropractors. The other group, called "mixers" by the Stanford Research Institute and "expansionists" by Lin, have extended their range of treatments to include light, heat, electricity, vitamins, air, water, exercise, and physiotherapy as modalities. Much controversy exists between these two groups, to the point at which they form somewhat separate organizations within chiropractic.

Traditionalists tend to practice alone with little office assistance and are committed to maintaining chiropractic as a form of practice distinct from medicine. The mixers or expansionists tend to hire more office assistants, engage in a wider range of therapies, and lean toward viewing chiropractic as a specialized practice that must eventually become part of a team of health professionals. Compared to traditionalists, mixers make more referrals to physicians. This group may be the vanguard of a movement to make chiropractic a medical specialty (but again we emphasize that this is a speculation that needs sociological research).

There are two separate national organizations of chiropractors, the American Chiropractic Association (ACA) and the International Chiropractic Association (ICA). Both originated in an older organization, the Universal Chiropractic Association (UCA), which was founded in 1906. The mixers began agitating for change within the UCA and in 1922 split off to form the ACA. The traditionalists in an attempt to "clean house" and expel the mixers, founded a caucus within the UCA, the Chiropractic Health Bureau in 1926, which eventually became the International Chiropractic Association in 1942. Thus the two groups reflect the ideological split. The ACA is an organization of mixers and the ICA an organization of traditionalists. Each now presses its own point of view, and except for occasional issues such as the eligibility of chiropractic patients for Medicare benefits, they do not coordinate activities.

The case of chiropractic is hence a fascinating one. It seems likely that it will split into two separate occupations and that at some future point those supporting the ACA group will become part of the mainstream of health occupations. The study of this process can reveal much about social movements, professionalization, and other similar phenomena.

PHYSICIANS AND PATIENTS

As an occupational group, physicians have become sophisticated in their knowledge of human biology and in modes of intervening in life processes. Historically they have developed from a major social menace to an effective source of cure. As noted in Chapter 1, this change has been accomplished at some cost, the primary one being a shift in focus from sick people to diseases. In addition, the very success of medicine has complicated relationships between the physician and the patient. Medicine has become an alien culture, structurally rooted in a network that excludes patients from active participation. Encounters between patients and physicians now require more negotiation to establish a common universe of discourse. In short, although the technical capacity of medicine has vastly improved, the conditions for applying that capacity has deteriorated.

Medicine as an alien culture

A patient going to a physician increasingly encounters someone who thinks differently, speaks a different language, and lives in a technological world alien to everyday experience. As noted in Chapter 5, patients seldom go to the physician with a disease. Rather they are concerned about some change in the way they feel or in the activities they can do and want to understand what the implications of the change are and what to do about it. Physicians, on the other hand, are interested in converting the complaints of patients into a diagnosis. This is often done by subjecting patients to a series of tests that may involve taking samples of body tissue. The reasons for these tests are self-evident to those initiated into the world of medicine but are incomprehensible to the patient. Many patients conclude that their physicians are experimenting on them in ways unrelated to their complaints. Davis and von der Lippe (1967) have documented that most instances of discharge from the hospital against medical advice follow from this kind of misunderstanding.

Samora et al. (1961) have found that the language of the hospital is alien to patients. They asked 125 hospitalized patients to define fifty terms that are part of the everyday discourse on hospital wards. Less than half could define such words as bacteria, nutrition, digestion, cardiac, orally, tissue, dilate, nerve, malignant, terminal, and tendon. Only 56% understood "specimen," 69% understood "pulse," 70% understood "reaction," and 80% understood "abdomen." Since these are the kinds of words typically used by physicans in talking with patients, we must conclude that patients understand little of what is happening to them in the hospital. Even college graduates in the sample missed almost one fourth of the terms.

Systems of healing that are outside the mainstream of modern medicine, the most important being chiropractic, subscribe to theories of disease that are closer to common sense for many people. These same fields tend to talk in the language of the patient, leading to a better fit between lay and professional perspectives (McCorkle, 1961).

Structural contingencies in interaction

The physician and patient are enmeshed in different social structures that impose claims on their behaviors, limiting the freedom of each to adjust to the other. As described by Bloom (1963), the physician is part of the institution of medicine, often in an office with other physicians or in a hospital with physicians and a variety of other health personnel. The day-to-day interactions of physicians are controlled to some degree by the shared definitions of the profession as to what constitutes an adequate level of performance, what is appropriate behavior, and other role requirements. The standards upheld by this role set are generally different from those of patients.

The patient, as noted in Chapter 5, is also enmeshed in a role set that, except for the contingency of sickness, does not include the physician or other medical experts. The kinds of behaviors regarded as appropriate and the evaluation of the services provided may not correspond to those of the medical profession.

The contact between the patient and physician is a contact not only between two different cultures but also between two distinct social networks, each of which will have different, if not mutually exclusive, expectations for the encounter, different performance needs, and different standards of adequacy. For the interaction to succeed, the patient and physician must come to a common set of understandings as to the nature of the problem and the appropriate response. This must be accomplished against great odds.

The negotiation of reality

That such negotiation takes place has been documented by Balint (1957) who gathered case documents from a large number of general practitioners and discussed the cases at length in group seminars. He found that the typical interaction sequence was a process of bargaining in which the patient proposes an illness by describing his symptoms. The expected response is for the physician to agree to the significance of the complaint and to provide the patient with a name for the condition and a plan of therapy. If the physician investigates and disagrees with the patient's proposal, he then makes a counterproposal to which the patient must react. If they fail to agree, the relationship is terminated, and presumably the patient looks elsewhere.

The important point is that each one, operating within his own framework, must come up with a set of definitions acceptable to both. Failure in this regard is a failure of the relationship and consequently of treatment and cure, at least in that encounter. It is not known how frequently the patient is right when there is disagreement between patient and physician, but one study of a small number of hospitalized patients documented several cases in which patients who had been told that there was nothing wrong with them subsequently were found to have serious illness. It is a question in need of investigation (Sweet and Twaddle, 1969a).

CODA

In this chapter we have looked at the one occupation that more than any other is at the core of the institutionalized response to sickness in so-called modern societies. In a brief overview, a few facets of the development of the field were discussed, and the highlights of research findings on the selection, development, and organization of physicians were reviewed. It was also noted that there is a persistence of some competing occupational groups, most importantly in the practice of chiropractic.

It would be a mistake, however, to consider the physician as the only source of help for the sick. The point made in earlier chapters that most diagnosis and treatment takes place in an informal manner either from the sick person treating himself or from friends and relatives must be underlined. Also it is increasingly the case that physicians do not practice alone. There is a never-expanding number of other occupations, most of which developed later than medicine and that practice jointly with physicians. In the next chapter we turn our attention to the oldest of these, the nurse.

NOTES

1. The degree doctor of medicine, awarded for four years of medical training, is uniquely American. Other countries award a bachelor of medicine degree or a licentiate of medicine certificate. In some countries, such as the United Kingdom, a doctorate of medicine can be earned but only as a research degree contingent on completion of a doctoral dissertation. In the United States the title "doctor" was an attempt by a low-prestige occupation, medicine, to bask in the prestige of the doctor of philosophy. As a form of address, "doctor" is now applied to physicians throughout the world.

2. This is according to a reprint with no identification as to source and no date found in the files of the Kirksville College of Osteopathic Medicine library in Kirksville, Missouri, entitled "White Paper: AOA-AMA Relationships."

3. The AMA denies that it is a minority organization. In a pamphlet entitled "Where We Stand," it asserts that it represents over 100,000 members. It was from those figures that we calculated the membership of the AMA at approximately one third of all practicing physicians. The contention of the AMA is that all practicing physicians do not constitute the proper denominator and that based on all *eligible* physicians, it represents over two thirds. What this means is that approximately one third do not even belong to their county societies.

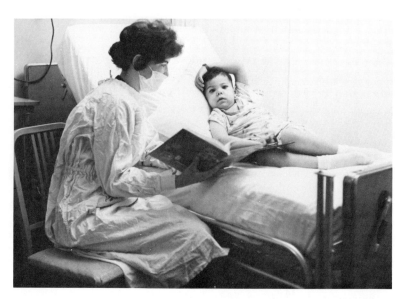

CHAPTER 8

Nursing

Some sociological characteristics of nursing as an occupation will be discussed in this chapter. Here we will attempt to discern the social organizational structure of nursing, including its status within the hierarchy of medical professions. Then some of the major historical antecedents to the contemporary nursing scene will be presented. The objective in this regard is to establish the relationships between historical developments in nursing and problems faced by nurses today. Finally, we will interpret some of the most recent changes occurring within nursing's occupational structure, analyzing them as strategies for resolving some of nursing's most troublesome dilemmas.

SOME SOCIOLOGICAL CHARACTERISTICS OF NURSING
Sex

The most striking and possibly most salient structural feature of nursing is its femaleness. Nursing is almost wholly a female occupation. This fact cannot escape one's attention, since the sexual discrimination in the society at large has permeated the medical professions and constrained the organization and growth of nursing to a large extent. In 1972 only 1.4% of employed registered nurses were men compared with 1.1% in 1966 (American Nurses' Association, 1974). In this sense, nursing as an occupation reflects society as a whole. The sex role socialization that portrays women as submissive and deferential to men in the larger society occurs in nursing where women continue to be subservient to men, the protagonists only incidentally having nursing or medical degrees.

Size

Compared with physicans, dentists, pharmacists, dieticians, physical therapists, and other members of the healing occupations, nurses far outnumber each of these occupations. For example, in 1972 it was estimated there were 794,979 employed registered nurses, with 1,127,657 registered nurses holding licenses to practice (American Nurses' Association, 1974).

Occupational diversity

In addition to its sheer size of numbers, nursing is the most heteromorphic of the healing occupations. From a lay perspective, "a nurse is a nurse is a nurse"; however, nothing could be more fictive! There are licensed practical nurses and registered nurses. Within the ranks of registered nurses, there are those who have baccalaureate degrees (B.S.); others who have diplomas from three-year, hospital-based training programs; and still others who have two-year associate of arts (junior college) degrees. Furthermore, there are nurses with masters and doctorates. The training associated with each of these degree programs is different, and the type of nurse produced in each program varies greatly in terms of career aspirations, orientation to professional striving, income, and other characteristics. Nursing is a complex, multifaceted health care occupation, let us make no mistake about it.

Work settings

Hospitals and nursing homes have been and continue to be the predominant employers of registered nurses. In 1972, 71.1% of all employed nurses worked in hospitals and nursing homes. This fact that a large percentage of employed registered nurses work in highly bureaucratic settings has

led to occupational-bureaucratic conflict. Nursing students, especially those in collegiate programs, are taught to think of themselves as professionals autonomous in certain sectors of their work. In training programs, student nurses come to value knowledge, innovation, individually tailored direct care for patients, and self-regulation of nursing work (Kramer, 1970). This training occurs in a setting far removed from the hospital bureaucracy where most nurses will enter as employees after graduation. The hospital, because it is highly bureaucratized, requires a highly specialized division of labor. To coordinate the resultant multitude of roles, a hierarchical control structure is imposed on nurses and other employees. The norms of this structure are external to the occupations thus controlled. Therefore the work setting can in fact be dialectically opposed to the training and expectations of nurse tyros, and conflict between these two worlds is inevitable. It should be noted that conflict between occupational groups and bureaucracies is not a process unique to nursing per se. Wilensky (1960) has argued that most careers no longer lead to the gradual creation of a plan for one's life. On the contrary, bureaucracies are being subjected to automation influences, and careers are no longer coherent progressions to upward mobility. In fact, Wilensky's research shows that many administrators are experiencing downward mobility during the height of their careers, victims of automation.

Professionalism

A major debate is raging currently over the question, "Is nursing a profession?" Even among nurses, there is disagreement, with many taking a negative or neutral position, whereas others attempt to lay claim to a professional place in the sun on the same stretch of beach occupied by medicine, law, the ministry, and university academicians. One fact for certain, the degree of doubt concerning professional status is directly related to the amount of talk about being a professional, and nursing seems to have the advantage over other health occupations in this regard.

Is nursing a profession? The answer is written on the other side of the occupational page, and it is written in the core characteristics that determine professional status. To list these core characteristics as structural-functional theorists have done (Goode, 1957; Greenwood, 1957; Pavalko, 1972) obscures the message because the list of characteristics such as a code of ethics, an association, a journal, knowledge base, commitment to the public, and others misses the most critical question: What is the most salient, important, distinguishing facet of an occupational group that clearly and unambiguously defines it as a profession?

First, the nature of the work must be identified by the public as a function that meets one of the high-priority, core needs of the society. Legal, religious, educational, and medical aspects of peoples' lives are considered top priority needs in United States society. Occupational groups whose works fulfill these needs are deemed vital by the society and are accorded enormous respect.

This leads to the second point regarding the key facet of a profession, that is, the degree of autonomy in decision making that an occupation enjoys (Freidson, 1970). Those occupational groups that possess control over tasks deemed most salient for health care or religious life are accorded the greatest prestige by the public, and subsequently, these groups have great freedom to define how their work will be organized, produced, and regulated. In short, the group with the greatest degree of autonomy by definition controls the means of production within its sphere of work and dominates all related occupations. Thus functional autonomy (Freidson, 1970) and the control over the means of production are distinguishing characteristics of a profession.

Within the sphere of medicine, many different occupational groups exist, forming a hierarchy of rank and prestige. At the top of the heap is the profession of medicine. Physicians control the knowledge base and the production of medical services, and are accorded high prestige and functional autonomy by members of society. With the exception of a few health occupations such as pharmacy, dentistry, optometry, and others, the vast majority of health occupations are organized with limited functional autonomy to serve the profession of medicine in the role of a supporting cast. They are the workers who carry out medical tasks under the direction and control of physicians, who accordingly claim possession of a body of theory and knowledge that makes healing possible.

Nurses are next in line to physicians on the ladder of medical professions, but it is not possible to say with confidence that nursing is a profession given the criteria mentioned earlier concerning what constitutes a profession. Functional autonomy and societal prestige are not possessed by nursing to the extent necessary to propel nurses into professional status and roles equal to physicians and other similar health professions.

Yet clearly nursing is engaged in a struggle to attain functional autonomy and prestige on a level with physicians. Some of the changes taking place in nursing as well as the barriers to change will be discussed later in this chapter. For the moment, suffice it to say that what one observes in nursing by way of this struggle can be defined sociologically as professionalization. Nursing is in the midst of a process designed to lead ultimately to the achievement of the label "professional" and to convince society that the label is legitimate and deserved. In short, this process of professionalization is similar to a social movement with attendant ideologies, rhetoric, disciplines, and strategies for change (Bucher and Strauss, 1961). The development of knowledge and skills is only part, perhaps even a minor part, of the development of a profession. Professionalization includes a realization on the part of those striving for professional status that they must be accepted by other occupational groups in their field, as well as by society at large. Durkheim (1933) identified this community of which professionals in a given field are a part as the "moral community." In this context, nursing must convince physicians, other health workers, and patients that its contribution to health care is to be fully recognized professionally as equal to the work performed by physicians.

NURSING EDUCATION AND SOCIALIZATION

How nurses are educated is of critical importance for understanding the process of professionalization. The struggle for professional status is intimately related to three factors inherent to nursing education: (1) the knowledge base nursing students learn, (2) the technical skills students acquire, and (3) the process of socializing students to a nurse role.

Focusing for a moment on the knowledge base, it is clear that there is no uniformity among nurses as to what that base should include. Habenstein and Christ's study (1955) found nurses who believed in the utility of formal rational knowledge (professionalizers) versus nurses who thought that informal nonscientific knowledge about tender, loving, bedside care is the distinctive knowledge base of nursing (traditionalizers). Alas for the professional strivers, there were nurses who cared not at all about developing nursing knowledge and who were concerned primarily with the technical and organizational details of work performance (utilizers).

It is reasonable to assume in the absence of enlightening research on the subject that the push for socialization of student nurses to expect to acquire a distinctive base of rational knowledge takes place in baccalaureate programs. Associate of arts programs tend to stress bedside-care knowledge, and diploma programs produce the utilizers.

Interestingly, although recruitment into all registered nursing programs has increased rather significantly in recent years, the largest number of admissions in the

1971-1972 academic year was in the associate degree programs (36,996), with the diploma programs pulling in 29,801 students and baccalaureate programs drawing 27,357 student nurses (American Nurses' Association, 1974). The percent increase in admissions from the previous year, however, was largest for baccalaureate programs (34%) and smallest for diploma programs (2.8%), although this reverses a ten-year, downward trend for diploma programs (American Nurses' Association, 1974). The trend is clearly in the direction of associate of arts programs, which have gained great popularity relative to baccalaureate and diploma programs (Fig. 8-2).

Similarly, the issuance of licenses to practical nurses has increased continuously over the years. In 1972, 46,004 licenses were issued to individuals who had never held such a license in the United States (American Nurses' Association, 1974). This represents an increase of 3,000 between 1971 and

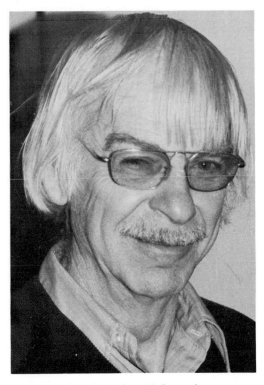

Fig. 8-1. *Robert Habenstein.*

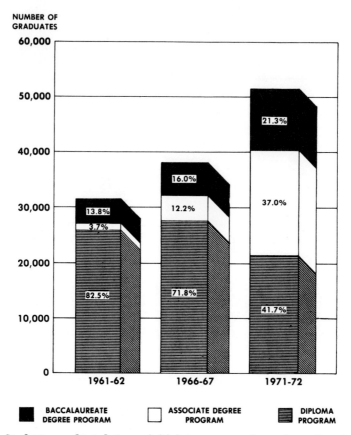

NUMBER OF
GRADUATES

Fig. 8-2. *Students graduated from initial programs of nursing education: registered nurses, academic years 1961-1962, 1966-1967, and 1971-1972.* (From National League for Nursing. *State approved schools for nursing—R.N., 1968-1973.* Kansas City, Mo.: American Nurses' Association, Statistics Department, 1973.)

1972 among the ranks of the approximately 500,000 licensed practical nurses in 1972.

Finally, the number of nurses enrolled in master's and doctoral programs in nursing has declined in terms of the proportion who attended full time, and the net gain has been relatively small compared to changes in nursing practice with regard to expanded roles and clinical practice. In 1972, for example, there were 6,342 registered nurses enrolled in master's degree programs and 402 doctoral candidates (American Nurses' Association, 1974).

These trends have rather serious implications for nursing education. That sector of nursing in which one anticipates the greatest commitment to and action on behalf of professionalization, that is, the baccalaureate and post-graduate degree programs, is numerically far outweighed by associate, diploma, and licensed practical nursing programs. Furthermore, a look at the baccalaureate socialization process per se leads one to assess nursing's drive toward professional status and functional autonomy with considerable pessimism.

First, baccalaureate nursing students are different from the general college population of females. In a study by O'Neil (1973), 465 nursing students in three baccalaureate programs located in the Midwest were surveyed using the Allport-Lindzey scale for measuring dominant values and Gordons' Survey of Interpersonal Values.

O'Neil found in comparing nursing and general female college population the following:

1. Nursing students attached greater importance to altruistic and philanthropic service, and they placed a greater emphasis on theoretical than on practical affairs of the business world.

2. The general college population attached greater importance to personal power, influence, and the domination of people.

3. On the "conformity" and "benevolence" values, nursing students placed greater emphasis on being generous and helping underdogs and less emphasis on following rules closely. Nursing students stressed the greater importance of being free to make one's own decisions and being treated with understanding. They placed less emphasis on the importance of achieving recognition than the general college population. However, medical students were even more attached to the value of being free to make one's own decisions than were the nursing students.

4. When analyzing class level differences among nursing students, O'Neil found that the "helping people" value was reinforced consistently throughout the four years of nursing school. Finally, the low leadership value scores of nursing students were similar across class lines.

When one looks closely at what actually transpires during the four years of baccalaureate nursing education, the dilemma of socialization, hinted at in O'Neil's research, emerges as a lighthouse of clarity. Kramer (1970) describes a strong example of this problem. Baccalaureate nursing students are the foot soldiers of the war on professional recognition. During their four years of nursing education, students are socialized to a nurse role that values individualized direct patient care, rational knowledge, and innovation, and they are taught to think of themselves as autonomous, professional persons. Like Odysseus, the hero of Greek mythology who successfully negotiated countless tribulations only to return

home to Ithaca where he was accidently speared to death by his son, Telegonus, so do nursing students graduate only to find that their role values are dysfunctional in the work world of bureaucratized medical care organization. Specialization of tasks or the increasingly complex division of labor in medicine demands external coordination and hierarchical control of work. In this highly bureaucratized structure, there is no room for nurses to function governed by their own individualized system of norms, and they are faced with the prospect of working in a setting that is antithetical to the one advocated by the socializing institution.

Do baccalaureate nurses hang on to their conceptions of their role as autonomous professionals or do they accommodate? Corwin (1961) found that baccalaureate nurses maintained high professional role conceptions more frequently than did diploma nurses. However, this created a high intensity of conflict for baccalaureate nurses. Kramer (1967) presents a different picture. Rather than hanging on to their role conceptions, neophyte nurses either increased their loyalty to bureaucratic values and consequently became less committed to functional autonomy, independence, and other such values, or they dropped out of nursing in lieu of accommodating to the bureaucracy. Simply put, role deprivation was experienced by neophyte nurses, and it increased after graduation over time until nurses accommodated by either giving up their visions of working as an autonomous professional or by dropping out of nursing entirely. This is consistent with the data on the values of baccalaureate nursing students (O'Neil, 1973), their background characteristics (Kramer, 1970; Wren, 1971), and the general and well-documented problems experienced by highly specialized workers in bureaucratic settings (Katz, 1968; Etzioni, 1969).

SOME HISTORICAL DEVELOPMENTS

The history of nursing holds clues that helps one understand nursing's current state of affairs. Actually the history of nursing should start with the history of women as healers, since it is no accident that nursing is primarily a female occupation today. Current developments in nursing may be viewed as logical extensions of a social movement in health care in which women once occupied positions of autonomy and influence as healers, were severely suppressed, and have reemerged in the occupation of nursing as we know it today.

Women were healers from the beginning of recorded history. In ancient Greece of Homer's time, women functioned as independent medical practitioners. They were known as "navel cutters" *(amphalotomai)* who assisted women with prenatal and postpartum care, throwing in the birth itself, of course, as a feature of their trade.

Medieval Europe witnessed a great expansion of the rolls of women healers. The first free hospital in Rome was established in AD 390 and was run by a patrician woman called Fabiola. One of her colleagues, a wealthy and powerful Roman woman named Paula, built hospitals in Palestine and Jerusalem around this same time period. Women were powerful and autonomous in public and private sectors of medieval Roman society, and there was one standard of sexual conduct shared equally by men and women.

Women healers developed and used herbal remedies and other curative techniques and achieved autonomy and independence in their work well into the fourteenth century. Then the roof fell in! Witch-hunting, spanning four centuries, was born in Europe. Witch-hunts were financed and organized by Church and State and were aimed primarily at exterminating women healers (Ehrenreich and English, 1973).

The reasons for witch-hunting are probably less moral and religious (witches consorting with the devil and sexually seducing innocent men) than political, since women healers had become the major source of medical care and comfort for the peasants. It is only logical to make the case that the peasant revolts against feudalism swept up the women healers who were singled out by the ruling classes as leaders of the rebellions. The female healing role was labeled "witchcraft," which legitimated persecution and destruction of women healers.

In the meantime, beginning in the thirteenth century, university-trained healers emerged and rapidly established themselves as a medical profession. They were able to gain full professional status, that is, to monopolize and control the medical field because the clients of these early physicians were wealthy and powerful members of the elite ruling classes. Freidson (1970) points out how professions in effect are creations of the ruling classes, dependent on their patronage and support. He states, "A profession attains and maintains its position by virtue of the protection and patronage of some elite segment of society which has been persuaded that there is some special value in its work."

These early physicians had no scientific knowledge base and relied heavily on bleeding, leeching, incantations, and quasi-magical rituals. The state of medical science was much less empirical and scientific than the state of witchcraft and its knowledge base.

Nevertheless, women healers were persecuted and murdered, and aspiring women physicians were denied places in universities. In the end, men physicians were able to gain complete dominance over healing, even to the extent that by the eighteenth century, they gained control over obstetrical practice among the middle classes. This was in earlier times the sole province of women healers cum midwives.

In America this process of dominance of one type of healer over all other practitioners occurred later than it did in Europe but occur it did, nevertheless. During the early 1800s, the United States experienced a rapid growth of diverse practitioners such as the thompsonians, eclectics, homeopaths, allopaths, and others. Also during this period, one group of so-called formally trained practitioners, calling themselves "regulars," gained a monopoly over middle- and upper-class patients. Certainly their training and treatments were no better scientifically or effective than those of the other types of healers, since there was no body of scientific medical knowledge at this time (Chapter 7).

Because of their frequent contact with the elite and powerful members of the society, the regular practitioners succeeded in getting legislation passed, so that by 1830 many states had licensing laws that made it illegal for all but regular healers to practice medicine. Partly in response to this medical elitism and legislation of morality and partly as a spin-off of the worker-feminist social movements, the Popular Health Movement (1830 to 1850) began. "Irregular" medical practitioners formed associations, medical schools, and denounced the regular practitioners. Women were firmly ensconced in the Popular Health Movement, heading up "ladies physiological societies" (Ehrenreich and English, 1973) teaching preventive medical practices, and functioning as healers. Women's medical colleges were established and other irregular medical schools admitted women to be trained as eclectic, homeopathic, or allopathic healers. This health revolution was fostered by a great new democratic wave that swept up the United States in Andrew Jackson's day. The thirties and forties were the decades of manhood suffrage, followed in the sixties by women's suffrage, which struck down property restrictions on voting. Cheap newspapers and periodicals appeared, with the *New York Sun* launched in 1833 by Benjamin Day followed two years later by the immensely popular *New York Herald.* The first popular magazine, *Godey's Lady's Book,* was established in Philadelphia in 1830, and Horace Mann was leading the battle for public education in Massachusetts.

During this period of intense democratization, women practitioners and other irregular groups could have emerged as dominant, autonomous, medical practitioners. Instead conflict within the ranks of irregular medicine, coupled with the failure of the working class to gain political power, allowed the regular practitioners the oppor-

tunity needed to establish once and for all a virtual monopoly over medicine in the United States. In 1848 the AMA was established, and the attack against the irregular practitioners, particularly women healers, was launched. In 1871, Dr. Alfred Stille said in his presidential address to the AMA:

> Certain women seek to rival men in manly spots . . . and the strongminded ape them in all things, even in dress. In doing so they may command a sort of admiration such as all monstrous productions inspire, especially when they aim towards a higher type than their own.

Some women healers, perhaps sensing the imminent decline of their irregular professions, attempted to join forces with the regulars in denouncing irregulars, including their sister midwives. By 1920 regular healers had become the unmitigated dominant medical profession through various licensing laws, and most of the irregular practitioners were outlawed. Women healers turned for guidance to physicians who, overloaded with Flexnerian recommendations for good hospitals and scientific training, readily suggested nursing as an option for women health careerists. The process of deprofessionalization of women healers was complete.

Nursing was ready to accommodate the increased demand. In Europe prior to the 1840s nursing was looked on as a disagreeable and vulgar form of domestic service. So-called nurses were often alcoholics or prostitutes who extorted money from hospital patients as often as they exhorted them to recover. Hospitals were pestholes, and nurses were neither paid enough, educated enough, nor sober enough to appreciate the need for some form of vocational spirit among themselves.

In 1840 Mrs. Elizabeth Fry founded the Institute of Nursing Sisters, which was the first organization of nurses to exist and to stress training. St. John's House Sisterhood, founded in 1848 in London, stressed practical training as well.

The Crimean War broke out between Russia and Great Britain in 1854. Medical care for the wounded became a great public issue in Britain (*London Times*, October 12, 1854), and public pressure was brought to bear to improve the status of nursing and medical care in general. The desperateness of the situation notwithstanding, the image of the new nurse needed was consonant with English males' images of the role of women in society. Nurturance, obedience, and the need to be protected from worldly excess and privation, all these female stereotypes were built into the new nursing image. For example, a *London Times* correspodent wrote:

Why have we no Sisters of Charity? There are numbers of ablebodied and tender-hearted English women who would joyfully and with alacrity go out to devote themselves to the nursing of the sick and wounded, if they could be associated for that purpose, and be placed under proper protection (*London Times*, October 14, 1854).

Florence Nightingale returned from the war a heroine because her nursing administration had cut the death rate at Scutari hospital from 42 to 22 per thousand. The Nightingale Fund was established in 1855 in London, and the Nightingale School of Nursing was established at St. Thomas Hospital under the direction of Nightingale. Later in 1859 Nightingale published the first nursing textbook, *Notes on Nursing*. None of these developments were received with any enthusiasm by physicians of the day. However, physicians accepted the development of nursing as long as control over nursing work rested with physicians.

From this era, nursing developed into a formal occupation. At the time, the central characteristics of nursing, which persist even to this day, included a hospital base of operations, control of functional decision making by physicians, questions about what could constitute a proper body of nursing knowledge, and an endless struggle to acquire prestige and support by society for professional status. Interestingly the blind obedience and subservience to physicians that some researchers (Ehrenreich and En-

glish, 1973) have argued Nightingale demanded of her followers is not accurate. Although elements of obedience and deference exist in nursing, a quick glance at Nightingale's "Annual Letters," which she sent to her trainees as a sort of policy statement on what nursing ought to be, suggests that Nightingale should not be blamed for these characteristics. As one can see in the following excerpts from her "Annual Letters," Nightingale was concerned about nursing producing the ideal lady, in whom character and not skills was emphasized:

A woman who takes a sentimental view of nursing (which she calls "ministering" as if she were an angel) is, of course, worse than useless. A woman possessed with the idea that she is making a sacrifice will never do; and a woman who thinks that any kind of nursing work is "beneath a nurse" will simply be in the way. . . . For us who nurse, our nursing is a thing, which, unless in it we are making progress every year, every month, every week, take my word for it, we are going back. The more experience we gain, the more progress we can make. . . . After all, all that our training can do for us is teach us how to train ourselves. . . . Do we look enough into the importance of giving ourselves thoroughly to study in the hours of study, of keeping careful "Notes of Lectures," and of type cases—and of cases interesting from not being type cases—so as to improve our powers of observation, all so essential if we are [in the future to have changed]. . . . It is not the certificate which makes the nurse or the midwife. It may [un-make] her. The danger is lest she let the certificate be [instead] of herself, [instead] of her never ceasing going up higher as a woman and a nurse (Nightingale, 1914).

The Nightingale plan for nursing and hospital organization spread to the United States where in 1873 a training school was established at Bellevue Hospital in New York. New Haven Hospital in Connecticut started a nurse training school 6 months after Bellevue, and the New England Hospital for women in Massachusetts developed its training school in 1873.

Recognizing the paucity of intellectual life in the hospital programs, Mrs. Hampton Robb and Adelaide Nutting who succeded Robb at Johns Hopkins Hospital established the first university-based department of nursing at Columbia University. The first collegiate school of nursing was established in 1909 at the University of Minnesota, and in 1933 the Association of Collegiate Schools of Nursing was established to coordinate the activities of a growing number of collegiate programs. In 1896 alumnae societies of training schools were united, and in 1911 the Nurses Associated Alumnae of the United States and Canada became the American Nurses' Association (ANA).

The development of nursing in the United States has continued to set a trend in which training is shifting away from the technical apprenticeship role of the hospital setting into the two-year and four-year academic settings. Throughout its history, nursing did not acquire an academic or scientific discipline to stand for a body of knowledge that is nursing's domain and not the property of physicians or other health workers. Nevertheless, nursing was a ripe and ideal health occupation for the displaced and would-be women healers of the future. Given its history and developments, the nurse role was a safe place to send women and be confident in the knowledge that the authority and professional dominance of physicians would not be challenged. The clinical management role for nurses, with limited medical care responsibilities, historically always was supportive of the professional autonomy of physicians, the primary beneficiaries of nursing's largesse.

NEW ROLES FOR NURSES

As mentioned at the beginning of this chapter, the issue most central to professionalization and professional status is the question of functional autonomy. Thus it is no surprise to find that the development of new roles for nurses, sometimes called "expanded roles" or "nurse practitioner roles," boils down to the stand that whatever the new nurse does, she will not continue in a dependent relationship to physicians. Regardless of whether one is concerned with the pediatric nurse practitioner, the family nurse practitioner, or the family planning nurse specialist, the common thread binding all these new roles is the push for functional autonomy, to get away from under the thumb of physicans and their orders, to transform the basic existing pattern of health manpower deployment, the structure of the health care delivery system, and to achieve full professional status.

Some of the new roles are not as new as one would like to think. Early in 1925 Mary Breckinridge returned to America from England where she had obtained a British midwife's license. She settled in Kentucky, her ancestral home, and established at Wendover, the Frontier Nursing Service (FNS), which today boasts the sixteen-bed Hyden Hospital, five clinical outpost centers, the School of Midwivery and Family Nursing, and a social service department. From the outset to the present, the Frontier Nursing Service has trained nurses to function as autonomous obstetricians without control by physicians (Fig. 8-3), even though many physicians have worked with the FNS and a physican serves as medical director (Frontier Nursing Service, 1974). The FNS nurse works relatively independently of physician control and utilizes knowledge and techniques usually reserved for physician-obstetricians (Breckinridge, 1952). This autonomy is owed in part to the fact that physicians have been unwilling to commit themselves to working with the rural, isolated population that FNS serves. This is autonomy born out of necessity but it is autonomy nevertheless in the form of independent medical practice.

The FNS and other similar precedents not withstanding, the potential for new nursing roles with functional autonomy is great in the 1970s. This potential is the result of four interdependent forces that are at work independent of physicians', nurses', or any other health workers' efforts to either foster or hinder them. These forces external to nursing are as follows.

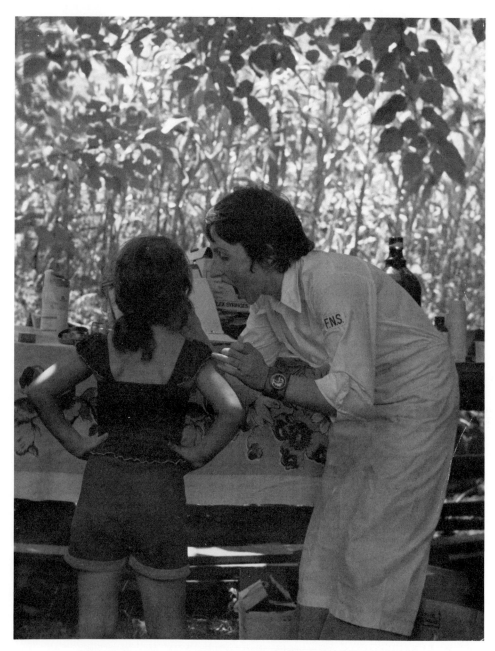

Fig. 8-3. *Frontier nurse providing medical care in rural Kentucky.*

(Courtesy Gabrielle Beasley and Frontier Nursing Service, Wendover, Ky.)

1. The change in the nature of disease from acute, short-term, infectious diseases to chronic, long-term diseases, called by some "diseases of civilization" (Dubos, 1965)
2. Increasing consumer demand for medical services coupled with health manpower shortages
3. Increasing specialization in medical care (e.g., highly specialized services such as breathing clinics for obstructive lung diseases)
4. An increasing cohort of aging people with chronic health problems associated with the biology of the aging process

The medical occupations that confront issues of care and whose focus of work and knowledge is on health rather than disease, on the social, political, and physical environment rather than on germs, and on the patient rather than on the disease process are the occupations with the greatest potential to meet the health needs of the future. Such is the fate of nursing.

Even more fundamental is the concept of the medical team. New roles in nursing, such as the nurse practitioner or family care specialist, deal with health problems so complex and the acuteness of the maldistribution of medical workers is so severe that the medical care team has become the logical context for the development of the new nursing roles. This is consistent with a national trend toward an increase in group medical practice and a decline in solo practice models.

In summary, the four societal forces mentioned earlier and the organization of medical practice, in this case the team approach, are major stimulants of professionalization in nursing, and changes taking place in the form of new roles for nurses are greatly affected by these factors.

If nurses are to succeed in developing new roles that have social and personal status, are functionally autonomous, and lead to professional status, the following developments must take place. These developments can be classified as elements of social organization that facilitates the process of professionalization. The resistance to changes in the role of nurses will be less both from within nursing as well as from other sectors of the medical care arena and the larger society if the following five elements of social organization occur.

Transfer of work

One must transfer work before medical teams can be developed (Banta and Fox, 1972; Beavert, 1974). The nurse practitioner to function as a clinician must give up some of the management or administrative roles historically associated with nursing work. Similarly, physicians must give up some of their clinical domain to nurses. This process involves changing the division of labor and the structure of control over the production of medical services. Rather than physicians maintaining sole control over production of services, some of this control would be shared with nurses in the transfer of work. Accountability would be transferred as well.

The problem of occupational uniqueness

At the same time that medical work is transferred, proponents of new roles for nurses must pursue the current attempt to distinguish the practice of nursing from the practice of medicine (Walker, 1967). If functional autonomy is to be a part of the new roles for nurses, then the legislative sector of society as well as the general public must be convinced that the new nursing roles are not merely carbon copies of physician tasks reduced in size but are contributions to the well-being of patients that are unique to nursing and that nursing can do best. Some of the most serious resistance to the new roles and functional autonomy have come as a result of attempts at introducing legislation that would legitimize the autonomous professional nurse practitioner. Where these attempts have occurred, it has been extremely difficult to secure the support of legislators because of their prevailing stereotypes and lack of knowledge about what nurses do (Driscoll, 1972).

Approval of higher status medical occupations

Resistance to change in nursing roles is less in those situations in which physicians or even nurses of higher prestige (e.g., deans of nursing schools, directors of nursing services) approve the change.

The organizational climate

Nurses will be more likely to develop functionally autonomous nursing roles in medical care organizations in which the climate encourages innovation and where high value is placed on experimenting with new approaches. Neighborhood health centers, outpatient services of large municipal hospitals, and preventive medical programs in areas of medical scarcity are potentially more favorable climates in this regard than community hospitals. Individual personalities play an important role in establishing climate.

Demographics and education

Finally, the number and background of nurses trained in a manner conducive to active support of the new roles for nurses and their occupational bases of employment are important facilitators. For example, in Walker's study (1967) of ritualistic nursing practices that prevented the nurse from giving patient care, she discovered that within the hospital structure, nongraduate nurses were more reluctant to give up facets of the management role to give direct patient care than were graduate nurses. Walker hypothesized that the larger the proportion of graduate nurses assigned to a ward the less extensive the nurses' participation in the management of patient care.

BARRIERS TO ACHIEVING FUNCTIONAL AUTONOMY IN NEW ROLES FOR NURSES

Two generic types of barriers face nursing's attempt to attain functional autonomy and professional status. One type is found within the nursing occupation per se, whereas the other barriers are located in the social order, external to nursing as an occupation. These barriers are closely associated with the five aspects of social organization just discussed.

The most powerful barrier to change

from within nursing is the nurse. The baccalaureate nurse is the most receptive to professionalism and changes in roles (Corwin, 1961), and the doctorate- and masters-level nurses are the major source of energy for the planning and action associated with developing new roles. However, as noted earlier in this chapter, baccalaureate and advanced degree nurses represent a relatively small proportion of all nurses. In fact, throughout nursing at large, the trend is developing in the direction of an ever-decreasing complement of graduate nurses relative to the need for direct patient care (Walker, 1967). The bulk of direct patient care will continue to be performed by associate and nongraduate nurses. Thus pressure will be on graduate nurses to continue in the management roles within hospitals that historically have proved to be an occupational deadend in terms of achieving functional autonomy.

Perhaps an even more perplexing problem within the ranks of nursing is the issue of who chooses nursing and the effects of socialization through nursing education. The occupational diversity in nursing is reflected in the wide range of social and cultural backgrounds among its recruits. Decisions to enter nursing are made much earlier than decisions about other careers (Williams and Goldsen, 1960). Nursing students, although representing all socioeconomic classes, tend to be upwardly mobile socially. Studies have shown that the percentage of nurses achieving higher economic status than their families of origin has grown systematically between 1940 and 1960 (Hughes et al., 1958; Williams and Goldsen, 1960). Corwin and Taves (1963) suggest that degree schools have more status, attracting upwardly mobile faculty with broader training backgrounds than faculty of diploma schools. Upwardly mobile students from working- or middle-class families possessing the economic means to afford a college education are likely to be attracted to the degree programs.

Wren (1971) studied the backgrounds of associate, diploma, and baccalaureate nursing students in all twenty-two state-approved schools of nursing in Georgia. In comparing the three types of students, he found that associate degree students tended to be older, were more likely to have had work experience in the health care field prior to entering nursing school, were more likely to come from families where the father had less than a high school diploma, had the lowest Scholastic Aptitude Test scores, were more likely to have entered nursing school by way of a licensed practical nursing school, and gave as their major reason for choosing nursing, to help people or that nursing was something they always wanted to do. The baccalaureate and diploma students tended to come from middle-class families and gave as their reason for choosing nursing, to help people and to achieve personal advancement.

Furthermore, an analysis of the values that nursing students possess on entering school would suggest that power, influence, and dominance over others, values necessary to achieve functional autonomy, are low on the priority lists of students and probably nurses as well, since there is no evidence to suggest that the educational process does anything save to reinforce the existing values. In a study of 465 students in three baccalaureate programs in the Midwest, O'Neil (1973) found that nursing students were higher on conformity, attached less importance to achieving recognition, were less interested in accumulating wealth than in helping others, and were less interested in domination over others, personal power, and influence than was the general college population of women at the three schools. Assuming that baccalaureate students learn to value nursing as a profession and to develop some degree of loyalty and commitment to the advancement of nursing, in her sample Kramer (1967, 1970) showed that collegiate nurses demonstrated a significant increase in loyalty to bureaucratic values after employment and experienced a significant decrease in the value of professional advancement. The nurses in Kramer's study who hung

onto their professional values were more likely to drop out of nursing than those who accepted the bureaucratic role conceptions. Similarly, nurses who adopted the bureaucratic role conceptions were judged "successful" by their employers, contrary to the nurses who had higher professional values.

Finally, the great diversity within nursing has made it difficult, if not impossible, for nursing leadership to mount a focused, consistent drive toward developing new roles and professional status. A new role that may appeal to baccalaureate nurses could have the opposite effect on diploma or associate degree nurses. Thus the new nurse is portrayed as a master clinician (National Commission for the Study of Nursing and Nursing Education, 1970), as a family nurse practitioner (Mussallem, 1969), as a nurse midwife, as a physician extender, and others. Rather than focusing on one new role with clearly defined functions and autonomy, what has emerged is a kaleidoscope of people, qualifications, and activities. The result is to blur any possibility of distinguishing a unique contribution of nursing in the delivery of health care. The movement toward professional status is diluted through diffuseness, which is a deterrent to clear legislation or effective practice.

External to nursing, forces have been at work limiting the success of nurses who seek functional autonomy. A major source of resistance to the new roles concepts rests with physicians and administrators of health care systems, two groups threatened professionally and fiscally. A recent study of physicians' attitudes toward an extended role of the nurse points out the reluctance of physicians to accept functional autonomy for nurses (O'Dell, 1974). Of the fifty-seven physicians sampled (thirty-five graduated between 1960 and 1970), the majority agreed to expanding nursing roles in functional areas that physicians could exert control over. None of the physicians accepted the concept of nurses doing complete physical examinations of patients or of nurses interpreting diagnostic findings to patients. In short, the physicians studied viewed the extended role of nurses as a form of assistance to the physician controlled by the physician. This finding is consistent with the increasing interest physicians are showing in the physician's assistant concept (Chapter 9).

A great increase in nonprofessional physician extender occupations represents another serious external barrier to the development of new professional nursing roles. The physician's assistant program is the best example, although several similar paraprofessional occupations must be included as threats to functional autonomy for nurses (Hessler and Griffard, 1976). Physician's assistants "are selected by physicians, trained by physicians, and report administratively directly to physicians . . . they interact at the physician-patient interface and are capable, under the direction of the physician, of performing functions now usually performed by physicians" (National Academy of Sciences, 1970). Given this widely accepted definition, it is clear that the physician's assistant theoretically will perform the same or similar health care functions as the pediatric nurse practitioner only without autonomy. The physician maintains full control and accountability over the work of the assistants. The new nursing roles are predicated on minimal supervision and control by physicians to achieve professional autonomy.

Physicians and health care administrators have shown a much greater interest in hiring physician's assistants than assisting in the development of new roles for nurses. This is due partly to sexism in medicine, since nurses are overwhelmingly women and physician's assistants are predominantly men. On the more practical side, the physician's assistants do not expect or seek functional autonomy. There is no agitation and movement toward professional status among physician's assistants, and this is enhancing to the beleaguered and skeptical physicians and administrators. Economics appears to play little if any role in the mat-

ter of preference, since physician's assistants are paid considerably more than nursing specialists even though the new nurse roles command greater training. In physician's assistants there exists a new source of exploitable, trouble-free labor.

Finally, the trend toward institutional licensure calls for eliminating individual licensure for nurses and other health professionals. With the exception of physicians and dentists who would continue to be licensed as individuals by the state medical and dental societies, hospitals, health centers, physicians' private offices, and other health care establishments would exert legal control over the functions of nurses and other health workers. State licensing agencies would oversee the process, but it would be up to the administrator of the specific health care facility to determine the appropriate use and functional autonomy of the health workers employed by the agency (Hershey, 1969). This proposal or others like it could maintain nursing in a dependent role vis-à-vis the expanded functions. The physician, with an administrative framework established by state regulatory bodies, would supervise and control legally the functioning of all health workers.

CONCLUSIONS

Nursing is facing the most exciting and difficult era in its entire history. Many factors exist to prevent nurses from achieving functional autonomy and attendant status as professionals. Demographics are against nursing. The tremendous diversity of educational background among nurses severely restricts any movement toward functional autonomy due to the limited appeal that professionalism holds among nursing's rank and file. The limited research on the appeal of functional autonomy shows that most nurses do not want the increased accountability associated with professional autonomy (Walker, 1967). Furthermore, sexism, multiple proposals for change, opposition from physicians, and the rapid growth of physician's assistant programs, which have preempted some of the functions unique to nursing, have retarded the development of nursing as a profession.

Historically, nursing's predecessors had cleared a path for an autonomous nursing profession. These early women healers had successfully carried out unique medical care roles the quality of which overshadowed the regular practitioners of the time. This momentum was lost, and modern nursing practice emerged as an oddly static, dependent, and exploited health care occupation.

However, increasing complexity of medical technology, the profusion of medical specialties, and the advance of chronic diseases linked with civilized, industrialized life-styles have converged as fructuous forces for the future of nursing as a profession. The time is ripe for nursing to seize the initiative and break out of its dependent role. The odds against nursing achieving functional autonomy and professional parity with physicians are great. However, the overriding question is not whether nursing can do it but whether the acquisition of autonomy through new roles will serve in the best interests of the consumer. The odds are stacked against the consumer, as the history of medicine teaches us.

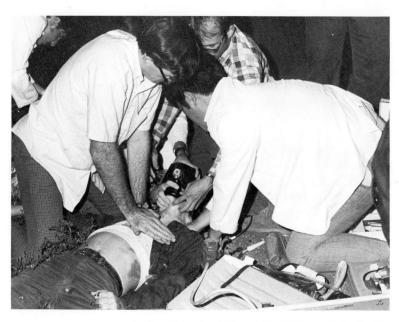

Courtesy University of Missouri Medical Center, Columbia, Mo.

CHAPTER 9

New health workers

EMERGENCE OF NEW HEALTH WORKERS: A QUIET REVOLUTION IN MEDICAL CARE

We are witnessing a quiet medical revolution worldwide, quiet because the revolutionaries carry stethoscopes rather than guns. The fighting over professional dominance in medicine is being waged by means of demonstrations of competence in diagnosing, treating, and even at times preventing illness by nonphysician community health workers who are willing to work in medically underserved areas of inner cities and rural areas. We shall look closely at this revolution by first analyzing the social, economic, and technological forces behind the emergence of community health workers. It is important that one be fully aware of these forces, since within this understanding lies the framework for resolving

the most important problem facing medical care providers and consumers. This is the problem of expanding, extending, and equitably distributing health services to all segments of society, rural and urban, poor and wealthy alike.

Four forces operate singly and in combination to encourage and nourish the development of nonphysician community health workers: (1) ideology, (2) technological developments, (3) medical manpower demographics, and (4) consumer demand. Each of these forces will be discussed to better understand how they affect the emergence of the health workers.

Ideology

The growing acceptance in the United States of the idea that health is a humanly rightful condition to which all members of society have a just claim is a powerful ideological force. Its power derives from the fact that once the members of a society accept the notion, then the society assumes a responsibility for achieving this goal.

Once the ideology "health care as a right" is accepted, then society is responsible for expanding, extending, and more equitably distributing health services to the people. Earlier in this book, the concept of health was defined to include aspects of life that extend well beyond but that affect the primary care of illnesses. Therefore the responsibility for bringing health care to all the people includes components such as consumer health education, adequate sanitation, nutrition, housing, schools, clean air and water, effective fertility control, and other preventive measures to ensure protection against communicable disease. In effect this commitment fairly guarantees the emergence of new health workers, given the complexity and scope of the task at hand.

Professionalism is a second component of ideology that plays a role in stimulating the development of new health workers. The idea of upward occupational mobility is as much a part of the health care system as in the business world. Medical work, even within the ranks of physicians, is stratified according to the level of training, the number of people trained to do the work, and the value that society places on the work through the demand for particular services. Rewards of prestige, power, and wealth are distributed differentially according to the position of a particular job within a hierarchy. Movement from jobs with less to more status, in short professionalism, is something for which all health workers strive. For new health workers, the concept of a "career ladder" is an integral part of their ideology.

Technological developments

The structure of occupations and the development of technology are highly interrelated. Technical innovations in the form of new machinery or new methods of delivery can mean that new types of health workers are needed to operate and manage the systems which technology has produced (Fig. 9-1). New medical technology results in more complex methods of treatment that require greater specialization of medical practice (Field, 1957; Geomet, Incorporated, 1972). For example, communication satellites and mobile laboratories are part of the Indian Health Service Units on the Papago Reservation in Arizona. Laboratory results and live video communications can be transmitted from the field to a medical center, and patient histories are computerized and available to the field staff from any location with electrical power (Garrett, 1972). This makes it possible for nonphysician health workers to function as primary care specialists under the supervision of a physician who may be many miles away from the site of actual medical care delivery. New chronic disease specialty centers are other examples whereby a new method of treatment gives birth to new medical manpower. Kidney dialysis units, physical rehabilitation institutes, and chronic lung disease centers are staffed with new types of medical care providers who treat patients with complex techniques and machines, and nonphysican health workers are assuming more responsibility in treatment.

Medical manpower demographics

Maldistribution and shortages of certain types of medical practitioners are factors that are stimulating the growth of new health workers throughout the world. Medical density (the number of physicians per 10,000 people) varies tremendously. Worldwide there are roughly 2.5 million physicians, which translates into a medical density of 8 physicians per 10,000 people (Dorozynski, 1975). Some regions or countries are well served in terms of having relatively large numbers of physicians, but there are vast areas, even in the United States, where there is less than one physician per 10,000 people and where people never see a physician at all. Many of these underserved areas are rural, such as in Africa where there are 1.4 physicians per 10,000 people or in rural

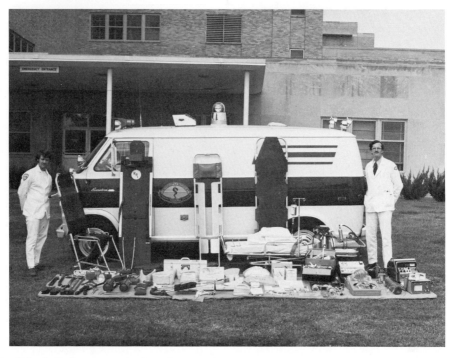

Fig. 9-1. *Ambulances, once thought of only as a fast means of transportation, are now emergency rooms on wheels.* (*Courtesy University of Missouri Medical Center, Columbia, Mo.*)

Missouri in the United States where several counties are without physicians entirely and where many others are served by aging physicians who are close to retirement.

The solution seems simple. Increase the number of physicians where there are shortages. Although attractive and simple, this strategy is impractical, particularly for economically developing areas. The length of time it takes to turn out a physican is great, and to keep pace with population growth, the number of physicians required must be multiplied by a factor many times the current number of physicians. The cost would far exceed the benefits.

For this reason, the training of tiers of new health workers represents the latest strategy for overcoming the manpower problem. In the United States the government has encouraged the development of new health workers through the Manpower Development and Training Act of 1962, the Health Professions Educational Assistance Act of 1963, the Nurse Training Act of 1964, the Allied Health Professionals Personnel Act of 1966, the Economic Opportunity Act Amendments of 1967, the Concentrated Employment Program of 1967, the Vocational Rehabilitation Act Amendments of 1968, and the Public Services Careers Program of 1970 (United States Department of Labor, 1971). It is estimated that allied health workers in the United States will number 1.3 million by 1980 (Pennell and Hoover, 1970). In China, Chairman Mao formulated the policy that medical care should extend first aid foremost to the underserved rural areas. This led to the growth of "barefoot doctors" who numbered over 1 million in 1975. They are trained in basic medicine, treatment, and prevention of common diseases, and they prescribe common Western drugs, herbs, and other traditional medicine, give injections, perform abortions, deliver babies, organize sanitation campaigns, and report on communicable disease incidences. Barefoot doctors receive training for periods ranging from 3 months to two years, depending on the needs of their specific region. Rural barefoot doctors function with minimal and occasional supervision of physicians, whereas urban workers are more closely associated with physicians usually from a specific hospital, and they are less autonomous in their medical work. Russian *feldshers* and *promodores* (health promoters) of Guatemala are similar to barefoot doctors. Many other countries experiencing the medical manpower squeeze are moving in similar directions of developing new health workers rather than attempting to increase the supply of physicians and thereby running the risk of incurring great costs in terms of time and money.

Consumer demand

Every health system throughout the world is experiencing rising demand for services. This increase in demand is responsible to a large extent for the rapid rise in the costs of medical care, and in countries that have achieved a delicately balanced national health system, increasing public demand is the one force that poses the most severe threat to fiscal viability. Nowhere in the health care system is demand more keenly felt than in the manpower section. One outcome of the rising demand is the emergence of new health workers.

Demand has two important aspects. First, the demand can arise in the form of new or different disease patterns within the society. For example, the United States and other postindustrial societies have populations that are getting progressively older and larger. This has led to an increase in chronic illnesses, which represents a new demand for specific types of health services. Second, demand is created by societal recognition and definition of the types of health problems considered problematic for achieving national goals (Parsons, 1958). Thus a group may believe that what were previously considered social problems should be redefined as medical illnesses. Child abuse and alcoholism are two examples of this. Previously legal problems in the United States, they

suddenly became medical problems, thereby introducing almost instant demand for new types of medical services. As demand continues to increase, the pressure to expand medical manpower builds, particularly when existing health workers are unable to meet those demands. The creation of new types of health workers is a method for reducing the pressure.

DESCRIPTIONS OF SELECTED TYPES OF NEW HEALTH WORKERS

In this section, several types of new health workers will be described by analyzing their functions, work settings, and the nature of their relationships with physicians and patients. The types of health workers selected by no means represents the vast array of what could be considered the universe of new health workers. Rather the selection is limited to those occupations that have been studied to the extent that empirical data about them exist.

The physician's assistant

The term "physician's assistant" is used generically to describe many types of health workers that have emerged as physician extender occupations. The following occupations are included under the term "physician's assistant": physician's assistant, physicians' associate, MEDEX, child health associate, PRIMEX, syniatrist, Flexner, clinical associate, and several similar designations. In an attempt to clear up some of the confusion caused by the myriad of terms, the AMA has defined the physician's assistant as a "skilled person qualified by academic and practical training to provide patient services under the supervision and direction of a licensed physician who is responsible for the performance of that assistant" (Todd and Foy, 1972). The National Board of Medical Examiners' Special Advisory Committee for the Evaluation of the Assistant to the Primary Care Physician has defined the physician's assistant as one who "capably performs those functions delegated by and with the supervision of the primary care physician."

The first physician's assistant–training program was begun at Duke University in 1965. Most of the ensuing programs have emulated the Duke program to a large extent. Students are recruited from those who have had previous health care experience, either in the armed forces as corpsmen or in civilian life as practical nurses or emergency medical technicians. In the Duke program, approximately 90% of trainees are men, who tend to be in their midtwenties or older and have families (Estes and Howard, 1970). The average trainee in most of the programs has one or more years of college.

The Duke program is two years in length and usually leads to a certificate rather than a college degree, although it is possible to attain a bachelor of science degree at Duke and in other programs as well. At Duke the first 9 months are didactic, with the trainees spending 6 weeks in lectures in medical terminology, medical history, and laboratory procedures. Six months are spent in lectures of anatomy, physiology, diseases, principles of therapy, history taking, the physical examination, radiology, and electrocardiography. The students spend the last 15 months in clinical rotations, working in inpatient wards, outpatient services, emergency departments, and out in the community working with a local physician in private practice. Medical school faculty do most of the clinical teaching, but graduate physician's assistants teach the students practical applications that have proved useful in their work experience.

Another example of a large physician's assistant–training program is the University of Oklahoma's Physician's Associate Program started in 1970. At Oklahoma there is a 10-month didactic phase followed by 14 months of clinical practicums (Godkins et al., 1974). Table 9-1 presents the courses and hours, and Table 9-2 presents the clinical practicums and the number of weeks spent on each clinical rotation.

It is interesting to note that during the clinical phase of training, primary care is

Table 9-1. Physician's assistant's training courses and hours (phase I—didactic courses)*

Course listings	Hours
Etiology and pathogenesis of disease†	216
Behavior dynamics	54
Anatomy	64
Chemistry	48
Physical diagnosis and clinical medicine	324
Laboratory medicine†	66
Pediatrics	26
Pathology	52
Obstetrics/gynecology†	38
Physiology‡	126
Nutrition	32
Radiology	16
Pharmacology	48
Parasitology	20
Dental seminar	18
Dermatology seminar	18
Emergency medicine	30
Laboratory procedures	20
Ethics of medical practice and introduction to health care services	20
Electrocardiography	10
Clinical medicine practicums	138
Total hours	1,384

*From Godkins, T. R., Stanhope, W. D., and Lynn, T. N. Current status of the physician's assistant in Oklahoma. *Journal of the Oklahoma State Medical Association,* 1974, **67,** 102-107.
†Sophomore Medical School Course.
‡Freshman Medical School Course.

emphasized by requiring rotations in rural practices. Prior to receiving the physician's assistant certificate, students must pass examinations that test clinical competency. Skills such as taking a complete history, doing physical examination, ability to handle medical emergencies, and ability to interact with patients are evaluated by pencil and paper tests and oral case presentations made before faculty members. On graduation the physician's assistant is supposedly trained to accept a position requiring the following skills and tasks:

Table 9-2. Physician's assistant's clinical practicums (phase II—clinical practicums)*

Weeks	Practicum
6	Medicine (inpatient)
6	Medicine (outpatient)
6	General surgery
6	Emergency medicine
6	Elective
6	Elective
6	Primary care†
6	Primary care†
8	Preceptorship‡
2	Vacation/leave
2	Review and testing

*From Godkins, T. R., Stanhope, W. D., and Lynn, T. A. Current status of the physician's assistant in Oklahoma, *Journal of the Oklahoma State Medical Association,* **67,** 1974, 102-107.
†Primary care is defined as a rotation with a physician(s) in the areas of family medicine, general practice, pediatrics, and/or obstetrics and gynecology whereby the physician accepts responsibility for initial and/or continuing general medical care and health maintenance of his patients.
‡Preceptorship—rotation with a physician of the student's choice or precertor associated with the PA Program.

Principal duties and responsibilities

The incumbent must be a graduate of an approved program for Physician's Assistants, and certified by the Oklahoma State Board of Medical Examiners. The incumbent will perform all duties listed below:

Professional

1. Perform history and physical examinations on new and return patients, both in the office and to a hospital, establish presumptive diagnoses, establish the general workup of the patient by ordering appropriate laboratory studies, and be responsible under the physician's supervision for the management of the patient's problem following diagnosis
2. Perform diagnostic tests such as insulin and IV glucose tolerance tests, gastric analysis, lumbar punctures, and other procedures in consultation and under the supervision of the supervising physician
3. Perform the following technical tasks
   a. Venipuncture and the starting of intravenous therapy
   b. Arteriopuncture and blood gas analysis
   c. Application and removal of orthopedic casts and traction apparatus
   d. Nasogastric intubation
   e. Nasotracheal intubation
4. Manage medical emergencies such as cardiac arrests, acute respiratory failure, and life-endangering traumatic injuries until the arrival of a supervising physician
5. Assist the physician in planning, organizing, and delivering orderly medical management programs for patients under the physician's care
6. Make specific nursing home, extended care facility, and home visits under the direction of the physician
7. Participate in appropriate continuing medical education programs
8. Assist the physician as directed in the training of health personnel in certain diagnostic, therapeutic, and clinical techniques (Godkins et al., 1974:104)

Clearly all these tasks have been performed by other health care personnel. However, in recent medical care history, no occupational groups trained in the manner of physician's assistants have performed these tasks routinely and legitimately.

Work settings. The original thinking behind the physician's assistant concept was to train a cadre of physician extenders who would provide primary medical care to people living in rural and inner-city areas of medical scarcity. A few studies of postgraduation employment are available to help determine the variety of work settings that physician's assistants find themselves in.

Of the first twenty-nine graduates of the Duke program fourteen stayed at Duke to teach and do clinical research (Estes and Howard, 1970). After the initial need for physician's assistant teachers was met, subsequent graduating classes tended to be employed in solo and group practices. Godkins et al. (1974) studied the location of University of Oklahoma graduates of physician's assistant classes 1970 to 1971. Table 9-3 presents the locations. The 1971 class has a greater percentage of rural locations than the 1970 class, with neither class locating in rural areas exclusively.

Table 9-3. Location of University of Oklahoma graduates of physician's assistants' classes 1970 to 1971*

Types of practice	Town/state	Population† (thousand)
Class of 1970		
Institutional/medicine	Oklahoma City, Okla.	>300
Primary care	Wakita, Okla.	<1
Primary care	Muscateen, Iowa	>20<30
Orthopedic surgery	Muskogee, Okla.	>30<40
Institutional/neurology	Oklahoma City, Okla.	>300
Primary care	Drumright, Okla.	>1<10
Institutional/primary care	Oklahoma City, Okla.	>300
Class of 1971		
Orthopedic surgery	Grand Junction, Colo.	>20<30
Primary care	Guthrie, Okla.	>1<10
Institutional/surgery	Muskogee, Okla.	>20<30
Primary care	Ada, Okla.	>10<20
Primary care	Granger, Iowa	<1
Primary care	Yale, Okla.	>1<2
Primary care	Ada, Okla.	>10<20
Primary care	Sapulpa, Okla.	>10<20
Primary care	Arkadelphia, Ark.	>1<10
Primary care	Memphis, Tenn.	>300
Primary care	Midwest City, Okla.	>40<50
Primary care	Stilwell, Okla.	>1<10

*Modified from Godkins, T. R., Stanhope, W. D.. and Lynn, T. A. Current status of the physician's assistant in Oklahoma. *Journal of the Oklahoma State Medical Association,* 1974, **67,** 102-107.
†Based on 1973 *Almanac Atlas and Yearbook* statistics.

Relationships with physicians and patients. The physician's assistant has a unique role. Schneller (1974) believes that the physician's assistant has achieved "negotiated autonomy" vis-à-vis physicians. The range of tasks performed by physician's assistants is extensive (Sadler et al., 1972), yet the physician's assistant's occupation is totally dependent on the physician for training, task assignments, and supervision. As Sadler et al. (1972) point out, physicians can delegate any task that they believe the assistant can perform.

Consequently, by remaining closely attached and under the authority of the physician, physician's assistants have not gained autonomy in the sense of control over the technological, organizational, and social facets of medical work (Freidson, 1970). However, they have negotiated a high level of autonomy for performing medical work as a result of the direct negotiation of standing orders with physicians for whom they work (Duttera and Harlan, 1975). Whereas nursing has gained control over the education and supervision of nurses, thereby reducing dependency on physicians and gaining autonomy over administrative and other nonmedical tasks, physician's assistants have accepted physician control and thereby have gained more medical responsibility and in growing measure greater financial rewards than general nursing. According to Sadler et al. (1972) "In responsibility and remuneration, they [physician's assistants] are coming to occupy the number 2 position on the health care team." Although this remains to be seen, it is interesting to note that nursing was approached by the AMA in 1969 and invited to develop a physician's

Table 9-4. Expressed willingness of sample populations to allow trained physician's assistants to perform various select medical services in their communities (N=253)*

Select medical services	Very willing	Somewhat willing	Undecided	Somewhat unwilling	Very unwilling
Routine physical examinations and histories	202	37	5	1	8
Simple emergency care including sewing up cuts	118	76	27	16	16
Prenatal care	64	57	65	31	36
Routine deliveries (sic)	35	41	48	38	71
Postnatal care including immunizations	104	70	46	18	15
Initial screening to determine whether patient needs to see the doctor or not	98	73	26	24	32
Patient referral	142	61	28	7	15

*From Litman, T. J. Public perceptions of the physician's assistant—a survey of the attitudes, and opinions of rural Iowa and Minnesota residents. *American Journal of Public Health*, 1972, **62**, 345.

assistant program. The offer was firmly rejected at that time (Sadler et al., 1972).

Acceptance of the physician's assistant by patients and the general public exists, but studies show that this acceptance is qualified by a few important factors. Litman (1972) surveyed a probability sample of 253 southern Minnesota and northern Iowa households and asked persons to state their attitudes about the idea of allowing specially trained former medical corpsmen to serve as physician's assistants in their communities under the supervision of a licensed physician. Perhaps the most interesting finding was that the public's acceptance of the physician's assistant rested heavily on the endorsement of the family physician. In short, the public would accept physician's assistants only if their family physician said it was all right. Whereas there was some disagreement over the specific duties that the public thought a physician's assistant should be allowed to perform, only 16.4% of those interviewed maintained that they would not allow a physician's assistant to take care of them or their families. In spite of the general acceptance (94%), Litman found

(Table 9-4) the public most opposed to the idea of physician's assistants aiding in prenatal care or with routine deliveries, even under the supervision of a physician. Litman suspects that this finding may reflect the sexual mores of rural people, and he concludes that attempts to utilize former medical corpsmen in this capacity would likely meet with stiff opposition and skepticism by the public.

A study by Pondy and Breytspraak (1969) revealed that patient acceptance has some relationship with income. Patients from the lowest and highest income groups were more reserved about accepting physician's assistants than the middle-income group. The lowest income group suspected that they were receiving the ministrations of the assistant because they could not afford to pay for a physician, whereas the highest income group expected to have the services of a physician exclusively. Also the higher the level of formal education the greater the acceptance of the physician's assistant. In general, Pondy and Breytspraak found uniformly high acceptance by patients.

In conclusion, although there are some

areas of skepticism and concern, the public and patients support the concept of the physician's assistant. This support is based on (1) a belief that physician's assistants would be well-trained, (2) a recognition that local physicians cannot continue to meet the growing demand for services, and (3) a strong trust in the judgment of physicians who employ assistants (Litman, 1972).

Community health workers

The community health worker concept was conceived as part of a larger strategy designed to break the cycle of poverty in the United States. The thinking behind this approach was that the poor get sicker and the sick get poorer and one way to deal with sickness is to provide jobs for the poor. Put another way, having enough money for the family's food and negotiating for power and participation in decisions that affect one's life may be much more useful in breaking the cycle of poverty than medical care per se. The New Careers Amendment (1967) to the Economic Opportunities Act was the primary legislation that authorized the training of the poor in human service jobs. Neighborhood health centers (Chapter 12) became the major health institution in which the new careers program developed and community health workers were born.

The community health worker model includes a full-time job, remedial education with release time to attend school, on-the-job training for medically related skills, and a career ladder to ensure occupational mobility and a continual source of new manpower (Riessman, 1969).

Functions. Recent studies of community health workers verify that the rank and file is recruited from the low-income neighborhoods served by the health centers (Smith, 1973; Hessler and Griffard, 1976). In contrast with physician's assistants, community health workers do not deliver primary medical services, and the functions they perform are not found specifically in the tasks and job behaviors of physician's assistants.

The major function of the community health worker is to serve as a liaison and bridge between professionals, on the one hand, and low-income consumers on the other. Health professionals, often from middle-class backgrounds and with middle-class life-styles, run up against a communication and confidence gap in attempting to serve low-income consumers with ghetto life-styles and values. The community health worker is seen as having one foot in the world of the health professional and the other one in the ghetto. As long as they keep their balance, these workers could provide that much needed link between the community and the health center. After all, health centers appeared not long after the major riots that wrecked ghetto areas across the United States, and communication with the community, however vague that was at the time, was one method of survival for the health centers. There is evidence that suggests that this function may be a problem for the community health workers who become marginal people, not quite of the community and not quite of the world of medical science (Levinson and Schiller, 1966; Meyer, 1969; Hessler and Griffard, 1976).

Another function which community health workers perform is that of change agent (Smith, 1973). It makes no sense to provide medical care for the poor unless the care is integrated with preventive programs such as sanitation, environmental improvement, and community organization and education. These programs involve changing the conditions of poverty that cause health problems and community health workers who perform these tasks can be considered social change agents. Digging clean wells; educating the residents of a community about birth control, sanitation, or home medical care; and organizing food cooperatives or political action groups are a few of the change functions performed by community health workers. There is some evidence that this function produces significant results, although the experience is highly variable depending on which neighborhood health center one is talking about. Geiger

(1969) writes that the Tufts-Delta Health Center, serving a rural population of 14,000 desperately poor people in Bolivar County, Mississippi, has benefited enormously from the efforts of community health workers. He attributes much of the large improvements in health to the community health workers who screened windows, dug wells, built privies, and organized a farm cooperative, thereby creating jobs and food for a severely malnourished population. In urban areas the social change efforts of community health workers have met with much less success than the Mississippi experience (Geiger, 1967a; New and Hessler, 1972).

Client advocacy is another function performed by community health workers (Smith, 1973). This is done at an internal level by guiding the patient through the bureaucracy of the health center or outside the center by seeing to it that patients are treated decently and fairly by other health and welfare agencies.

Finally, community health workers are hired by health centers to do aggressive case-finding. Frequently, the center's services are unknown to people in the community who have desperate, unmet needs, and it is a job of health workers to find these persons and to encourage them to utilize the services.

Work settings. Neighborhood health centers, community mental health centers, and other decentralized outposts of care in urban and rural areas such as group practices, clinics, and health stations are the types of work settings for community health workers. Their role is performed in media settings almost exclusively outside of hospital care.

Relationships with physicians and patients. Community health workers seldom if ever treat patients medically. The closest they come to giving medical treatment occurs during those instances when the worker gathers diagnostic data from the patient in the intake interview. Although there is an oblique, limited involvement with the production of medical services, the social and cultural activities of community health

workers make it extremely difficult for them to be under the direct supervision of a single physician. Instead, nurses, community health educators, or community organizers provide the direct supervision because the health workers jobs are closer in content to these nonphysician jobs in the outreach programs. For this reason, community health workers have an indirect relationship with physicians, which is filtered through nonphysician supervisors who become intermediaries of a sort. This is unlike health care programs utilizing physician's assistants. Studies have shown that when direct supervision is utilized, one physician per physician's assistant seems to be the most workable arrangement (Lohrenz, 1971).

Nurses, community organizers, and health educators do not establish relationshiships with patients that are as formal or as intense as the physician-patient relationship can be. When contact with patients occurs, it is usually at the request of a physician and is restricted to some limited aspect of the patient's total problem such as dietary needs or lead paint in the house. In as much as community health workers become involved with patients, they relate to even more limited aspects of the patients' problems than the supervisory professionals do. The patient-community health worker relationship is much more limited than is the case for physician's assistants.

Nurse practitioners

The largest development of new careers programs in the United States is occurring within the field of nursing. In 1973 and 1974 there were over eighty-three nurse practitioner programs for nurses, with additional training in pediatrics, geriatrics, cardiology, family medicine, and a host of other clinical specialties. Because of the current vast array of specializations, we will look at the pediatric nurse practitioner career in this section of the chapter. In addition to the practical side of studying one example, the pediatric nurse practitioner program was the first modern nurse practitioner development, although it has several historical antecedents, particularly the Frontier Nursing Service (Breckinridge, 1952), urban ambulatory settings (Connelly et al., 1966), and the New York City Nurse Midwifery Program established in 1931 by the Maternity Center Association (Harris, 1969; Harris et al., 1971). Soon there will be evaluative data on the various nurse practitioner specialties, particularly on the family health practitioner.

The pediatric nurse practitioner concept began out of a desire to provide health care for children who are medically underserved. Perhaps the best known program in the United States is the one developed jointly by the Department of Pediatrics of the School of Medicine and the School of Nursing at the University of Colorado. This was established as the first formal training program in the country, although there were historical precedents (Chapter 8), particularly the Frontier Nursing Service (Breckinridge, 1952; Connelly et al., 1966). This and other similar training programs are designed to place nurses in an expanded role to provide comprehensive health services to children in low-income areas. In this capacity, nurse practitioners perform medical tasks that formerly were the sole responsibility of the physician. As of 1971 twenty-four training programs for pediatric nurse practitioners were listed in the Directory of Training Programs, and approximately 200 graduates had been registered. The ANA and the American Academy of Pediatrics (1971) have established guidelines for pediatric nurse practitioners–training programs.

In general, nurses from diploma, registered nursing, or master's programs enter the training program and spend several months studying the theory and practice of pediatrics. Training occurs in the classroom, hospital wards, clinics, and nurseries. Students are taught to perform a complete physical examination and to design immunization schedules, but the greatest effort is spent learning how to interview a patient, studying the psychosocial issues associated with growth and development, and developing the art of counseling parents about child-rearing. It is important to recall that the pediatric nurse practitioner is a nurse with additional training, not to be confused with the physician's assistant who may have a baccalaureate degree but who is a non-nurse. The nursing profession has opposed the physician's assistant concept, as mentioned earlier in this chapter, because the nursing profession is unwilling to be dependent on physicians or institutions and is unwilling to give up accountability for providing care for patients (Lewis, 1974).

The training programs that prepare registered nurses for expanded roles award a certificate, and some programs award a master's degree. In 1973 to 1974 there were eighty-three training programs offering a certificate to registered nurses for expanded roles and fifty-four programs offering a master's degree for expanded roles (American Nurses Association and United States Department of Health, Education, and Welfare, 1975). This list includes many different clinical roles in fields such as cardiology, psychology, gerontology, child psychiatry, and others, but the vast majority of the expanded role training programs are directed to pediatric nurse practitioners.

Functions. Mauksch and David (1972) argue that the nurse practitioner is a new product. Nurse practitioners possess different knowledge and function differently from the traditional nurses. According to Mauksch and David, nurse practitioners use nursing theory and process to set up practice in such ways that decisions are made and risks are taken interdependently with other health workers, yet nurse practitioners remain accountable only to themselves and to the consumer of the services.

Cleland (1972) has undertaken the task of differentiating the diverse tasks or functions that nurse practitioners perform, including the pediatric nurse practitioner. However, the rapid emergence of the new roles, which are partially institutionalized at this time, make it extremely difficult to develop a systematic, categorical scheme describing the functions of pediatric nurse practitioners. The functions are changing too fast for this.

Silver and Hecker (1970) describe the functions of the pediatric nurse practitioners trained at the University of Colorado. In the course of their training, they provide total well-child care, including giving mothers instruction in formula preparation, bathing, toilet training, and psychological counseling. Pediatric nurse practitioners do routine physical exams and immunizations, and they manage a host of minor illnesses. Interestingly Silver and Hecker (1970) report the results of a survey of the pediatric nurse practitioners in actual practice and found that in less than one fourth of their cases was referral to a physician deemed necessary.

Work settings. Suffice it to say that pediatric nurse practitioners primarily engage in ambulatory care modes of medical practice in which they deliver primary pediatric medical care. This is in contrast to other clinical nurse practitioners who by dint of their specialized training (e.g., cardiac, neonatal) deliver hospital inpatient services as part of a multispecialty medical team.

Nevertheless, there is a large variety of employment conditions and work settings for pediatric nurse practitioners. All the various work settings can be grouped into private practice and agency practice settings. A study of work settings by Yankauer et al. (1972) found that nurses in private settings tend to see more children, well or sick, than those in agency settings. They reported no differences across settings with regard to the types of cases handled, but the activity profiles of nurses working in private and agency settings differed substantially. Nurses in private settings made a relatively larger number of hospital visits to see newborns, and they handled proportionately more office telephone calls about medical problems. On the other hand, the agency nurses did more home visiting.

Relationships with physicians and patients. The type of work setting determines to a large extent the nature of the interaction between pediatric nurse practitioners,

physicians, and patients. Health stations that are located miles from a physician or other health facility may be run by a pediatric nurse practitioner, with only occasional visits by a physician. This stands in sharp contrast to a family medical care setting in which the pediatric nurse practitioner interacts daily with physicians and other members of a health care team. Perhaps because there are so many different types of work settings or possibly because the pediatric nurse practitioner is a relatively recent development in medicine as well, there are few studies of the patient– and physician–pediatric nursing practitioner relationships. These few studies suggest that pediatric nursing practitioners have succeeded in gaining support and approval from their patients from physicians.

Silver and Hecker (1970) carried out an opinion survey of parents who took their children to a pediatrician who employed a pediatric nurse practitioner as an associate in his office. According to the investigators, there was a high degree of parent satisfaction, particularly with the idea of having both a pediatrician and a pediatric nurse practitioner on the case, a sort of medical double-teaming effect. Fifty-seven percent stated that the care given jointly by the pediatrician and nurse was better than they had received from a physician alone, and 95% favored the concept because they saw it as a strategy for providing comprehensive care to a larger number of patients.

In another study by Yankauer et al. (1972), twenty-six pediatricians were asked to evaluate the pediatric nurse practitioner's working with them. Generally, the physicians were enthusiastic about these nurses' performance. Two instances of mothers choosing a pediatrician precisely because a pediatric nurse practitioner was associated with the practice were reported. Twenty-two of the twenty-six pediatricians believed that the medical care delivered to the children in their practices had improved in quality, and four reported a drop in quality. Three physicians reported parental objections to the pediatric nurse practitioner and in these cases one or both parents were health professionals. Physicians were equally divided between those who thought that pediatric nurse practitioners allowed for an increase in the volume of patients and those who claimed that pediatric nurse practitioners freed their time that they might spend it more productively on fewer patients. However, among those physicians reporting an increase in patient load, most were unwilling to cite the pediatric nurse practitioner as the cause of this increase, which ranged from ten to seventy-five cases a week. In this same study, it was found that pediatric nurse practitioners in agency settings were somewhat underutilized, a problem that they attributed to the structure of the agency and some physician resistance.

Pediatric nurse practitioners relate to their patients as a physician does, assuming full accountability for the care delivered. There is much more professional autonomy from the direct control of physicians for pediatric nurse practitioners than for physician's assistants. However, pediatric nurse practitioners appear to be dependent on physicians in the sense of using physician approval and association with physicians as a point of entry to gaining patient acceptance. This appears to held true even for nurse midwives who are the most autonomous of the nurse clinicians (Record and Cohen, 1972). Finally, although pediatric nurse practitioners have fought physician control and have achieved independence in this regard, there is no evidence that this has led to greater medical responsibility or better salaries than the physician's assistants, for example.

SOME ISSUES CONCERNING NEW HEALTH WORKERS

There is much debate and conflicting data about the roles and functions of new health workers. Two issues loom above all the rest in importance for the future of the new health worker movement: (1) the functions of new health workers are determined more by the way medical care is organized than by ideological or formal statements about what the role ought to be, and (2) expectations among health workers are escalating.

Determination of function

In treatment organizations, particularly in the more bureaucratized and centralized medical centers, one finds two contradictory lines of authority affecting the roles of new health workers. There is a general assumption made that the physician will supervise directly the work of various new health workers and thereby represent the topmost layer of clinical authority. On the other hand, the complexity of medical tasks and division of labor makes it almost impossible for physicians to supervise the new health workers and still meet their own obligations to their patients. Out of sheer necessity, new health workers are diagnosing and treating independently or jointly with physicians, and tensions exist along the two lines of authority. Physicians want to maintain clinical dominance but are torn by the realities of the work load, and new health workers seek autonomy and resent the physician's presumed control. Role opacity or the state that exists when roles have no clear meaning through their enactment in the real world characterizes the situation facing new health workers as they negotiate their future in the health care system. Where the new health workers fit on the temporal sequence of medical care and what the scope of their responsibility and accountability to the patient will be are the big unanswered questions.

This structured role opacity has led to some legal confusion that in turn has resulted in premature closure of particular new health workers' chances of gaining more autonomy and control over the production of health services. For example, the Colorado Child Health Associate Law was passed in 1969 by the Colorado General Assembly. This law restricts child health associates from practicing autonomously by requiring that the physician be readily available at all times to supervise directly primary and follow-up care of patients. The law restricts the physician's authority to delegate responsibility to the child health associate, and it requires the physician to maintain legal responsibility for patient care provided by the associate. The law specifies that no more than one child health associate shall be employed at any one time by any one physician and only physicians whose practices include a large percentage of children can have an associate in their practice. Finally, the associates must complete at least fourteen hours of postgraduate study in pediatrics each year to renew their certification.

Proponents of this law favor strict legal regulation of nonphysician health workers in general. The concern of those in favor of legal regulation is stated clearly by Silver (1971) who sees the Child Health Associate law serving as a model for the legal regulation of all new health workers. According to Silver (1971:305):

If the legislature does not establish its own specific controls, there is an increased possibility that the new practitioners will extend their activities beyond their capabilities and beyond any reasonable limits envisaged by the legislature . . . Clarification of their functions, activities and role would minimize the possibility that they would over extend themselves, thereby discrediting the allied health professions, as well as their supervising physicians.

Critics of strict legal regulation (Coleman, 1970; Curran, 1970) are opposed to the concept of minutely regulating by law the activities of any group of medical professionals. Curran (1970) states that child health associates are "now tightly locked into a highly detailed piece of legislation that regulates their activities comprehensively and minutely . . . it is an excellent model of what should not be done with any licensed group of professionals."

Finally, the issue of two lines of authority associated with bureaucratized and centralized health care organizations poses a highly practical question for new health workers. Should new health workers be at-tached to complex organizations and physician practices or should they work in decentralized community outreach capacities as autonomous health professionals? The choice will affect the growth and development of new health worker careers and ultimately will determine the availability, cost, and types of health services delivered in rural and urban areas where current medical care shortages exist.

Escalating expectations

One of the much ignored and least understood factors behind the crisis-level decline in the number of physicians practicing medicine in rural and inner-city areas of the United States is the state of expectations that physicians have concerning the amount of time they want to devote to medical practice in light of a life-style that includes activities other than medicine. Few if any young physicians or medical students are willing to go into a rural area like their older predecessors and practice medicine nonstop for the rest of their days. In ever-increasing numbers, young physicians and student physicians are more and more concerned about personal and family needs, and they have decided that they need time away from medical practice to pursue these interests. In large measure, the physician shortage is due to the physician's unwillingness to be the only physician in an area where the practice of medicine means a 24-hours-a-day, 7-days-a-week commitment (McAllister, 1975).

New health workers are not immune to the same needs and desires that their standard-bearers, physicians, have expressed. The glamour and awe associated with new medical careers wears thin after the careerists have had time to live with the job through the everyday life issues such as working hours, autonomy, occupational mobility, and salary. A good example of this process taking place is within the ranks of emergency medical technicians (Fig. 9-2). Although the excitement of emergency medicine continues to draw new recruits into the emergency medical technicians' fold, the

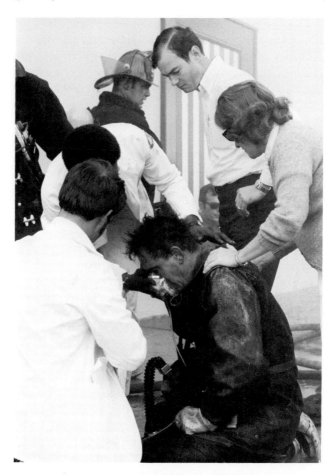

Fig. 9-2. Emergency medical technicians provide medical support for high-risk occupations. Here they administer oxygen to a fireman at the scene of a fire.

(Courtesy University of Missouri Medical Center, Columbia, Mo.)

everyday exigencies of the job have led to rapid turnover and widespread job dissatisfaction. Many emergency medical techicians are beginning to look to medical or nursing school as a strategy to move onward and upward away from emergency medicine work. Needs and expectations of new medical workers are rising relentlessly, much to the concern of those who expect the new health workers to deliver more and less expensive medical care. Studies of new medical workers in general dental practice in Holland show no increase in medical productivity. However, relief from the pressures of working with chronically ill patients and from long hours occurred as a result of physicians and new health workers sharing the work load (Council on Dental Education, 1969). Indeed placing new workers in medical outpost settings where they are working alone and in isolation from other medical colleagues may affect the quality of medical care adversely by decreasing the social dimension thwarting the rising expectations of medical workers and thereby creating a situation in which the patient's needs are neglected.

PART FOUR

THE ORGANIZATION OF
HEALTH SERVICES

Having explored the experience of disease and sickness from the perspective of the patient in Part Two and the health occupations in Part Three, they now must be brought together. This section deals with the organization of health services by focusing on the settings in which health care takes place and the relationships among those settings.

We begin in Chapter 10 by looking at medical practice as it is organized in office settings. Trends in practice organization are noted, comparing solo, partnership, group, and hospital practices. The implications for control of medical practice are then explored in some depth, leading to the inescapable conclusion that efficiency is being purchased at the expense of client alienation. The dynamics of this process, including quality control in medicine, are discussed.

In Chapter 11, we examine a complex organization peculiar to medicine, the hospital. Historical, ideological, and ecological discussions provide a background for description of hospital organization, linkages between hospitals and other organizations, the motivation of hospital behavior, and the perspectives of staff and patients on the hospital as an organization.

The neighborhood health center is a reemerging invention that has received considerable attention in recent years. Accordingly, a case study of this mode of organizing health care is presented in Chapter 12. These centers were designed in part to serve as entry points for preventing sickness and disease by changing the social, political, and economic forces in society that produce ill health. Consumer participation is very much a part of this strategy, and it has become a vital part of health center organization. The effectiveness of consumer participation is evaluated against its great promise as a key to unlocking the door to a more equitable and healthy society.

In Chapter 13 we turn our attention from discrete health care organizations and consider the organization of health services at the national level. Several factors that influence the organization of health services at this level are noted and described, including ecological, social, economic, and technological factors, the latter in the context of the cost of care. Some major ways in which national health systems differ are then described, and the impacts of the economic system and ideology on the organization of health systems are singled out for detailed analysis. Examples are drawn from the United States, the United Kingdom, the Soviet Union, China, Cuba, and the Scandinavian countries.

This part completes the analysis portion of the text, having presented an overview of the key variables and processes that not only order the provision of health services but are the raw materials of social policy in the health field.

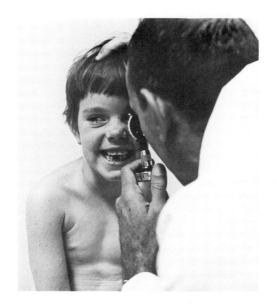

Courtesy University of Missouri Medical Center, Columbia, Mo.

CHAPTER 10

Medical practice

The delivery of medical service (as differentiated from health service and care, which are delivered mostly by nonphysicians) is influenced by the organization of medical practice. Chapter 7 outlined the selection and training of medical practitioners and the political organizations that represent medicine in the national political arena. This chapter will consider how the practice is organized, with emphasis on the influence of organization on the physician-patient relationship. It is important that there are major changes taking place in the organization of medical practice which have implications for the control of medicine. Hence the organization of practice is a currently "hot" political issue within medicine itself.

THE SHIFT FROM SOLO TO CORPORATE PRACTICE

The prototype for medical practice is the solo physician who operates as a private entrepreneur, charging patients a fee for ser-

vices rendered. It is a type modeled on classical liberal capitalism, assuming that there is market competition that will allow patients to make a choice based on the quality of results and price. It is a model that is somewhat romanticized as being the way things once were. In fact, things were never quite that way.

The reality component in the image is solo practice. Overwhelmingly physicians in the nineteenth century and a majority even today practice alone in an office. In this sense, medicine has been described as a "cottage industry." The solo physician is his "own boss," engaged in a business that is acknowledged to require some special restraints with regard to ethical conduct. He may employ a nurse or a receptionist, but he makes all the decisions while providing a needed service to a grateful clientele.

The unreality is with respect to the degree of competition. Most physicians in the last century enjoyed virtual monopolies in their local areas, since few communities had

219

more than one physician. The patient's choice was often to either accept the services of the local practitioner or to do without. Also by the early part of the twentieth century, specialization was well underway, making general practice less viable (Davis, 1916).

Since World War II in the United States, there has been a tremendous growth of practices that depart from the solo model. Partnerships, in which two or more physicians share some common facilities and divide income according to a formula, are more common. Such an arrangement allows more flexibility in the coverage of the practice. Partners can alternate weekends "on call," for example. Partnerships almost always consist of physicians who practice the same kind of medicine (e.g., general practice, pediatrics).

Even more spectacular has been the growth of groups in which two or more physicians incorporate, creating a limited liability legal entity. Single specialty groups are similar to partnerships. Multispecialty groups differ in that they often attempt to provide comprehensive medical care. That is, the physicians who constitute the group represent a number of specialties and by referral within the group meet all the needs of the patients they serve.

Between 1945 and 1967 the number of primary care physicians available for children in the United States increased by 48%, and general practitioners decreased by almost 10% (Council on Pediatric Practice, 1971). From 1946 to 1969, almost the same period, the number of medical groups (both single specialty and multispecialty) increased by 1,576% and the number of physicians practicing in multispecialty groups increased by 697% (Stevens, 1971).

This shift is one that will be discussed below in terms of its consequences for both physicians and patients.

THE SHIFT FROM GENERAL TO SPECIALIZED PRACTICE

The shift from general to specialized practice is too well known to require much documentation here. In the nineteenth century the physician "working alone and with the equipment he could carry with him . . . was able to provide most of the medical care his patients needed" (Coe, 1970). He was a generalist, providing all the services performed today by all physicians and dentists.

With the growth of medical knowledge and especially after its implementation in medical training following the Flexner report, medical practice became increasingly specialized. In the United States, ophthalmology became a recognized medical specialty when they founded a board to examine specialists in diseases of the eye in 1917. By the end of the 1930s, fifteen such boards had been established, and by 1967 there were nineteen. In addition, the number of specialty societies was growing. In 1972 there were 128 such societies, six of which accounted for one third of the membership of all specialist societies. In decreasing membership, these were the American Academy of Family Physicians, the American College of Surgeons, the American College of Physicians, the American Psychiatric Association, American Society of Internal Medicine, and the American Society of Anesthesiologists (Theodore et al., 1968; Vahovich, 1973).

In 1945 almost three out of four physicians were in general practice. By 1973 this had declined to under 16%; the remainder were about equally divided between medical, surgical, and other specialties (Martin, 1973). Specialization has also affected the nature of physician-patient relationships, and this will be systematically considered in this chapter.

TYPES OF PRACTICE

There are basically four types of medical practice organizations: solo practice; partnership, group practice, and hospital practice. The research literature on practice organization, however, is most uneven. In the United Kingdom there have been a large number of studies of the solo physician who functions as a general practitioner. In the United States, studies that have focused on general practice have been specific and limited to particular problems. On the other hand, in recent years in the United States there has been an explosion of literature on group practice, especially as this is currently seen by government authorities as a panacea for problems in health care delivery. Literature on other countries or on other forms of practice is sparse indeed (Weinerman, 1966).

Solo practice

Solo practice is different in the United Kingdom and the United States. In the United Kingdom solo practitioners are almost inevitably general practitioners, whereas in the United States they are more likely to be specialists. In the United Kingdom solo practice is overwhelmingly ambulatory care, since general practitioners do not have access to hospitals except by referral to other physicians. In the United States perhaps a majority of general solo practitioners and almost all specialist solo practitioners conduct a large part of their practices in hospital settings (Cartwright, 1967; Mechanic, 1968a, 1975a).

Solo practice in both countries is considered to have some distinct advantages. Primary among these is that physicians are freer to treat the "whole patient." This means that their concerns will not be narrowly limited to the disease process, but rather they can consider "the implications of health and disease for work, family life and the patient's general welfare" (College of General Practitioners, 1965; Royal Commission on Medical Education, 1968; *Patient Care*, 1971; Mechanic, 1975b). In the United States physicians also widely believe that in solo practice they will have higher incomes, provide better continuity of care, and have more freedom to make decisions than in group practice (*Patient Care*, 1971).

The extent to which this is true is unknown. Some data from the United Kingdom, however, suggest that a concern with total patient care is not characteristic of all general practitioners. Mechanic (1975b)

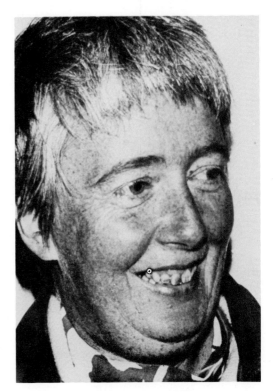

Fig. 10-1. *Ann Cartwright.*

classified physicians according to their use of diagnostic tests (an indicator of scientific orientation) and their expressed interests in treating a variety of nondisease problems (an indicator of social orientation). More than one third of physicians were classified as "withdrawers" (low on both measures), only 17% were "moderns" (high on both measures), and 19% were "technicians" (high on diagnostic tests, low on social interests). Presumably a similar case would hold in the United States. Peterson et al. (1956) found that general practitioners in North Carolina tended to perform poorly in physical examinations and to underuse diagnostic tests. This finding has been replicated in other parts of the United States and Canada (Taylor, 1954; Clute, 1963; Jungfer and Last, 1964, Cartwright and Marshall, 1965).

The disadvantages of solo practice are generally considered to be professional isolation, lack of colleague support, and greater difficulty in obtaining hospital appointments.

Partnerships

Partnerships differ from solo practice in that two or more physicans share office facilities and have an agreement by which they divide income and facilitate time off while providing continuous coverage of the practice. Although no research deals specifically with this type of practice, it would presumably lessen professional isolation.

Group practice

Group practice is a relatively new development in the United States and is usually defined as three or more physicians "formally organized to provide medical care, consultation, diagnosis and/or treatment through the joint use of equipment or personnel, and with income from medical practice distributed in accordance with methods previously determined by members of the group" (American Medical Association, 1971). Groups have been in existence since at least 1920 and have been vigorously opposed by organized medicine until recent years. Early the AMA warned that groups might violate ethical principles and during the 1940s called them "medical soviets" (Saward, 1970; Mahoney, 1973). Clearly the AMA, representing the solo practitioner, felt threatened by this new development.

Groups vary greatly by size and the professional mix of participating physicians. In addition, they can be classified along two major dimensions: (1) whether they contain one or several medical specialties and (2) whether they are financed on a fee-for-service or prepayment plan.

When one speaks of a prepaid multispecialty group practice, the protoype is the Kaiser-Permanente Health Plan, which pioneered this style of organization. That plan began as an emergency mechanism to provide medical care for shipbuilders during World War II. By 1960 in Portland, Oregon, the plan had three major components. The Kaiser Foundation Health Plan was a nonprofit organization that colletced dues and contracted for medical services on a capitation basis. The Permanente Clinic was a partnership of full-time specialists who provided all medical services to the enrolled population. The Bess Kaiser Hospital was a community hospital reimbursed by the plan on a capitation basis. Essential elements were prepayment, group practice, integrated health facilities, an emphasis on preventive medicine,[1] and dual choice[2] (Saward et al., 1968).

The Kaiser-Permanente Health Plan has demonstrated that high-quality medical care can be delivered at a cost much below that suffered by the population at large. As financial pressures on medicine have mounted in recent years, governmental authorities have enacted legislation to encourage other such plans to develop. Mistakenly (we think) believing the emphasis to be on preventive medicine, prepaid groups have come to be known as "health maintenance organizations."

A great deal of rhetorical literature deals with the advantages and disadvantages of group practice for physicians, but there is little supporting evidence on either side. Advocates of groups claim that groups provide regular hours and colleague support. On this opponents do not disagree (*Patient Care,* 1971). However, it is further claimed that groups provide services that are more accessible and are of higher quality, greater continuity, and greater efficiency. On all these points, the evidence is equivocal (Graham, 1972). Overall, groups seem to be no worse than solo practices on most measures but no better either. Differences on any given measure are small in either direction.

Major disadvantages cited for group practice are that groups limit earnings, the physician has less freedom in choosing to whom to refer patients, prepayment encourages overutilization of services by patients, and groups provide less continuity of care for patients. Again there is no unequivocal evidence to support any of these claims, although to some degree they are shared by both group and nongroup physicians (McElrath, 1961).

About the only finding that is documented with reference to group and nongroup practice is that group physicans tend to handle increased patient loads by increasing the number seen in a given time period, whereas nongroup physicans tend to increase the number of hours at work (Mechanic, 1975a). Also the power of administrators is greater in consumer-owned groups than in physician-owned groups. The power of the medical staff does not vary with type of ownership (Schwartz, 1968).

Hospital practice

Apart from studies of hospital organization, which will be reported in Chapter 11, little work has been done on the organization of medical practice in hospital settings. What has been done has concentrated on the physician in training: the intern and resident. There is no literature on the full-time hospital physician in the United States.

The bulk of hospital admissions in the United States would seem to be patients of private physicians, who then follow their patients during the course of confinement. House staffs provide services for those who are too poor to have private physicians. Duff and Hollingshead (1968) found four types of organization of physician services in the Yale New Haven Hospital: committee, semicommittee, casual, and committed. These were presented as forms of sponsorship of patients that characterized physicians.

Committee sponsorship was characteristic of wards in teaching hospitals. A group of physicians had responsibility for the ward. The patient had no single physician who was consistently in charge. In this system, physician-patient relationships were at their worst. The degree of disease severity typical of patients in such a setting, the socioeconomic status gap between patients and physicians, and the mass production character of work, which was usually done on "rounds," led to maximum patient alienation and anger. At the same time, the technical quality of work was generally high.

Being a teaching setting, the ward was a place where staff were most up to date. Care under such a system tended to be expensive, however, because of the reliance on technology, particularly the extensive use of laboratory tests.

Semicommittee sponsorship was more characteristic of the semiprivate service in which a private physician was nominally in charge, but most of the work was delegated to the house staff. Technical quality was lower than on the ward service, and there were few additional amenities. In addition, the patient bore the cost of the private physician.

Casual sponsorship was found in all services of the hospital and was characterized by three features:

1. The physician looked upon the patient as his own and he remained in the forefront of the doctor-patient relationship.
2. The physician focused his attention upon the presenting symptom . . . and treated the symptoms by recourse to technical knowledge he had about the real or assumed disease of the patient.
3. The physician allowed little time for the patient to question him about the illness (Duff and Hollingshead, 1968:139).

Committed sponsorship was found mostly on the private service and occasionally on the semiprivate service. It was characterized by the assumption of responsibility by a single physician whose interest in the patient extended beyond the disease process. This sponsorship allowed the best opportunity for "the physician and patient to join in the diagnosis and treatment of health problems" but also was the one in which pathological relationships were most likely to get out of hand. Physicians were also most likely to be out of date, and technical quality suffered.

CLIENT VERSUS PROFESSIONAL CONTROL

In one of the most important books on the medical profession, Freidson (1970) argued that professional autonomy is a core characteristic of medical practice. He developed arguments first stated in his earlier works to the effect that medical practices could be classified according to the degree to which they could be influenced by the wishes of patients (Freidson, 1960, 1961). Some practices are organized in such a way that they are dependent on patients enmeshed in a *lay referral network* (Chapter 5) to provide new patients. Such practices are *client dependent* and must satisfy patients to remain viable. Such an organization gives patients a good measure of power. At the other extreme are practices that are more specialized or otherwise organized so as to be dependent on other physicians for referrals. These are part of a *professional referral network* and can be considered *colleague dependent*. Such organization keeps power concentrated in the professional community and out of the hands of patients.

In the United States, there has been a trend toward consolidation of power in the hands of physicians (Freidson, 1972). As noted in Chapter 7, this began long before professional authority could be said to be based on real expertise, much less tangible benefits to patients. A shift from solo practice to group and hospital practice has furthered professional autonomy. At the same time a not insignificant consumer movement has emerged in the health field, some aspects of which are discussed in Chapter 12. In recent years the growing "third parties" in medicine, the insurance industry and government, have begun to intervene in the organization of medical services in an effort to hold down costs. By restricting the entrepreneurial freedom of the physician, third parties may be providing a counterbalance to professional autonomy.

Practice organization and professional control

The shift from solo practice to group and hospital-based practice has served to increase professional autonomy and control. Standards of practice both with respect to the technical quality of service and the conditions under which the services are dispensed have increasingly been determined solely by physicians. From another perspective, changes in the organization of practice have been at the expense of the power of the patient.

It should be acknowledged that the notion of solo practice is somewhat of a myth. Although there are communities that have only one physician, these are increasingly uncommon. It is probably only in that kind of isolated practice that one can talk about a true solo enterprise. Most practices called "solo" are actually to some degree either client or colleague dependent (Freidson, 1972). As Freidson (1970, 1972) has argued, solo practice is inherently unstable. It must either become client dependent, which limits the physician's options in one way, or colleague dependent, which limits them in another. At the least, the physician must make arrangements for time off during which his practice is covered by another physician. Hence his work is visible and subject to some constraints. In fact, most physicians have ongoing relationships with other physicians, making the practice a cooperative one short of partnership. The conception of solo practice, then, is as much an ideological as a descriptive state. It emphasizes the personal autonomy of the practicing physician.

The opportunity for client control is higher in solo practice than in other forms. Relative to partnerships, groups, and hospital practices, solo practitioners are insulated from colleagues. They are relatively more dependent on their reputation in the lay community. To attract and keep patients, they must satisfy them that they are getting good treatment, and to do this, these physicians must "give them what they want." Hence the incidence of giving antibiotic drugs for viral infections (antibiotics have no effect on viruses) is much higher among solo general practitioners than among other physicians.

A partnership shifts the practice from one insulated from colleague observation to one in which professionally trained colleagues can oversee a great deal. Hence this kind of practice places more constraints on the physicians to conform to professional standards of good medicine and to pay less attention to the wishes of the patients. The extent to which this improves the technical quality of medicine is problematic, since physicians of roughly equal competence tend to practice together. There can be little doubt, however, that the power of the patient is reduced.

In group practice, control is further removed from the patient. The physician not only works with a relatively large number of others, but referrals are made within the group. Hence each physician is more intimately aware of the activities of the other physician. Furthermore, the practice of each member of the group affects the income of the others directly, and each physician has an interest in what the others do. In some groups such as the Kaiser-Permanente group in Portland, Oregon, this is reflected in an ongoing program of research in which each patient contact is computerized for a sample of patients and monthly printouts enable the system to monitor its internal behavior. Those who practice outside the norms of the group are easily identified and called to account. Such a practice is even more professionally controlled than are partnerships, and the patient has even less power in a system in which physicians are formally held accountable by colleagues.

The power of the patient is almost completely eroded in the hospital. In addition to a high density of colleague interaction and peer control on the part of physicians, the patient has been moved into a setting in which he is under constant supervision and in which virtually everything is done for him. Even such elementary decisions as going to the bathroom are reinterpreted to be "privileges" conferred by the hospital staff rather than natural functions.

It is necessary to reemphasize that in the United States, hospital practice is not distinct from the other forms. Solo practitioners often have admitting privileges to hospitals and spend a portion of their practice time in hospital settings. Differences in the practice mix of physicians would make these distinctions somewhat less sharp than presented here, but we would argue that the general point holds true.

In other countries such as the United Kingdom, there is a sharp distinction between community physicians, or general practitioners, and hospital physicians, who are specialists. There the distinctions may be even sharper than presented here.

Third parties and consumer control

In recent years there have been a number of third parties involved in medical practice. The term "third party" refers to any agency or organization that has become involved either by means of direct provision of care or the financing of care. Several labor unions, including the International Ladies Garment Workers and the United Mine Workers, have established their own health centers to provide service to their memberships. In many instances, they become the employers of physicians and the owners of facilities. There has been a rapid growth of health insurance, with varying effects on the physician-patient relationship depending on how the insurance program is organized. In recent years, various governmental agencies have become involved either to provide direct service or as insurers of special populations.

Both the United Mine Workers and the International Ladies Garment Workers have opened a number of health centers. The facilities are owned by the unions, and the staffs are hired by a board of directors composed of union officers. Physicians are salaried. In this framework, considerable control is in the hands of people directly answerable to the consumers of the service. The aggregate wishes of the union members must be taken into account, although on a case-to-case basis the patient has little power. The union intervenes most frequently in administrative matters and with reference to the organization and terms of service delivery. Medical judgments are left to the physicians (Schwartz, 1968). It is likely that being relieved of the need to attend to the business side of practice, physicians can devote more time and effort to the purely professional aspects of medicine. Within the realm of diagnosis and treatment, they may have even more autonomy than private practitioners. At the same time, areas are reserved for consumer decision (Freidson, 1972).

The impact of insurance programs on the control of medical practice has varied with the type of program. As Freidson (1972: 351) has indicated:

The third party at its best has the client's welfare in mind and, unlike the client himself, also has available expert guidance in determining a policy which advances the health of community members. Thus, it can be better equipped than individual clients ever could be to counterbalance the material interests of the practitioner without detracting from the scientific quality of practice.

For the most part in the United States, however, the rapidly growing health insurance industry (Somers and Somers, 1961; Somers, 1971) has concentrated on the reimbursement of physicians fees or hospital charges. This has reinforced the fee-for-service system, and although it has improved physicians' incomes, it has had little impact on medical practice itself (Field, 1961).

Increasingly, insurance companies are finding it difficult to work with the fee-for-service system. As costs of medical care rise, it is increasingly important for those who pay those costs to have some control over expenditures or at least to have them made predictable. The fee-for-service system suffers, from the point of view of insurers, precisely because it is too open-ended. It is difficult to predict expenditures. Most would prefer some arrangement in which physicians are paid a set amount for each patient (called "capitation") or they are paid a set salary (Field, 1961; Somers and Somers, 1961; Freidson, 1972).

Roemer (1962) has suggested that the fee-for-service system is expensive for yet another reason. It encourages the delivery of a large number of services, many of them unnecessary, because this enhances physician income. By comparison, both capitation and salary eliminate the incentives to give unneeded service and hold down costs. Hence these methods improve the quality of care, as well as increase administrative convenience.

More attention is being given to prepayment schemes, whether through capitation or by placing physicians on salary. This requires some organization of the system so that it becomes possible to identify responsible physicians and link them with a patient population. Accordingly most of the experiments with alternative financing are taking place in settings with a regular clientele such as group practices and neighborhood health centers (Schwartz, 1968).

The fee-for-service system is much less important as a mechanism for financing health care in other countries. In the United Kingdom, patients register with a community physician who is paid on a capitation basis depending on the number of enrolled patients. Hospital physicians, who are the specialists, are paid a salary. In Sweden there is a complex system in which physicians are paid a salary, plus there is reimbursement for specific service. In Eastern Europe almost all physicians are on salary as government employees.

In fact, in most countries the third-party input of insurance programs and more direct governmental input overlap. Most governments are to some degree involved in the provision of health services, most often by intervention in the financing schemes of the health care system. Many own the hospitals and have the community physicians on salary. Others use capitation schemes. For some, such governmental programs constitute the health system of the country, with other financing being a small residual part of the system.

In the United States the government is involved directly in only three programs that serve limited populations: the military medical corps, the Veterans Administration hospitals, and the Indian Health Service. The first two programs have provided high-quality service, whereas the Indian Health Service has been faulted for its inability to surmount cultural differences between providers and consumers and suffers from a level of underfunding that suggests strong anti-Indian bias on the part of the Congress (Kane and Kane, 1972).

In summary, the changes in practice organization and specialization have served to enhance professional autonomy. Although physicians are more under the control of colleagues than in the past, they are better insulated from client pressures. Consumer movements and the recent growth of third-party interventions into the health care delivery system have acted in the direction of restoring the balance by providing for organized consumer inputs. To date in the United States the growth of professional autonomy has vastly outstripped the growth of consumer control.

Practice organization and patient flow

The question of how physicians develop a case load of patients, hold them, and refer patients to one another is of great practical interest to the practicing physician. Many journals that aim at an audience of young physicians devote several articles each year to giving practical advice, almost all of which is the shared wisdom of older practitioners rather than the findings of empirical research.

As noted at some length in Chapter 5, the initial decision to see a physician is the result of a series of decisions made by or on behalf of a symptomatic person. Included in these decisions is the choice of a physician or location for medical care. These decisions lead to a source of primary care through the choice of a client-dependent physician (Freidson, 1961).

Hall (1946) noted the importance of sponsorship for the young physician. It is through the active interest of established practitioners that necessary hospital appointments are obtained and patients are referred. Building and maintaining a practice then is a matter of "connections" or "who you know." Von der Lippe (1968) confirmed that in the communities where Hall did his work (Providence, Rhode Island, and Toronto, Ontario) the need for sponsorship had not diminished in twenty years. Furthermore, the likelihood of obtaining a powerful sponsor was to some degree a function of ethnic and religious background.

Increasingly, physicians are entering practices that are less client dependent and more colleague dependent. That is, a flow of patients is obtained by referrals of other physicians. Here sponsorship takes a different form. It is not enough that colleagues be willing to help out by sending patients; they must have confidence that the special expertise needed is present in the receiving physician. Thus to maintain a practice one requires a good reputation for skill. Other physicians need to be satisfied, not only patients.

Since patients are the capital of medical practice, physicians are reluctant to make referrals. Peidmont (1968) found that general practitioners see many patients with psychiatric symptoms but make few referrals to mental health specialists. Referrals are more frequent when the physician receives reports from specialists on the patients referred. This suggests that the fear of losing patients contributes to the reluctance to refer.

In a study of three group practices, Penchansky and Fox (1970) found that referral rates were influenced by several patients characteristics. Young and old patients were referred less frequently than middle-aged ones; internists referred married patients less frequently than single or other (widowed, divorced, or separated) ones; general practitioners referred single people less than others; whites were referred more often than blacks; and among pediatricians, patients under group prepayment were referred more often than fee-for-service patients, although there were no differences among other physicians.

Among internists in private practice in the northern suburbs of Chicago, high-status physicians referred to each other, whereas lower status physicians tended to refer to higher status ones (Shortell, 1973). Physicians also referred more often to colleagues who were personal friends. Distance was not a strong factor, since more than 90% of referrals were not to the closest colleague. Almost all referrals were to colleagues with appointments at the same hospital.

An aside: the issue of free choice

In the United States, there has been much discussion about what is called "socialized medicine" (which seems to refer to any form of corporate practice, government involvement, or both and has little to do with socialism) and the issue of "free choice of physician" on the part of patients. It is contended that any major third-party involvement will result in the assignment of patients to physicians, and patients lose the right to select their own physician.

Aside from the fact that this loss of freedom has not occurred in any country with a socialized payment scheme, the issue of free choice may be ephemeral.

First, the patient is typically not well enough informed to establish criteria for evaluating the technical quality of the care given, much less to make a good selection on a priori grounds. There is some evidence, however, that patients know when they are getting poor care and do change physicians under those circumstances (Sweet and Twaddle, 1969b). Rather, prospective patients must rely on the reputation of the physician in a technically inexpert population (Freidson, 1961).

Second, the growth of group practice and specialization have made an increasing number of patient-physician encounters a matter of referral from one physician to another. The selection of a physician is increasingly physician dominated.

Hence patients' choice is already limited, and what exists may be irrelevant to the quality of care provided. Furthermore, considering that most communities originally had only one physician, it is doubtful whether such choice ever existed.

THE QUALITY OF MEDICAL PRACTICE

Considerable attention has been given recently to the quality of medical practice. This is partly motivated by the recognition that poor technical quality of physician performance is not infrequent, the demand of third parties for better controls over medical practice, and (perhaps) an unarticulated recognition that the lack of patient choice places an ethical burden on medicine to police itself. Medical codes of ethics have recognized the inability of consumers to judge quality and enjoined the physician to maintain reasonable skills. In part the rise of malpractice litigation has forced the hand of practitioners.

Quality can be divided into the following two components: *technical quality*, bearing on physicians' knowledge and skill in making a diagnosis and organizing a plan of treatment; and *quality of care,* bearing on the extent to which patients trust their physicians and cooperate in a course of treatment. These dimensions roughly approximate the "science" and "art" of medicine, and both are important in their effects on patient health and treatment outcome.

Need for quality control

The perceived need for quality control comes from two sources: the inherent nature of the physician-patient relationship and documentation of the widespread existence of poor quality practice.

The physican-patient relationship shares the qualities of any professional-client relationship. The client is typically someone needing help and unable to provide it for himself. The professional has expert knowledge. Hence there is a competence gap that makes it mandatory that the client be able to trust the judgment of the professional. Relative to other professional-client relationships, the problems of the client are more consequential in medicine than in any other field with the possible exception of criminal law. In addition, the sick person is to some degree incapacitated and unable to exercise even normal lay controls over the encounter (Parsons, 1951).

More immediately important is the evidence for poor quality. Peterson et al. (1956) studied eighty-eight general practitioners in North Carolina to assess their performance. They found that the physicians could be classified into five quality ranks. This done, only seven fell into the highest category and sixteen into the lowest. More than half took totally inadequate medical histories. Only a bare majority had the patient disrobe sufficiently to carry out a physical examination; most did no examinations or incomplete examinations (e.g., incomplete ear examinations). Most did not make adequate use of laboratory tests. In short, most of the physicians studied were not performing adequately to identify disease in their patients. There was some tendency for the better medical student to make a better physician, but this was not consistently the case. More important was the amount of training received in internal medicine in medical school. Practice was worse among physicians who were older, had poor laboratory facilities, or practiced alone.

Subsequent studies have either confirmed these general findings or have focused on different dimensions with the same result. A poor mortality picture and a preponderance of unnecessary surgical operations are two such indicators (Abse, 1969; *Medical World News,* 1971; Donabedian, 1972).

Factors influencing quality

Quality is difficult to assess. It is inescapably a value judgment that involves approximation of one or more normative standards.

"Technical quality" is generally used to refer to the skills of the physician, that is, his level of knowledge and facility in reaching a reasonable diagnosis and deciding a course of treatment. High technical quality tends to be associated with the approximation of medical practice to medical norms. Hence it is almost uniformly found that high technical quality is associated with

profession-dependent practices. The results of all the studies cited in the previous section are consistent with the findings that higher quality physicians follow procedures in physical examination that correspond to the teaching of the medical schools, they have hospital appointments, they have served in residency training beyond the internship year, and they practice in settings where there is peer review (i.e., their work is seen and reviewed by other physicians).

"Quality of care" is generally used to refer to the skill of physicians in relating to patients. They are able to establish rapport with patients, demonstrate concern, and inspire trust and confidence on the part of sick people. Although this aspect has received much less study, it is widely assumed in medical circles that high quality of care is associated with solo practice in which there is an ongoing, one-on-one, physician-patient relationship. Furthermore, it is more characteristic of primary care specialties than of disease-oriented specialties. Hence family practice is considered to be more oriented toward quality of care (Figs. 10-2 and 10-3) and surgery toward technical quality.

The language of medicine often distinguishes between the science and the art of medicine, which seem to be similar dimensions. Although both are considered important, physicians differ in their emphasis, and many assume that the two are somewhat mutually exclusive. That is, too much attention to art diminishes the quality of the science and vice versa. There is some evidence that is consistent with this viewpoint, although we would contend that it is an artifact of definition and practice.

It seems to be true that most measures of technical quality are associated with specialization, hospital practice, and university appointment. These are the places where knowledge is most up-to-date, there is more peer review, and the emphasis is on disease and technology. The fact is that such settings have deemphasized the art of medicine in favor of the science, which has become the sole criterion for evaluation. Fur-

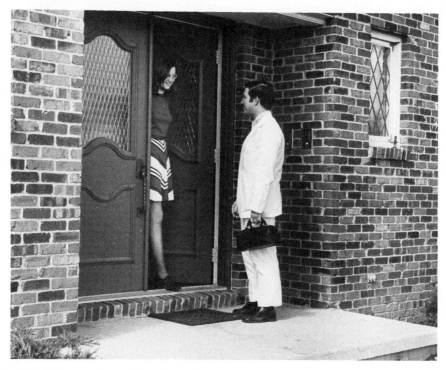

Fig. 10-2. *House calls are largely a thing of the past, although the new specialty of family practice has produced a small revival.*

(*Courtesy University of Missouri Medical Center, Columbia, Mo.*)

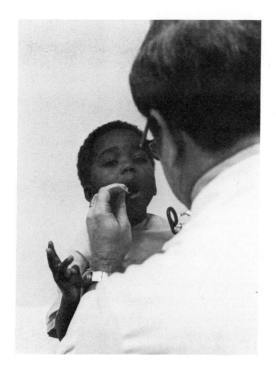

Fig. 10-3. *Routine screening examinations are an essential part of family practice's commitment to health maintenance.*

(*Courtesy University of Missouri Medical Center, Columbia, Mo.*)

thermore, participants define the science of medicine as important because they know that they will not be faulted for bad art. The reality has followed the definition. Emphasis is on diseases and laboratory tests rather than people, and quality of care and technical quality appear to be inversely related.

There is some evidence to suggest, however, that this emphasis has been one-sided and costly. In a study of admissions to the Massachusetts General Hospital in Boston, designed to develop a method for identifying preventable admissions, it was found that a large proportion of admissions were preventable in that either the disease was one that could have been avoided (e.g., rheumatic fever can be prevented by diagnosing and treating streptococcal infections) or a different course of treatment may have avoided the need for hospitalization (Twaddle and Sweet, 1970). A search for the failures that explained preventable admissions yielded suggestive information that inadequate history taking, poor patient-physician rapport, poor communications among physicians, and lack of patient understanding were consequential. In a setting of unquestioned technical excellence, there were serious defects in the art of medicine that had serious consequences for the patient. Hence high-quality medicine must pay attention to both. Correct diagnosis and treatment are worthless if the patient cannot follow them.

Existing mechanisms to ensure quality

As discussed in Chapter 7, Freidson has made a rather compelling argument that the formal mechanisms of control in medicine are not used and the most extreme sanctions of the quality of medical practice are informal talks and the refusal to refer patients. In effect, internal professional mechanisms are weak and do nothing to eliminate low-quality practitioners.

Currently peer review has been advocated as a mechanism for quality control. The prototype for this procedure in the United States is the Utilization Review

Committee established under the Medicare legislation. Each hospital is required to have a committee that reviews every Medicare patient by the twenty-first day of admission to certify that continued hospitalization is necessary. The intent is to reduce length of stay and hence the expenditures of the Social Security Administration, which administers the program. The actual effects on length of stay have been minimal. Kolb and Sidel (1968) have shown that there is a slight increase in discharges on the twentieth day at the Massachusetts General Hospital which results from the operations of the Utilization Review Committee, specifically physicians avoiding review. However, relatively few patients are hospitalized long enough for such a change to have any appreciable aggregate effect.

Recent legislation has called for the establishment of Professional Service Review Organizations (PSROs), which are to be composed of community groups who will conduct medical audits of the performance of various components of the medical service system, including the practice of private physicians. Physician organizations have the first chance to create PSROs, but if they fail to do so, other community groups will have a chance. It is possible that consumer groups may have an occasional chance to monitor the system and influence it, although this remains to be seen.

Many government-sponsored health services require that there be community participation in governing the system. Since these have applied to neighborhood health centers more than other organizations, discussion is deferred to the next chapter.

Another mechanism that is inefficient and expensive is private litigation, primarily through malpractice suits. In the United States malpractice litigation has increased dramatically in recent years. Although no systematic evidence has been found, it is reasonable to suspect that much of this activity stems as much from failures in the art of medicine as in the science. It is the only way that many patients have to retaliate for abusive personal treatment from physicians as well as to seek compensation for crippling mistakes. Whether the threat of higher premiums for malpractice insurance will generate pressures for physicians to police themselves remains to be seen.

POLITICS AND THE FUTURE OF MEDICAL PRACTICE

The issue of who is going to control medical practice is a real one. As we have seen, the situation has changed from one in which patients had considerable say and physicians were client dependent (this is relatively speaking, since there was probably not as much choice of physicians as commonly believed at any historical time) to one in which a large proportion of practices are colleague dependent. The increasing scale of organization, the specialization of practice, and even the intervention of third parties have served to increase professional autonomy (Freidson, 1970). With greater power in the hands of the medical profession, physicians have done little to police the quality of practice, leaving discipline to informal and ineffectual channels. In addition, costs of medical care have risen so rapidly, even in comparison with other services, that the third parties, who pay a good share of the bills, have begun to feel the need to exercise their own controls. In some areas, patients have become restive, feeling that their needs and wishes are ignored by the medical establishment. Hence there is a countermovement to the increasing autonomy of the professional.

Within medicine, broadly conceived to include all interested parties, the control of medical practice is a political issue, with different groups taking different positions. In closing this chapter, we will briefly outline three positions and offer a guess as to what the future may hold.

Professional, public, or consumer control: the AMA, government, and MCHR

The student will recall from Chapter 7 that the AMA was founded in the mid-nineteenth century to protect the interests of regular physicians against the claims of competing health care movements. It represented the private practitioner in solo practice. Furthermore, it has continued to represent this group and has ignored the emerging interests of physicians practicing in other modalities. In fact, it led the fight against group practice, calling them "medical soviets;" campaigned vigorously against social security legislation in the 1930s; and opposed every form of national health insurance.

The position of the AMA with regard to the control of medical practice has been that it should be in the hands of physicians. The organization has consistently held that only physicians can judge the quality of medical work or set reasonable fees. Furthermore, all patient-physician encounters should be a matter of private contract, with no intervention from any third party. One way of viewing the AMA then is as a political organization dedicated to physician control of medical practice (Harris, 1966; Ribicoff, 1972).

All the third parties and consumer movements have in common the position that the medical profession must be held accountable to some outside group. The Board of Health of the City of Chicago, for example, has become involved in direct service and is now operating a number of neighborhood health centers financed through city taxation. The position of the Board of Health is that the government must control medical care by becoming the employer of physicians and the provider of facilities. Although limited at the present time to providing services to low-income groups, the city's arguments would lead eventually to a more comprehensive system. The argument is heard that government control is a method of ensuring public accountability on the part of a vital service.

A third alternative is advocated by the Medical Committee for Human Rights (MCHR), an organization of health professionals and citizens devoted to the proposition that "health care is a human right," which is in opposition to the AMA position that it is a privilege. MCHR initially developed as the medical arm of the civil rights movement and organized to provide a medical presence at places where conflict between groups was likely to result in injuries. They have been active in efforts to expand medical services to disadvantaged populations and have opposed any financial or social barrier to care.

One activity has been the support of a free clinic movement in low-income areas. Skills are provided to neighborhood groups for organizing their own community-controlled medical services. Ideologically they mistrust both city governments and the AMA. The contention is that health is too important to be left to the experts and that the clients should control the system.

In Chicago an enormous power struggle is taking place among these three contenders, with results yet to be seen.

The future?

It is of course impossible to predict the future. For the United States, however, several assumptions seem relatively safe.

First, the AMA will continue to fight its historical rearguard action, passionately opposing any and all change in the organization of medical care, losing, and embracing the result. At least in the short run, they will continue to represent the interests of the solo private practitioner.

Second, group and hospital practices will continue to grow, with the result that physician services will be less and less financed by the fee-for-service method. Third parties will encourage this trend as sound administrative practice.

Directly or indirectly consumers will gain more power in the physician-patient relationship, either through organized consumer groups or through governmental channels. Power will likely be split between practitioners, who will retain control over technical medical processes, and the third parties, who will have more control over the range of services provided and the conditions under which they are delivered.

NOTES

1. Saward et al. (1968) claim that the financing plan placed an emphasis on preventive care and early case finding as a mechanism for holding down costs, hence increasing income for the group. In a visit in the spring of 1970, one of us (A. C. T.) saw no evidence for any difference in the practice of medicine there and in more traditional settings. Preventive medicine seemed to have no greater emphasis there than elsewhere. Instead the program differed in consistently carrying out treatment in the cheapest possible setting. That is, nothing was done in the hospital that could be done in the clinics. Although not affecting unit costs, this procedure effectively held down the total cost to the system. Hospitalization rates are impressively lower among Kaiser-Permanente subscribers than for the population at large.

2. By this is meant that subscribers should have a choice as to enrolling in Kaiser-Permanente or another plan such as Blue Cross. This is important, since the major source of subscribers are the payrolls of local industries.

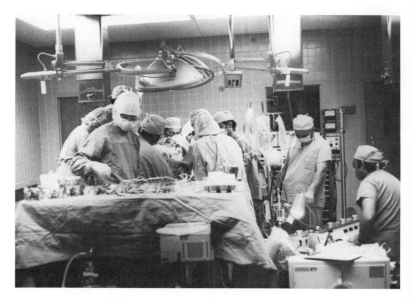

Courtesy University of Missouri Medical Center, Columbia, Mo.

CHAPTER 11

Hospitals and clinics

The hospital is a complex medical organization that has captured the imagination of modern people, professional and nonprofessional alike. It is seen as a modern shrine at (or in) which proper obeisance to technology will result in miraculous cures. It is certainly a power center in which the medical community can mobilize to do political battle. The hospital is a primary center for training health professionals. For these reasons along with the romanticization of the hospital on television and in the popular press, the hospital is seen by the public and health professionals alike as being "where the action is" in modern medicine.

In fact, there is a fit between the hospital and the values of such Western societies as the United States. The hospital is an impressive organization from the standpoint of its technical capacities. There all the most impressive equipment is to be found, creating a strange environment of machinery

that is properly mysterious. Dress symbolizes power. The language is arcane. People bustle about on errands that often involve life and death. It is the secular cathedral that displays the wonders of science and inspires awe in its believers.

The hospital is where the most sophisticated tools of medicine are brought together. There is little doubt that it is more effective in preserving life than any other organization yet devised. At the same time, the tools present dangers. They are extremely expensive. In fact, nothing has served to drive the cost of medical care up faster than the hospital. Many services are priced out of the reach of all but the wealthiest citizens. Furthermore, the machines and drugs with the power to heal also have the power to kill. The hospital is an organization that needs watching.

For all this, in spite of the facts that the hospital is symbolic of the Western cult of technology, that it preserves life, and that

234

people have been willing to invest in it to the point of their own bankruptcy, we must raise the question: is it important? In any given year, only a minority of the population will enter a hospital. Most of those who do could be equally well treated outside were it not for features of hospital organization and health care financing that encourage inpatient treatment. Also there is reason to believe that the volume of hospitalization cannot be explained solely by the technological superiority of the organization. Events are happening in other parts of the society that make hospitalization more likely irrespective of efficacy. At the same time, many hospitals are becoming superspecialized in the care of the supersick, confining their efforts to a smaller and smaller portion of illness experience in the society.

In this chapter, the nature of the hospital will be explored: its social origins, its distribution and utilization in the society, its organization and behavior, and the way in which it is viewed by both staff and patients. With this background, we can return briefly to the public policy questions alluded to here. As a general orientation, one must consider the hospital as a social movement with ancient origins and a modern development and have some appreciation for the types of hospitals that are to be found.

THE HOSPITAL AS A SOCIAL MOVEMENT

As discussed in Chapter 1, hospital-like organizations were present in ancient times. The ancient societies of India, the Middle East, Rome, and Greece had some provision for the care of the sick in facilities separated from homes. Generally, these were small scale operations with no special technical facility, and they were designed to serve special groups of people such as pilgrims.

The modern hospital as a communal institution began with the Roman Catholic monastic orders in the Middle Ages, experienced a spectacular growth and secularization in the nineteenth century, and became a technological center for the treatment of disease only in the twentieth century.

The medieval hospital

The hospital as a community organization emerged in the early Middle Ages as a religious phenomenon. The Christian focus on salvation through good works led the monasteries to set aside cells for the care of the sick. By the late fourth century, fairly large organizations had been founded in Cappadocia and Constantinople. By 1136 many elements of the modern hospital were already to be found, including an outpatient department, surgical and infectious disease wards, and a medical staff (Rosen, 1963). By the end of the fifteenth century, hospitals could be found all over Europe, with more than six hundred in England alone.

Most hospitals were directly agencies of the church, although a growing number were founded by guild organizations. In either case, all but a few provided little beyond nursing services in the hands of monks and nuns. All provided spiritual services, with a daily round of religious activities for both patients and staff. Also established was a tradition of giving donations for the care of the sick, a form of "good works as a means to salvation." The medieval hospital was important to the public as a means for giving charity (Rosen, 1963).

In the late Middle Ages, economic upheavals resulted in massive unemployment and the movement of populations from rural to urban areas. In addition to an increase in sickness, many persons feigned illness to improve their luck at begging. At the same time, there was a move afoot to challenge ecclesiastical authority. For these reasons, municipal authorities began to take over the administration of hospitals and to establish barriers to admission. The character of the hospital changed but little. What emerged was the modern "two lines of authority" wherein a lay or governmental body assumed responsibility for administration and another group was responsible for providing patient care (Rosen, 1963). The second group was still composed of churchmen for the most part.

The nineteenth century hospital

The rise of mercantilism in the seventeenth century led some people to view health as an important part of national policy. A healthy population was necessary for economic competition. The English poor law of 1601 set a structure for the identification of populations that were in need of medical service, and by the eighteenth century, local authorities were constructing hospitals at an increased rate (Rosen, 1963).

According to Rosen (1963:22-23), two main causes of expansive growth could be identified:

The great scientific outburst of the sixteenth and seventeenth centuries laid the foundation for the application of science to medical care, and increasingly knowledge of the structure of the human body was provided through dissection and observation by Vesalius, his contemporaries, and his successors . . . profound alterations in the economic life of the country necessarily disturbed its social structure and gave rise to a new attitude of mind toward problems of community life. Representing essentially the views of the middle classes, this distinctive ethos was characterized by two dominant facets: an insistence on order, efficiency, and social discipline, and a concern with the conditions of men.

In the United States, the first successful hospital was established in Philadelphia in 1751 by a group of Quakers led by Benjamin Franklin. In arguing for the creation of a public hospital, Franklin (1754) identified the following needs:

1. Poor people coming to the city in search of medical care had no place to stay.

2. The housing of the resident poor was such that they were "badly accommodated in sickness."

3. Those who had "lost their senses" had a tendency to wander about and terrorize their neighbors, and they could not be confined except in the prison.

4. It would be cheaper to care for the sick in one place rather than send help to their residences.

5. The middle class would be relieved of having to watch the poor die in the streets.

Two important developments were consolidated in the nineteenth century and have had a continued influence on the modern hospital. First, the type of hospital that was created differed from the earlier church- or government-owned model. Instead concerned citizens donated money and formed corporations that ran the hospitals as a public service on a nonprofit basis. Membership in the corporation was voluntary, and hospitals organized in this way became known as "voluntary hospitals." By the end of the nineteenth century, the voluntary hospital was the dominant form in the United States and of major importance in Europe.

Second, the voluntary hospital specialized in the care of acute, short-term illness. Partly because the knowledge base of medicine first allowed intervention in infectious disease at a time when the number of available hospital beds was limited, the decision was made to concentrate on those people who were curable. Those with incurable illnesses were denied admission and became the responsibility of governmental hospitals (Rosen, 1963; Stevens, 1971). The hospital became the source of specialist services for the poor; the rich saw specialists outside the hospital, and the middle class relied on general practitioners, being too poor to afford the specialist and not eligible for the voluntary hospital because of the means test that became almost universal (Stevens, 1971).

The twentieth century hospital

The modern hospital still shows its medieval origins. As discussed later, the organization of medical services is basically a feudal structure; medicine still has religious overtones in the ideology of service, the low pay traditional for hospital workers (although this has changed in recent years), and the monastic model used for medical training. From the nineteenth century, the voluntary model has been retained as the core of hospital organization, although other types are increasing in importance. The emphasis on acute illness and organization toward that end also remains a characteristic of the modern hospital, even in the face of dramatic changes in the pattern of disease outlined in Chapter 3.

What is new is that the hospital has become effective. As late as the turn of the century, hospitals provided a place where sick people could be housed. Although some knowledge about the human body and disease had been gathered, little was disseminated to the practitioner or the hospital. A large proportion of those who were hospitalized died in the hospital, frequently from diseases contracted as inpatients. Only within the last four decades has the hospital become an instrument of cure, in which most people admitted expect to get well and medical knowledge can be effectively mobilized. The remainder of this chapter will focus on the modern hospital.

TYPES OF HOSPITALS

The hospital is an organization that provides for people to have a place to sleep while being treated for a disease. Beyond this there is little that can be said that would apply uniformly to all organizations called "hospitals." That is, hospitals can be organized in many ways. Different investigators have tried to come to grips with the different organizational forms that are called "hospitals" by developing typologies. Hospitals have been classified according to their size, ownership, range of services offered, types of patients treated, type of financial support, and other dimensions (*Hospitals,* 1970; Croog and VerSteeg, 1972). Since we will be discussing hospitals as if they were a single entity at many points in this chapter, some important ways in which hospitals differ should be identified. Then the student will be better forearmed against overgeneralization.

Size

Hospitals range from organizations with only a few beds and one or two nurses to huge complexes with over a thousand beds and several thousand people on the staff in a large number of different occupations.

In general, the smaller the hospital and the fewer the services offered the more it is dependent on direct payment by the patient as a means of financing and the more personal are the services. Larger hospitals tend to be more bureaucratic, more dependent on third-party payment mechanisms, and more impersonal and provide a greater range of specialized services.

Ownership

Hospitals have been classified into three broad groups in response to legal needs arising from the increasing role played by third parties such as insurance companies. *Government* hospitals are those owned and operated by some unit of government, federal, state, or local. *Proprietary* hospitals are owned by a private corporation or partnership and are run so as to make a profit. *Voluntary* hospitals are run by a corporation on a not-for-profit basis (American Hospital Association, 1968).

Countries differ in the mix of these types. In some, all hospitals are governmental, as in various nationalized health services. In the United States at the federal level, military hospitals, Veterans Administration hospitals, and a few Public Health Service hospitals constitute the extent of government involvement. Most states have a system of mental hospitals and specialized facilities such as tuberculosis sanitoriums. Local governments differ, but most cities of over 100,000 population have either a municipal or county hospital.

Services

The range of services offered can also be used to classify hospitals. *General* hospitals provide a full range of general and specialty services, whereas *specialty* hospitals limit services to certain problems (obstetrical hospitals, tuberculosis sanitoriums, psychiatric hospitals) or to certain age groups (pediatric hospitals, geriatric hospitals) or to certain populations (veterans, merchant seamen).

Some caution must be used with reference to the term "general." Some hospitals that are called "general" do not deliver all types of medical and surgical services. The famous Massachusetts General Hospital in Boston, for example, does not provide obstetrical services. Most have some superspecialized services available but farm out others to avoid needless duplication of expensive equipment and personnel in any given area.

Training status

Some hospitals are teaching hospitals, whereas others are not. This usually means that the hospital has an affiliation agreement with a medical school and is used as a site for training medical students. Generally, many on the medical staff are the clinical faculty for the medical school. In addition, such hospitals may either have their own nursing school or have an affiliation with a university nursing school.

Biographical interest in patients

Rosengren and Lefton (1969) have classified hospitals according to their lateral and longitudinal interest in patient biographies. "Lateral interest" refers to the number of aspects of a patient's life that are considered relevant, in other words, to what extent they need to work with the whole patient. "Longitudinal interest" refers to the length of time they are typically in contact with a patient. Table 11-1 shows the four categories that this classification produces and gives examples of hospitals in each category. Rosengren and Lefton show how each of these categories has implications for "work

in hospitals, the substance of hospital life as it unfolds on a day to day basis, and for the hospital's relations to its external environment." Some of these findings are noted later in the chapter.

Our classification

Although in many ways the Rosengren and Lefton classification would be preferable and will be used from time to time, our discussion about hospitals will be based primarily on a modification of the American Hospital Association (AHA) classification. This is the one most frequently found in the literature and is selected for that reason. Four types of hospitals will be referred to as follows:

1. *Government.* This refers to any hospital that is owned and operated by any governmental agency be it national, state, county, or local. For the most part, these are general hospitals supported by tax revenue in addition to patient fees. Most are moderately large, are not affiliated with medical schools, and offer a broad range of commonly needed services.

2. *Community.* These are voluntary, nonprofit hospitals. Most are nonteaching, and the size range is across the full spectrum, from the smallest to the largest. Most teaching hospitals fall into this category.

3. *Proprietary.* These are like the community hospital except they are run for profit. Almost none are teaching hospitals. On the average, they are smaller than community or government hospitals.

4. *Specialty.* These are generally single

Table 11-1. Classification of hospitals by biographical interest in patients*

	Longitudinal interest	
Lateral interest	*Yes*	*No*
Yes	Long-term therapeutic hospital, some chronic illness hospitals	Short-term therapeutic psychiatric hospital
No	TB hospital, rehabilitation hospital, public health department, medical school	Acute general hospital emergency room

*From Rosengren, W., and Lefton, M. *Hospitals and patients.* New York: Atherton Press, 1969, p. 125.

service hospitals that limit practice to a single disease entity or a single age group.

IDEOLOGICAL ORIGINS OF THE MODERN HOSPITAL

The hospital at first glance seems to have been with us always in its present forms. Because the modern hospital has become such a powerful and autonomous determiner of the health care system, it is easy to lose sight of the fact that the modern hospital is the result of organizational evolution. The social and cultural environment of the hospital has had a profound effect on its modern forms, and perhaps the strongest yet least understood cultural force is ideology. Public notions about the nature of human responsibility to society, the causes and cures for disease, and ideas about the existential purpose of life are rooted in a culture and form the basic ideologic stance of a society.

As Glaser (1970) has pointed out, religion embodies these ideological stances; therefore religious ideology or dogma becomes an important determinant of the growth of modern hospitals. Ideological origins of the hospital can be found in religious beliefs and ideology.

Religious ideology concerning the causes of suffering and human accountability for the welfare of one's fellow traveler may lead religious groups within a society to assume responsibility for the care and cure of sick individuals. Indeed ancient Judaism expressed the ideology of disease as something mysteriously perpetrated on a powerless people by God who is seeking atonement for sins by means of physical suffering. Intervention is called for by Judaic ideology through which God commands adherents to love one's neighbor and to distribute good fortune among all needy people, including the sick. Since the treatment of the sick person's morals was considered necessary, given the idea that disease and sin were interrelated, hospitals were developed within Jewish societies even though Jews were living in tenuous circumstances without a homeland. Once Jews returned to Israel, modern hospitals developed rapidly in harmony with Jewish religious dogma.

Western Christianity embodied the same charitable and social commitments as Judaism. A key difference in the two religious and a major ideological force of Western Christianity was the idea of religious conquest. Conversion of non-Christians was, and still is for that matter, a major ideological thrust of most Christian denominations. This was related intimately with the involvement of Church organization in the political processes of the state.

Conversion and the establishment of religious beachheads within hostile countries provided the stimulus for Christian churches to establish institutions, including hospitals, to protect the converts and to attract new adherents. For example, the Congress of Vienna in 1814 had created a situation in which hundreds of thousands of Rhineland Catholics suddenly found themselves in the enlarged Protestant state of Prussia. Hostile relations between Prussia and the Church developed, which led to a six-year face-off between elements of the papal, Austrian, and French armies in the Papal States. Under these types of threatening conditions, religious orders assumed the role of protector of the health and welfare of their adherents.

Furthermore, the rise of Calvin and Lutheran ideology appealed along class rather than national or even religious lines. This ideology fitted nicely with the rising aspirations and expectations of the burgeoning middle class. It became evident that the good life, that is, material success, was enhanced if disease was controlled. Hospitals grew out of religious commitment to promote wealth seeking, and thus religious orders built hospitals along the trade routes and commercial areas of Europe during the sixteenth and seventeenth centuries.

Christianity was most successful in repressing the ideological basis for folk medicine among the converts in Europe and early American society. This had the effect of increasing the importance of scientific medicine and hospitals by decreasing the salience of folk curing in the home.

In contrast to the tight organizational linkages between Christianity and hospital growth, Buddhism and Hinduism profess ideologies that stress the autonomy of the individual. The individual is responsible for self-improvement, which is seen as the path to Nirvana. Furthermore, poverty and the rejection of worldly possessions is a major facet of Buddhist and Hindu ideology. This made it difficult for believers to engage in the kinds of financial and political processes necessary to organize and maintain hospitals.

Finally, the rigid caste system of Hinduism coupled with ideological taboos preventing cross-caste interaction made it exceedingly difficult for hospitals to be organized. Workers from different castes would have great difficulty working together, and the patient-healer relationship would be strained severely if caste differences intruded. Indian hospitals appeared occasionally out of political necessity or edict but eventually they disappeared.

Religious ideology and correlated political and social exigencies helped to foster hospital growth, or it served as an impediment as in India, for example. In most industrial countries the religious ownership of the hospital eventually transferred to local, state, or federal government, if not to private corporate entities. In several countries, notably Ethiopia, one or more religious denominations run the majority of the country's hospitals. This is usually a facet of the missionary activities of the church.

Nevertheless, religious ideology has played a major role in the development of the modern hospital. Even today concepts of charity and neighborly accountability provide an important impetus for the maintenance of hospital organization as a central component of the health care system.

THE ECOLOGY OF THE HOSPITAL

In this section, some patterns that characterize hospitals as they relate to their physical and social environments will be described. This descriptive ecology of the hospital is important, since it helps one discover explanations of why hospitals behave as they do. In looking at the ecology of the hospital, data are presented on location, changes in hospital size and type, changes in utilization, and the hospital labor force.

Location

There are over 7,481 hospitals in the United States (National Center for Health Statistics, 1974). The geographical distribution of these hospitals reflects the structured inequality endemic to the American medical care system. Many communities and entire regions of the country are underserved or not served at all medically due in large measure to the dearth of hospitals in these areas. Rural and inner-city areas are where the most serious shortages of medical manpower and hospitals exist (Hassinger and Hobbs, 1972). Two major reasons for the unequal distribution of hospitals are as follows: (1) difficulty in attracting medical professionals to a given area because of economic and/or cultural barriers, and (2) the economic variables associated with hospital support, particularly the economic potential of the residents of the area and the financial resources of the community decision elites responsible for generating and maintaining hospital support at the community level. In rural and inner-city areas, it is difficult to attract health practitioners, and economic factors equally are problematic.

Table 11-2 presents the hospital distribution by geographic area for the United States. This table examines states in terms of the number of beds per 1,000 population. With a few exceptions such as West Virginia, Wyoming, and South Dakota, the heavily populated industrial states such as New York, District of Columbia, and Massachusetts have the highest total bed rates. This is in marked contrast to the rural states, which rank the lowest in terms of hospital beds per 1,000 population. Suburban areas on the fringes of large cities have captured a lion's share of hospital services because the pattern of location for

Table 11-2. Hospital beds per 1,000 population by state: 1972*

State	Total hospital beds†	General medical and surgical	Specialty				
			Total	Psychi-atric	Chronic disease	Tubercu-losis	Other‡
United States	7.0	4.9	2.2	1.8	0.1	0.1	0.2
Alabama	7.2	5.0	2.2	2.0	—	0.2	0.0
Alaska	5.4	4.6	0.7	0.7	—	—	0.0
Arizona	5.5	4.8	0.7	0.6	—	0.1	0.0
Arkansas	5.7	5.3	0.4	0.3	—	0.1	0.0
California	5.6	4.4	1.2	0.8	—	0.0	0.4
Colorado	6.4	5.0	1.4	1.1	—	—	0.3
Connecticut	6.2	4.0	2.3	1.7	0.4	—	0.1
Delaware	7.8	4.2	3.6	2.0	1.0	—	0.6
District of Columbia	16.5	10.1	6.3	5.0	—	—	1.4
Florida	6.7	5.1	1.6	1.4	—	0.1	0.0
Georgia	7.1	4.7	2.3	2.2	—	0.1	0.1
Hawaii	5.8	4.0	1.8	0.5	0.3	0.4	0.7
Idaho	4.9	4.3	0.6	0.5	—	—	0.0
Illinois	7.1	5.1	2.0	1.6	0.2	0.1	0.1
Indiana	6.3	4.3	2.0	1.7	0.0	0.0	0.2
Iowa	7.0	5.9	1.0	0.9	—	0.1	0.0
Kansas	7.6	6.2	1.5	1.4	0.1	0.0	0.0
Kentucky	5.9	4.6	1.2	0.9	—	0.1	0.2
Louisiana	6.7	4.9	1.8	1.3	—	0.1	0.4
Maine	7.7	5.5	2.2	2.0	0.2	—	—
Maryland	6.7	3.6	3.2	2.4	0.4	0.1	0.3
Massachusetts	9.1	4.9	4.2	2.7	1.0	0.0	0.4
Michigan	6.4	4.6	1.8	1.7	0.1	—	0.1
Minnesota	7.5	6.0	1.5	1.2	—	0.0	0.2
Mississippi	7.7	5.3	2.4	2.3	0.0	0.1	0.0
Missouri	7.7	5.7	2.0	1.6	—	0.1	0.4
Montana	6.8	6.1	0.7	—	0.3	0.4	—
Nebraska	7.6	6.7	1.0	1.0	—	—	0.0
Nevada	5.7	4.6	1.1	1.0	—	—	0.1
New Hampshire	7.1	4.7	2.5	2.5	—	—	—
New Jersey	6.7	4.0	2.7	2.5	0.1	—	0.1
New Mexico	5.7	4.5	1.3	0.8	0.3	—	0.2
New York	8.8	5.0	3.9	3.3	0.3	0.0	0.3
North Carolina	6.4	4.3	2.1	1.8	0.0	0.2	0.1
North Dakota	8.4	6.9	1.5	1.5	—	—	—
Ohio	6.6	4.6	2.0	1.8	0.1	0.0	0.1
Oklahoma	6.6	5.0	1.6	1.4	0.1	0.1	0.1
Oregon	5.6	4.3	1.3	1.3	—	—	0.0
Pennsylvania	8.5	5.1	3.4	2.5	0.2	0.1	0.6
Rhode Island	8.3	5.3	2.9	2.2	0.5	—	0.2
South Carolina	7.2	4.7	2.5	2.3	0.0	0.1	0.0

*From National Center for Health Statistics. *Health resources statistics.* Washington, D.C.: United States Government Printing Office, 1974, pp. 364-365.
†Preliminary data.
‡Includes eye, ear, nose, and throat hospitals; epileptic hospitals; alcoholism hospitals; narcotic hospitals; maternity hospitals; orthopedic hospitals; physical rehabilitation hospitals; and other hospitals.

Continued.

Table 11-2. Hospital beds per 1,000 population by state: 1972—cont'd

State	Total hospital beds	General medical and surgical	Specialty				
			Total	Psychi- atric	Chronic disease	Tubercu- losis	Other
South Dakota	9.4	6.7	2.7	2.6	—	—	0.1
Tennessee	7.4	5.4	2.1	1.7	0.2	0.2	0.1
Texas	6.5	5.0	1.4	1.2	—	0.1	0.1
Utah	4.4	3.9	0.5	0.3	0.2	—	0.0
Vermont	7.7	5.1	2.6	2.6	—	—	—
Virginia	7.1	4.7	2.4	2.2	—	0.1	0.1
Washington	5.3	4.1	1.2	1.1	—	0.1	0.0
West Virginia	9.1	6.3	2.8	2.4	0.3	0.1	0.0
Wisconsin	8.2	5.4	2.8	2.4	0.0	0.0	0.3
Wyoming	8.2	5.6	2.6	2.6	—	—	—

inner-city hospitals has been to follow the exodus of people and money from the inner city to the suburbs.

Changes in hospital size and type

Perhaps the most dramatic changes in hospital organization and ecology have to do with hospital size and type. Since 1967 there has been a large decrease in the number of hospitals with a corresponding decrease in bed capacity. Between 1967 and 1969 there was a decrease of 371 hospitals; tuberculosis, geriatric, psychiatric, and other specialty hospitals were losing ground fast in terms of loss of both hospitals and beds. However, although general hospitals are losing facilities, they are gaining beds. This leads to an important point regarding changes in hospital size. The greatest loss of hospitals is occurring among those with smaller bed capacities. In fact almost all the losses are occurring in hospitals with less than a hundred beds. Conversely, hospitals with a hundred or more beds are on the increase, with the trend moving in the direction of ever larger hospital facilities.

The greatest decrease in hospitals is occurring in proprietary hospitals with less than a hundred beds. Nonprofit hospitals with less than a hundred beds also are on the wane but at a much slower rate than proprietary hospitals. On the other hand, the largest increases in hospitals are with government-operated facilities, either municipal, county, state, or federal. There has been little change in proprietary hospitals with a hundred beds or more, and nonprofit hospitals with 100 or more beds gained sixty-four hospitals between 1967 and 1969. During 1973 the average number of beds for community hospitals rose 26% from 123 beds to 155 beds (American Hospital Association, 1974). In 1963, 37% of all community hospitals had less than fifty beds, and only 9% had 300 or more beds in 1963. However, in 1973, 15% had 300 or more beds, which is a 60% increase (American Hospital Association, 1974). Therefore it is important to recognize that hospital size is a vital factor in stabilizing or promoting change among hospitals.

Changes in utilization

Are Americans increasingly becoming prone to illnesses that require hospitalization, or has third-party medical insurance (Medicaid, Medicare, Blue Cross) created a climate in which it is all too easy and convenient to hospitalize patients? These questions are salient because the decade 1963 to 1973 has witnessed unparalleled increases in admissions to hospitals. In 1973 admissions to AHA-registered hospitals totaled 34.4 million, a 3.3% increase over 1972 and a 24.9% increase over 1963 (American Hospital Association, 1974). Much of this increase occurred in community general hospitals. At the same time, the number of inpatient days decreased 8.4 million days from 433.7 million days in 1963. This means that there are more admissions all the time but that patients are staying in the hospital for much shorter lengths of time.

Again hospital size is an important factor, since community general hospitals with less than fifty beds experienced decreases in average daily inpatient censuses, whereas all other types of hospitals, including community hospitals, showed increases if they had fifty or more beds. Furthermore, the average length of stay is related to hospital size; one finds an increase in length of stay from small hospitals (7.1 days) to large hospitals (10.3 days). In short, the larger the hospital the longer the patients stay (National Center for Health Statistics, 1974). However, ownership enters the picture. Smaller hospitals decrease their average lengths of stay as they move from voluntary to governmental ownership, whereas large hospitals increase their average lengths of stay for the same types of ownership.

Although inpatient admissions to AHA-registered hospitals increased by 3.3% between 1972 and 1973, the increase in outpatient visits rose to 233.6 million in 1973, a 6.6% increase over 1972 (American Hospital Association, 1974). Almost 75% of all the visits were to community hospitals

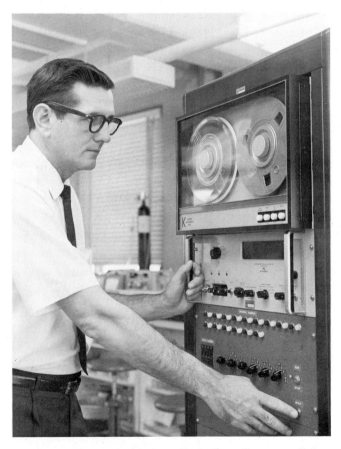

Fig. 11-1. *The computer has improved the technical quality of medicine, although for some it symbolizes the depersonalization of care.*

(Courtesy University of Missouri Medical Center, Columbia, Mo.)

where outpatient clinic visits represented 31.5%; referred visits, 33.1%; and visits to emergency rooms, 35.4%. For noncommunity hospitals, outpatient clinics take almost 79% of outpatient visits and emergency rooms get only 7.5% outpatient visits. For community general hospitals, the fastest growing services are abortion services (the second most frequently performed surgery in the United States in 1974), genetic counseling, renal dialysis, speech therapy, and social work services.

Clearly the trend among hospitals is toward larger, short-term, community- and government-owned hospitals. The growth of hospitals follows a pattern in which facilities and services are added and hospitals become more and more complex. Over the past several years this has been a trend, particularly in community hospitals, to offer more varied services and facilities. The services in turn require even more complex

technological equipment (Fig. 11-1), more physical space, and increased medical personnel of all types, particularly technicians.

There is a strong correlation between the bed size of hospitals and the types of facilities and services offered (Berry, 1973). The larger the bed size of the hospital the more likely it has particular facilities and services. For example, in a forty-five–bed, basic service hospital, it would be unlikely to find physical therapy services or other services that require complex technologies and highly specialized personnel. Fig. 11-2 portrays this relationship between bed size and facilities and services. For example, only 1.9% of hospitals with six to twenty-four beds offered occupational therapy services as compared to 78.2% of those with 500 or more beds. This relationship holds true for all services and facilities that require advanced and complex technologies and specially trained medical personnel.

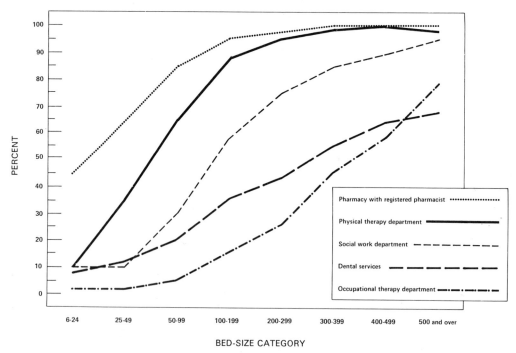

Fig. 11-2. *Percent of community hospitals reporting selected facilities and services by bed-size category, 1973.* (**From American Hospital Association.** *Hospital statistics.* **Chicago: The Association, 1974.**)

The hospital labor force

The fact that health care in the United States is one of the largest industries should come as no surprise in light of the fact that more than 3,045,515 persons, full-time and part-time, were employed at AHA-registered hospitals in 1973 (American Hospital Association, 1974). This number does not include interns, residents, and other trainees. The number of full-time equivalent (FTE) employees was 2.8 million in 1973.

The number of FTE personnel has increased greatly every year since 1967, except in hospitals with less than fifty beds. As the size of the hospital increases, the number of FTE personnel per 100 average daily patient census increases also. The larger the hospital the fewer the number of part-time workers in proportion to full-time employees.

The increases in FTE personnel have occurred in general community hospitals and noncommunity hospitals at a slower rate. The increase in the number of employees has been greater than the increase in the average daily patient census, and the ratio of full-time employees per patient has been steadily increasing.

A hospital is a labor-intensive organization. This means that labor costs represent the largest category of expenditures for hospitals. Salaries for hospital personnel have risen steadily since 1967 (Table 11-3). The increase for 1973 was 4.5%, the lowest in several years, and this lower rate is the probable result of the wage-and-price controls instituted as part of the fight against inflation and recession in the United States. Over the years, larger hospitals show greater percentage increases in salary, perhaps reflecting the fact that larger hospitals are usually located in metropolitan areas where the cost of living is high and inflation is more keenly felt by the hospital employees. Also larger hospitals have a greater need for specialized and highly skilled personnel to run the complex technology. This inflates the labor costs as well.

HOSPITAL ORGANIZATION
Hospitals and the model of bureaucracy

In the nineteenth century Max Weber noted the emergence of a new form of social organization that seemed to be becoming dominant in modern societies irrespective of political ideology. This organization type was characterized by several features that were markedly different from those typical of feudal organizations. "Bureaucracies," the name given to these types of organizations, were ordered into a set of offices, or positions. Each office had a fixed jurisdiction governed by a set of rules. Offices were ordered into a system of authority in which

Table 11-3. Percentage increase in average annual salary of employees in community hospitals, by bed-size category: 1968-1973*

Bed-size category	Percentage increase					
	1968-1969	*1969-1970*	*1970-1971*	*1971-1972*	*1972-1973*	*1968-1973*
Total (all beds)	9.4	10.1	10.3	8.0	4.5	49.8
6-24	4.0	19.5	10.6	0.5	3.3	42.7
25-49	6.9	12.3	8.9	4.1	4.0	41.5
50-99	12.0	8.0	7.8	5.7	4.3	43.7
100-199	8.7	9.4	8.5	7.1	5.6	46.0
200-299	10.4	10.0	8.6	7.3	4.5	47.8
300-399	10.2	9.2	10.8	8.4	2.7	48.4
400-499	8.0	10.3	11.8	7.3	5.4	50.6
500 and over	7.4	10.6	11.7	9.3	4.2	51.0

*From American Hospital Association. *Hospital statistics.* Chicago: The Association, 1974.

each was responsible for the supervision of a set of lower offices and reported to a higher one. The work of the office was recorded in and to some degree governed by a set of files. The person occupying each office was selected on the basis of qualifications obtained by special training and was expected to give his full working capacity to the position. Finally, management of the office followed a set of finite and learnable rules (Gerth and Mills, 1946).

Thus according to Weber's model, bureaucracy is a hierarchical system of offices in which power is centralized, final decision making is concentrated at the top of a pyramid, and job specifications are routinized and codified (Beavert, 1972). Several investigators have noted that this model is limited, and much of the work of any large scale organization is accomplished through "bureaucracy's other face," the informal structures that emerge from interpersonal relationships on the job and that have little to do with the official organizational chart (Blau, 1955, 1956; Litwak, 1961). As observed by Rosengren and Lefton (1969:49-50), the bureaucratic model is concerned with organization for work rather than the performance of work:

Hence a parody of such a study of hospitals would yield a description of a hospital unrelated to the larger social order in which it resides, which operates with reference to uniformly applied criteria of efficiency and rationality, which contains no doctors or nurses except as they are involved in the administration of work rules, and finally, a hospital which has no patients.

Hudson (1971) has delineated two models of complex organization that parallel to some degree the work reported by Litwak (1961). One of these approximates the Weberian model and is called a "serial structure." Serial structures are characterized as a one-dimensional communication structure in which messages flow up and down a hierarchy. Authority is vested in positions, and the failure of any member of the work group becomes a failure of the whole group. The activities of groups organized in this

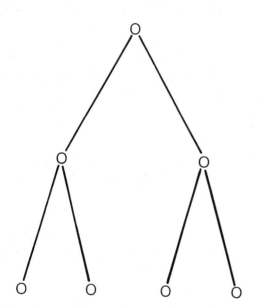

Fig. 11-3. *Serial structure.* (From Hudson, J. B. *Innovation and creativity.* Presented at the meeting of the Eastern Sociological Society, New York, 1971.)

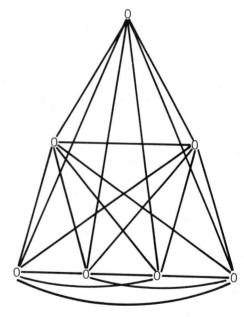

Fig. 11-4. *Parallel structure.* (From Hudson, J. B. *Innovation and creativity.* Presented at the meeting of the Eastern Sociological Society, New York, 1971.)

way tend to be routine, incremental, and repetitive as on an industrial assembly line (Fig. 11-3).

The other model, called a "parallel structure," represents the other polar extreme. Although there may be a hierarchy, its existence does not prejudice the flow of communications. Any member of the group is free to communicate with any other member in either a horizontal or vertical direction (Fig. 11-4). Authority does not vest in positions but in the occupants of those positions, placing the emphasis on personal competence rather than location in the hierarchy. Failures of individuals are less consequential, since the success of any member of the group is a success for all. These structures tend to be found when the product is not routine or repetitive and when close coordination and control are not crucial to the continuity of operations.

Both these models are approximated by different parts of the typical hospital irrespective of type. Where the models are found in the activities of the organization and the relations among different sectors of the hospital are strongly influenced by their joint operation.

Hospital administration: serial structure

Certain tasks in the hospital are routine and repetitive. Housekeeping chores, food preparation, billing, the filing of insurance forms and reports, the scheduling of elective surgery, the processing of laboratory specimens, and purchasing fit this category, and all approximate a serial model. Hence the hospital administration tends to be adequately described by Weber's characterization of bureaucracy. There is a hierarchy with an objective of "communication, control, and the centralization of information for effective decision making and for the operationalizing of central decisions" (Rosengren and Lefton, 1969).

One important consequence is that the whole hospital seems to the administrator to be based on this model as illustrated in Fig. 11-3. It is also important that efficiency, accountability, and cost control are central concerns of the administration, all of which require routinization and the orderly adherence to rules.

Medical services and wards: parallel structures

The hospital looks different in the settings where patient care is carried out. With regard to organization, the presence of patients demands a different strategy (Rosengren and Lefton, 1969). For one thing, the product is not standardized. Patients can be admitted with virtually any disease, some of them rare. The staff must be able to differentiate its response and tailor its activities to the needs of each patient. Furthermore, how each patient responds to treatment, holding disease process constant, is variable, calling for adaptability in the way in which each is handled. Relative to administrative activities, the staff activities are holistic, nonsegmented, and unstructured (Beavert, 1972).

On most hospital wards there is a hierarchy. The chief resident in charge of the service (e.g., medicine, surgery) has responsibility for patient care but seldom directly intervenes in the management of cases. Under him,[1] is the assistant resident, who supervises the interns, who give orders to the head nurse. In most settings, there is a good deal of communication among all these positions, and all participate in making decisions relative to patient care (Coser, 1958).

Communication patterns differ between medical and surgical services. The medical service is more likely to have extended discussion about patients and the alternatives for treatment, and all medical staff tend to participate in that discussion. At the same time, there is less communication between physicians and nurses. Much more interaction between physicians and nurses is typical of surgical settings, but there is less discussion of patient care alternatives among physicians (Coser, 1958).

The authority patterns of the hospital ward are not easily summarized. From a legal point of view, the chief of service and the chief resident are responsible for the care of each patient. In fact, authority is delegated downward. Again medical and surgical services typically differ. Decision making on the medical service is more of a collective process, with the final decision being delegated to the intern or resident in charge of each case. On the surgery service, decisions are made by fiat passed down from the chief resident, who reserves for himself the most interesting cases and allows the assistant resident and intern to participate only in the more routine procedures. Coser (1958) argues that "decision by consensus is time consuming," and surgery requires quick decisions as compared with medicine.

Further complicating the picture, it is often difficult to tell who has the right to make what decisions just from knowing formal positions in the hospital structure. Although it is true that certain decisions such as prescriptions are reserved to physicians by law, it is frequently the case that medication changes will be first suggested by nurses, or physicians will leave standing orders that give nurses considerable discretion in the use of drugs. Furthermore, among medical personnel, senior staff members observe the behavior of junior staff members and delegate to them tasks that they seem capable of handling. Authority is thus elastic, depending on demonstrated competence (Stelling and Bucher, 1972), and occupants of the same formal position may vary considerably in what the informal system allows them to do. The greater delegation on medical services makes the situation among junior staff more competitive, whereas the greater centralization on the surgical service results in a "negative democratization," which produces greater colleagueship among junior staff and between staff and nurses (Coser, 1958).

The reward structure is such that any staff member who comes up with a treatment that works has produced a success for the ward as a whole. Hence no occupation values individual responsibility and autonomy more than physicians (Freidson and Rhea, 1963; Freidson, 1970). The name of the game is prestige, which comes from the esteem of colleagues. This in turn requires successes that cannot be achieved without some willingness to take risk.

In summary, medical services of the hospital are totally under the control of physicians who act as a collegial body on decisions affecting the treatment of patients. The formal organization of treatment activities of the hospital is in terms of services such as medicine, surgery, psychiatry, and pediatrics, which have a physician head who supervises colleagues. Authority, which varies by service, rests with the medical profession, and a separation of treatment from administration exists not only in terms of personnel but also in terms of organizational models.

The interplay of structures

As Litwak (1961) has suggested, the simultaneous existence of two organizational models is typical of professional bureaucracies. Furthermore, whenever this dual model situation exists, it is necessary for there to be some "mechanism" for relating the two "conflicting forces" so that they can be "harnessed to organizational goals." He suggested four such mechanisms: (1) role separation, in which different people performed different tasks or there was agreement that different models would apply to different activities; (2) physical distance, in which some activities are spatially removed from others; (3) transferral occupations, which specialize in communication between the two models without contaminating either; and (4) evaluation procedures, which allow decisions to be made on a case-to-case basis as to which model is most appropriate.

Role separation has been the most common mechanism in the hospital, and evaluation is becoming increasingly important. Administrators are responsible for the routine functioning of the physical plant, the processing of routine reports, and other similar activities. They have no role at all with reference to the treatment of patients. The medical staff, on the other hand, takes no interest in the hospital routine and concentrates solely on patient care. This produces a unique situation, since costs and activities of the hospital become defined as outside the purview of the administration. More than anything else, this differentiates hospital administration from other organizations. Administrators are responsible for a budget, although they have no control over either the income or expenditures of the organization, which is determined by the medical activities.

This is increasingly an untenable situation. With the rapid escalation of costs, it has become necessary to gain control over medical activities to avoid bankrupting the system. Increased use is being made of evaluation procedures in which some form of medical audit is made of activities. Generally, a committee of professionals is created to exercise peer review. This keeps control in the hands of physicians while mandating some attention to the economics of patient care. Whether such procedures will be effective remains to be demonstrated, although there is reason to doubt that they will have a great impact. The claim of therapeutic need is compelling in any hospital. Failing that, the claim of emergency is unanswerable. Hence it seems doubtful that administrators will be more than marginally successful in asserting budgetary authority.

As Osler Peterson observed to one of us (A. C. T.) several years ago, "The hospital is not an organization as you might expect. It is a loose confederation of feudal barons."

LINKAGES TO THE OUTSIDE

Hospitals are linked to the communities in which they are situated in two principle ways. One is through those services which interface with the community and constitute the points of entry into the hospital by the populations being served. Outpatient clinics are the main vehicle for this linkage. The other is in the relationships between the hospital and other organizations that provide human services which either are jointly used by the client population (welfare agencies, the judicial system) or which directly support the patient in seeking medical care (insurance companies, departments of public health).

Outpatient clinics

There are two basic types of clinics in most large hospitals: the emergency (or accident) room, which is designed to meet acute crisis needs but is increasingly a source of general practice; and the ambulatory care clinic, which provides the kinds of services usually found in office practices but is oriented toward low socioeconomic status populations.

Emergency rooms. Emergency rooms of large hospitals are designed to provide for crisis management of serious, sudden onset, medical and surgical problems, such as accident-induced trauma (Gibson, 1974). How different hospitals do this is highly variable. Emergency rooms range from elaborate trauma centers, which mobilize the most sophisticated technology available to stabilize and treat persons with severe injuries, to those consisting of a single room with virtually no equipment. The lack of standards has posed some serious practical problems that are now being addressed by various groups (American Medical Association, 1971; Boyd et al., 1973; Gibson, 1974). Although several plans are being tried, no studies of their effectiveness have yet been published.

An important recent development is a shift in the use of emergency rooms, particularly in urban hospitals in the United States, creating a disjunction between the intended purpose of the service and its actual application (Weinerman et al., 1966). Increasingly patients are visiting the emergency room for routine care that might be expected in either a physician's office or an ambulatory clinic. Although this has caused much unhappiness among emergency room staffs, the reasons are apparent. In many parts of the country, including the inner cities, physicians are increasingly scarce. Those that are available are increasingly in bureaucratized practices with regular hours, and there are periods of unavailability, most notably in the evenings and on weekends. As a result the emergency room is for many people the only place in which physicians can be found at times when people are free to seek care. It is a reflection of the changes in the medical care system that have not adequately taken into account the needs of the population served.

Ambulatory clinics. With the decline of private practice in many areas, there has been an expansion of outpatient departments, or ambulatory clinics, in an attempt to provide comprehensive care to certain populations. In this, the hospital is developing an important interface with the surrounding community that helps to blur the boundaries at the hospital door by providing a direct service to people who are not inpatients. This can be seen as an effort of the hospitals to fill the gap left by the abdication of private physicians in caring for the poor. As an exercise in providing relatively complete medical service, however, the ambulatory clinic faces important limitations rooted partly in its own history and partly in the organization of most clinics relative to the rest of the hospital.

The ambulatory clinic was designed in the nineteenth century as a device for providing the hospital-based physician with a pool of cases for teaching purposes. Such a pool allowed for selective admissions to the hospital of interesting cases that could most benefit from inpatient treatment. Hence the physician could ensure more successes, have the subjects available for research, and create an adequate supply of teaching material. Patient care was low on the list of priorities (Abel-Smith and Pinker, 1964; Goodrich et al., 1972).

In most hospitals, ambulatory clinics remain the stepchild of the inpatient services. Staffing for the most part is by physicians who have their major commitment to in-hospital treatment but are required to spend a limited amount of time each week in a clinic run by their specialty. Much of the work of such clinics is given over to follow-up care of former inpatients. Clinic work is considered to be less interesting and important, particularly in university, teaching hospitals where clinic work receives less recognition (Nathanson and Becker, 1973). Partly because of this, physicians are willing to surrender more control of activities to other staff in such settings, making clinics a center for innovation in the organization of health services. For example, it is in clinics that nurses have often been demonstrated to be equal to if not superior to physicians in the management of patients (Lewis and Resnik, 1967; Gordon, 1974).

The continued movement of private practice out of the central cities and rural areas coupled with increasing costs of health care exert pressures toward the expansion of hospital-based ambulatory services. Such services can greatly reduce the need for hospitalization (Bellin et al., 1969), which is the single greatest source of inflation in medical prices. It is to be expected that changes in the status and organization of outpatient departments will be increasingly frequent, and they should be monitored by sociologists interested in social change.

Resource control

One of the most important but least understood sociological issues concerning hospitals is the question of the relationship of the hospital to the network of health care organizations in the external environment. How does the hospital fit within the environment of other hospitals, clinics, pharmacies, and other health care facilities? The survival of the organization depends on how well this issue of fit with the environment is met. Ultimately survival becomes a question of developing a strategy for resource control in a threatening environment made up of scarce resources.

The hospital can respond to this challenge of resource control by relating to external organizations in one of three basic ways: cooperating, coordinating, or differentiating. Hospital mergers and the sharing of services among two or more hospitals are examples of cooperation and coordination. For example, two hospitals in fairly close physical proximity can effect large savings if they share the cost of laundry or kitchen services rather than attempt to maintain their own separate facilities. By merging, hospitals can consolidate administrative costs and increase bed capacity without a costly building program.

Whereas cooperation and coordination are reasonably clear-cut processes in which an organization negotiates with the external environment for survival, differentiation is much more difficult to study and to understand. Differentiation as a strategy for survival is the opposite of coordination and cooperation. Here the response to social or economic threat in the external environment is to emphasize those qualities of the hospital which set it apart from other health care organizations. Rather than take the view that "we're all in this together so let's cooperate," the hospital that chooses the strategy of differentiation views other health care organizations as competitors for the scarce resources available. Differentiating means that the hospital strives to distinguish itself from all the other organizations.

One way to do this is for the hospital to develop unique, highly prestigeful, and highly complex technological services. This is discussed later as the theory of conspicuous production wherein the hospital attempts to outclass its competitors by having the biggest and the best.

Another approach, one that usually occurs alongside the conspicuous production strategy, is the management or control of the hospital support structure (Elling and Halebsky, 1961). This support structure consists of community power elites who, because of their wealth, high status, and influence, are able to generate dollars, investment opportunities, and public support for the hospital. Through the process of differentiation, the hospital seeks to become tied to the destiny of community power elites. This is accomplished by having elites on the hospital board of directors and by the hospital administration publicly representing the core ideologies of these elites. The overall purpose of the hospital is to strive for dominance over other health care organizations, and the most powerful members of the community become part of the means by which the hospital dominates and controls local health care resources.

MOTIVATIONS OF HOSPITAL BEHAVIOR

The question "What motivates organization decision makers to make the decisions they do?" is much more difficult to answer for hospitals than it is for business organizations. Hospitals do not produce a product that can be governed by the economic processes of efficiency, supply, and demand. Rather hospitals produce services that must be delivered at the local level, since the health care service market is a local market. In this sense, hospital services cannot be exported long distances as compared to business products. For this reason, hospital behavior is first and foremost motivated by the need to bring producers and consumers of the services together, face-to-face, and under one roof. This means that the size of the hospital market is always limited by the time and distance it takes to bring producers and consumers together. The factors that motivate hospital behavior revolve around the issue of producers and consumers. The major explanations of hospital behavior involve the producer or consumer of the services or both in their calculi.

Income and revenues

The income and revenue approach to explaining hospital behavior simply states that hospital beds are used the way they are because of consumer demand and the hospital's desire to maximize revenues and profits. An example of this school of thought is Rice's sales maximization model (1966) of the hospital, supported by Davis' study, in which hospitals strive to maximize profits by concentrating on the demand and the quatity of output. This approach measures the worth of hospital activity in terms of beds, average daily patient census, and profits. According to this approach, supply is determined by consumer demand, which is driven by biological need (Normile, 1969).

Complexity

But do hospitals maximize revenues and profits? Does the hospital build bed capacity in response to consumer biological needs? Recent research suggests that hospital behavior is not driven by these factors, and consequently the income and revenue approach is a partial explanation of hospital behavior, at best. One study was unable to demonstrate that consumer health or disease was a determinant in the demand for beds (Rosenthal, 1964), and Ro's excellent analysis of hospital use (1969) arrived at the same conclusion. In fact, Roemer and Elling (1963) concluded that there is no ceiling on demand, and the more beds there are the more people are hospitalized to fill them. Roemer and Elling studied a county in the United States that for years had a hospital bed supply of 2.8 per 1,000. At this rate, the occupancy rate was 78%. The bed supply was precipitously increased to 3.2 per 1,000, the utilization rate rose 38%, and length of stay increased for forty out of fifty-three diagnoses. "You build a bed, you fill a bed, "as long as the third-party economic incentives are viable. In short, the supply of beds creates the demand (Newell, 1964).

As bed capacity increases, hospital facilities and services become more complex. Furthermore, this complexity reaches a stage at which revenues are high but profits and particularly efficiency are reduced. Berry (1973) concluded that one is able to predict, given the number of beds in a hospital, at which point specific facilities are added and the scope of the services provided. Berry defined the hospital as a multiproduct firm of teaching, research, and patient care, and hospital behavior, seen as the mix of the products, can best be explained by identifying the complexity and scope of hospital facilities and services.

Berry discovered that there was a pattern to the growth of facilities and services. For example, five services are established by all hospitals early so that by the time a hospital has six facilities, chances are good that it will already offer an x-ray diagnostic service, clinical laboratory, emergency room, operating room, and delivery room. According to Berry's research, these basic-service hospitals have small capacities of around forty-five beds. It is not until a hospital has twenty-five or more facilities that a big jump in the complexity of services occurs. These are 230-plus–bed hospitals that offer, in addition to all the basic services, more complex services such as outpatient care, physical therapy and rehabilitation, home care, social services, and others.

More importantly he found that the complexity of hospital services is related to several efficiency factors. As the product mix changes from basic-service hospitals to more complex community-service hospitals, that is, as hospitals became more complex the following efficiency factors are affected:

1. Increase in number of patients treated (admission and total patient days)
2. Increase in mean number of patient days
3. Increase in average length of stay
4. Increase in occupancy rates
5. Increase in labor and capital required per unit of labor

In contrast to smaller ones, larger, more complex hospitals cost the medical care system more in terms of dollars and time for patients and medical personnel alike.

The complexity approach is useful for describing the process whereby supply creates its own demand over and above questions of profit maximization and efficiency. What this approach does not explain is what in fact motivates hospitals to expand acute inpatient facilities at technological and and human cost untempered by considerations of benefits. Why do general hospitals expand exotic technologies within a medical care arena where the vast majority of the population needs more mundane health services for chronic disease, emotional problems, and health maintenance?

The answer may lie at least in part in the theory of status gap minimization.

Status gap minimization

The income and revenue approach and the complexity approach to explaining hospital behavior assume that the hospital is a firm motivated by profit maximization, and inputs are acquired to meet the production functions necessary to ensure top profits. An alternative theory of hospital behavior has been developed by Lee (1971, 1975) who challenges the traditional neoclassical economic approach that has formed the basis for so much research on hospital behavior. Lee's approach is much more sociological, since it is assumed that hospital decision makers operate to produce conspicuously to maximize status and prestige rather than profits. This idea is based on organizational theory, which argues that the salary, prestige, power, and status of the organization's decision makers are important determinants of the functions of the organization (Thompson, 1961; Simon, 1965; Barnard, 1968). Lee assumes that the status and prestige of the hospital becomes a goal among hospital administrators and medical decision makers that produces competition among hospitals, not for profits but for status. Drawing on Veblen's concept of conspicuous consumption, Lee describes hospital behavior as conspicuous production representing a drive for self-esteem on the part of hospital administrators. According to Lee (1971:49):

The status of a hospital is an abstract, nonmeasurable concept. It is a relative concept which exists in the minds of people who pass a judgment on a hospital. Since a judgment of this nature is concerned with the status of a hospital as a producer of hospital care, it is usually based on visible objects or symbols. For this reason, attention of hospital administrators has been focused on the variety, quantity, and complexity of the inputs available in the hospital. Thus, the status of a hospital is assumed to vary directly with the range of services available and the extent to which expensive and highly specialized equipment and personnel (including M.D.'s) are available.

Hospitals compete for complex medical technology to attract and maintain medical staffs and to enhance the public image. In this sense, hospital administrators are responsive to the demands of their medical staffs and trustees, which often place equipment, facilities, services, and personnel in the role of status symbols. The acquisition of these inputs is done without adequate regard for the degree to which they will enhance production. In the final analysis, hospitals are engaged in a process of creative waste in which more resources are used than are required to produce given services; either expensive equipment is infrequently used, higher quality technology and personnel are used than required to meet the medical problems, or appropriate resources are used in greater quantities than required. Hospitals compete with each other to minimize the status gap that may exist among them. Expenditures and prices may increase without any change in output or productivity, and the motivating force for an increase in prices may be the desire to become the hospital with the most status in a region. The costs of this conspicuous production are passed on to patients.

PERSPECTIVES ON THE HOSPITAL

Each participant in the hospital tends to view the organization and other participants from different perspectives, depending on location in the structure. Each participant has by virtue of location in the structure a set of interests that influence attitudes toward organized activities. If the activity has no perceived effect on those interests, the stance is often indifference; if it is perceived as enhancing the interests, then the stance is advocacy; and if detrimental, opposition. Almost any change in procedures will differentially affect different participants, making conflict a normal part of organized life and negotiation a continuous feature of the social order (Strauss et al., 1963).

In this section we will discuss some interests typical of three important occupational groups in the hospital and how those interests affect the ways in which the participants perceive each other and the hospital. The contrasting perspectives of the patients will then be briefly considered.

Staff: a place to work and learn

Although there are many occupational groups in the typical hospital, most have not been studied at all. Hence this discussion is limited to three groups: administrators, physicians, and nurses.

From the standpoint of the administrator, the hospital is a complex organization that requires coordination of effort and a routine to make life predictable. It is a rational structure that must be managed through budgeting, directives, and accounting. Administrators must focus on the needs of the hospital as an organization. Primary among these is fiscal solvency. The hospital must have an adequate patient load, fees must be collected, funds solicited, and costs held down.

The major problem of hospital administrators, which differentiates them from administrators of other organizations, is that they have no control over either costs or expenditures. These are determined by the activities of the medical staff, who admit patients, order tests and therapeutic procedures, and try to directly influence policies of the hospital, including the ordering of high-capital equipment. Accordingly the administrator tends to view the medical staff with a somewhat jaundiced eye. Physicians are seen as not fully responsible. The "hospital incurs debts, runs less efficiently, and puts less emphasis on the care of patients than might otherwise be the case" (Duff and Hollingshead, 1968).

Physicians tend to consider the hospital as a "doctor's workshop" in which they treat patients, having the advantage of sharing costly facilities. In university hospitals, physicians think of administrators as people who "do not understand the importance of teaching and research" (Duff and Hollingshead, 1968). Private practitioners view the

administration as overly bureaucratic and insensitive to the individual needs of patients. Physicians tend to focus on the unique features of each patient, and require flexibility in reaching a diagnosis and planning a course of treatment. They want the hospital to provide the necessary support services when they are needed and with a minimum of "red tape." They tend to be intolerant of routines regarded as essential by the administrator, and it is not infrequent that they perceive the hospital as frustrating therapy.

The problem is one of conflict between parallel and serial structures, the physician committed to the first and the administrator to the second. The commitment of each is understandable, and the two types of structure differently serve the needs of each. It is hence built into the social structure and is not a matter of personalities as is often suggested by the participants.

Of special interest in this regard is the position of the nurse, who is caught between these two structures, which are frequently thought of as "two lines of authority" (Smith, 1955; Mauksch, 1969, 1972). The nurse is simultaneously responsible to the administration for the orderly management of the ward and to the medical staff for the implementation of patient care. To the administrator, nurses are "their agents in supervising patient-care divisions," whereas to physicians nurses are "administrator(s) of medical orders and assistant(s) to the doctor" (Duff and Hollingshead, 1968). Neither group provides much support to the nurse in what many nurses regard as their core concern, providing humane care to "distressed ward patients."

The demands on the nurse are often intense and laden with conflict. Nurses feel that there is not enough time to carry out all the obligations assumed to be theirs by people in power. Furthermore, the demands are frequently mutually exclusive such as when a treatment order is inconsistent with administrative routine. Although this has not been explicitly studied, it might be expected that nurses have a critical role in negotiating the conflicts between medical and administrative structures. Furthermore, they occupy a position in which role strain is particularly intense, which would partially explain the high turnover of nursing personnel described in Chapter 8.

Common to all the occupations that are housed in a hospital is the notion that the hospital is a place to work. Whatever they do, whatever interests they have, and whatever perspectives they share with particular subgroups, it is "part of the job." In this, all hospital personnel are differentiated from patients.

Clients: a lousy place unless you're sick

The hospital is a much different place to patients. It is not a familiar work environment in which they can exercise power and engage in interaction with familiar people. Instead patients typically enter the hospital in an existentially vulnerable state, being to some degree incapacitated by disease and apprehensive about the outcome. The hospital adds to this vulnerability by enforcing additional dependencies, intensifying the helplessness of patients and making them passive participants in a drama in which they have little to say about events that are more than usually consequential (Parsons, 1951; Taylor, 1970; Tagliacozzo and Mauksch, 1972).

When asked what they think of hospitals, patients most often respond that they are "lousy places to be" but "the only place to be when you are really sick." The hospital is a risky place to be, being the only place where there is adequate knowledge and resources to produce a cure but where it is difficult to know whether one is getting good care.

Patients tend to be relatively unconcerned about the occupational struggles and do not see the conflicting perspectives of the hospital staff. Instead they have an overriding concern with their own condition and the care they receive. Core concerns of patients are with safety and seeing to it that they get the services they need (Tagliacozzo and Mauksch, 1972). Surrounded by powerful people who may withhold needed services, the patient feels the need to show cooperation, trust and confidence, and not be too demanding.

Patients differ, however, in the extent to which they behave in accordance with these concerns. The sicker patients perceive themselves to be the more they will demand service rather than passively wait for it. Men place less concern on personal service and more on cooperation with nurses than do women (Tagliacozzo and Mauksch, 1972). Older patients see the service as more technical and less personal than do younger ones (Griffin, 1975).

HOSPITALS AND HEALTH CARE PLANNING

The hospital as a social institution is at a major turning point. Although it has an important place in the history of medicine, economic necessity is forcing a rethinking of the role of the hospital in medical care. For a century, the trend has been toward increased use of an increasingly sophisticated organization in which vast technical resources can be mobilized in the fight against disease. More and more the hospital has become *the* source of treatment.

The cost of medical care is rising faster than any other part of the economy, and most of that increase is a reflection of the charges for hospitalization. The addition of new diagnostic and therapeutic equipment has increased labor intensity as well as capital outlay. Greater use of these technological arms has increased the cost per patient day beyond the capacity of most people to pay. Cost per se has become an important issue.

At the same time the increasing complexity of the hospital places it more and more beyond the realm of common sense. It is no longer an organization that its users can understand. Its complexity even baffles the people who work there. Increasingly the errors in treatment and patient care are traceable to the organization rather than to technical judgment of individual practitioners. Size, scope, and complexity make elementary communication a major problem and coordination a nightmare.

The result is that hospitals are under increasing pressure to change. The role of the hospital as an organization also requires rethinking. The principle pressures have been toward increasing the efficiency of the hospital so as to reduce the unit costs of delivering service and reducing the use of hospitalization in situations in which alternatives are identified.

Economic choice and the cult of efficiency

The process of status gap minimization leads to a situation in which every hospital trys to become a comprehensive source of medical care. Even rarely needed services tend to develop in geographically close hospitals, leading to expensive duplication of services. With the advent of the Bingham Associate Fund in Maine in 1936, there has been an increasing move in the United States toward the regionalization of services. "Regionalization" refers to the coordination of hospitals' services within geographical areas to avoid duplication, cooperation between hospitals to reduce costs by sharing facilities, and other similar measures.

The problem is particularly acute in the United States where voluntary hospitals have been dominant. In England, Denmark, and other countries with more nationalized health schemes, regionalization is much more advanced. Pressures from major insurance companies and the internal threat of bankruptcy have been major forces for this kind of change (Roemer and Morris, 1959).

Another attempt to improve efficiency has been internal. Hospitals have looked to industry for models that will hold down costs while increasing productivity. The result has been increasing division of labor and specialization into departments. This move has served to increase complexity and to compound problems of communications to the extent that it is unclear whether efficiency has been enhanced or diminished

(Titmuss, 1958). Closely related, the hospital has adopted assembly-line procedures such as scheduling all clinic appointments at the same hour and mass processing as rapidly as possible.

The drive for efficiency is undeniable but raises the following important question.

Efficiency for whom?

It seems probable that certain attempts by hospitals to increase internal efficiencies have made the hospital more inefficient for its clients. One example is the scheduling of clinic appointments.

Most hospitals with large clinic structures schedule appointments by having all patients show up at the same time, for example, at 7:30 in the morning. This is efficient from the standpoint of the hospitals. If a patient fails to keep an appointment, expensive staff are not kept idle waiting for the next to show up. Patients can be processed one after another with no slack time.

From the standpoint of the patient, however, this is a most inefficient way to handle appointments. Patients spend many hours waiting to be seen, and many of them are losing income if they are paid a wage. In some cases extended waits are detrimental to their health, the added stress complicating conditions. This is one instance of efficiency in whch the perspectives of the organization and client are in conflict.

On a larger scale is the issue of specialization. Here one must differentiate patients. Those with serious, complicated, or rare diseases have different interests than do those with more so-called ordinary diseases. For the seriously diseased, there are advantages in having a physician who is a specialist, an expert on the precise difficulties that are at issue. More expert treatment should improve the likelihood of recovery. On the other hand, the seriously sick patient often has more than one disease at a time and frequently must be managed by two or more physicians simultaneously. Hence there is greater danger of error from problems of communication and incompatible treatments.

For the patient with an ordinary disease, the advantages of specialization are less obvious. Generally, the great expertise of the specialist is not needed, and someone with broad training would be preferable. Where generalists are not to be found, which is increasingly the case, the patient must first properly identify the disease type so as to be able to find the right physician. Once found, the specialist too often takes little interest in the case because it is not complicated enough to be interesting.

Although specialization is at best a mixed blessing for patients, it is undoubtedly in the interest of the physicians and the hospital. Prestige comes from expertise, which specialization allows. Furthermore, early specialization has been noted to be a way in which the student physician can manage the volume of knowledge to be absorbed (Becker et al., 1961). The consequent departmentalization of the hospital is a way of improving cost accounting for the administrator. Again the interest of the organization and the client conflict.

To date the cult of efficiency has considered only the internal interests of medical care organizations and professions. Continuing on this course will result in further alienation of the clients. External efficiencies have been sacrificed and must be taken into the accounting.

NOTES

1. The pronoun "him" is chosen deliberately. The overwhelming majority of physicians in the United States are men, which reverses the situation in Eastern Europe where most are women. Furthermore, as Mauksch has pointed out, it is impossible to understand medicine without first understanding sexism. A physician is thought of as male, irrespective of gender, and a nurse is female, also irrespective of gender. This underlies the widespread suspicion that women physicians and men nurses must be sexually abnormal.

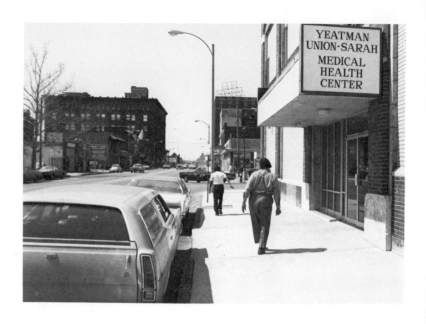

CHAPTER 12

Neighborhood health centers

In the midst of national affluence, the overwhelming degradation of the urban and rural poor caught the attention of the people of the United States in the early 1960s. Battle lines formed, and the United States government, principally through the Department of Health, Education, and Welfare and the Office of Economic Opportunity (OEO), launched the War on Poverty. At the time, little did the planners and Congress know that the war would become a skirmish and would ultimately be abandoned by the Nixon administration of the 1970s. Similarly, few if any of the poverty warriors foresaw the tremendous impact that their efforts to eliminate poverty would have on the organization and delivery of health care services. Although there was no precedent in the United States for providing comprehensive health care for the poor, the problems of poverty and health are so intertwined that the antipoverty campaign produced the neighborhood health center program, which was designed to provide comprehensive, primary, and preventive care to the poor and to remove the economic barriers to health care with the expectation that the cycle of poverty could be broken.

This chapter examines the neighborhood health center as a strategy for intervention and change in the social order. We will describe the core characteristics of these centers and will attempt to evaluate their effectiveness and contribution to the poor, to their communities, and to medicine by discussing two of their innovative aspects: consumer participation and the community health worker program.

BEGINNINGS

During the early 1900s, the United States possessed a highly decentralized medical care system. Residents of inner-city neighborhoods had their own health care team usually located in the middle of the neighborhood residential area. Public health and communicable disease, particularly the dreaded tuberculosis and venereal diseases, were pressing problems, and neighborhoods organized small, storefront health centers to meet these needs. Thus at the turn of this century, many neighborhoods had their local physicians, nurses, and other health workers living and practicing in the community (Stoeckle and Carnib, 1969).

Health services have been increasingly centralized over the past twenty-five years. Somehow in the post-Flexnerian scramble to implement the technical, specialized, and scientific aspects of the medical role, highly centralized medical bureaucracies emerged as the most efficient and effective standard of medical practice. These medical centers offered a wide range of advantages, including the economy realized by means of a standardized form of medical practice and increased power in diagnosis and treatment gained by incorporating many medical specialists, some quite exotic, under one roof and organization. Furthermore, the medical center bureaucracy was a most effective method for protecting health professionals from the demands of the consumer, since as the medical setting became more impersonal and complex, the patient found it increasingly more difficult to see a practitioner without first negotiating with bureaucratic gatekeepers. The overspecialization of personnel, inflexible formal rules of procedure, and the absence of client control over decision making are problems of bureaucracy that tend to make medical care less available, less accessible, less acceptable, and, most importantly, less accountable to the consumer. Although these problems are by no means limited to bureaucratic forms of medical organization, it is highly probable that they are highlighted and focused in the bureaucratic context.

In addition to the bureaucratic thrust, medicine turned more of its attention to disease rather than health. Within the walls of the most sophisticated medical centers, one would be hard pressed to find a health professional working to prevent disease or to improve health. On the contrary, much of the activity of modern bureaucratic medicine is designed to cure disease appropriately from the perspective of one afflicted with an infection or cancer. To some extent the issue of prevention must take the backseat in light of pressing acute illness.

Nevertheless, a startling paradox developed. Scientific medicine found itself superbly able to diagnose a child with infectious dysentery, rehydrate the child, destroy the germs, and then send the child home to drink from the same filth-laden drainage ditch. The medical center was incapable of dealing with the social, political, legal, and economic forces that play a major role in the cause and prevention of diseases, and yet it had become the predominant health care institution in our society.

Thus it was that the pendulum swung back slightly, and the neighborhood health center program began within the confines of the War on Poverty.

The War on Poverty established programs designed to intervene in and treat the cycle of poverty. The OEO and later the USPHS introduced legislation that established comprehensive neighborhood health centers located in areas where the poor were concentrated. The theory behind these centers was that poor health and poverty are old and fast acquaintances and that therefore the creation of health care institutions would provide one with multiple entry points to improve the quality of life and ultimately to erradicate poverty. If people do not have enough to eat, live in environments with rain coming through the roof and freezing on them, and suffer through repeated acute and chronic breakdowns, they will be unaffected by attempts to improve their level of education to enrich their lives with items from middle-class culture. The poor get sicker and the sick get poorer, and neighborhood health centers were a response to this vicious circle.

The underlying mix of three powerful forces—the government, the provider of services, and the consumer—converged at a point in history when medicine and government recognized at least in part the utility and possible humaneness of delivering health services to the poor to break the cycle of poverty.

Organization

The manner in which the centers were organized and run changed as they grew in size and weathered the passage of time. We will discuss the predominant early form of organization for OEO and USPHS centers and follow some of the changes to the present time. The reason our attention is centered on the government-funded centers is because they represent the earliest modern centers in terms of development and numbers, easily making up the majority currently in existence.

For the most part, these centers are located in urban inner-city areas, although there are several rural centers, and they serve low-income white, Native-American,

Spanish-speaking, black, and other minority racial and ethnic groups. Generally, these centers are managed through organizational linkages with medical schools, departments of public health, hospitals, or other health care facilities and resources (Sparer et al., 1970) (Fig. 12-1). In fewer instances, the centers are managed by neighborhood associations or corporations, and health services are provided through contracts with health facilities. In rare instances, the center is its own corporation, and it receives and manages the federal funds with which outpatient services are provided on site and inpatient services are contracted (Fig. 12-2).

Services offered vary from center to center, but in general, a patient can obtain primary health services, including laboratory work, x-ray examinations, and minor surgery under one roof. Many centers provide dental care and mental health services, in addition to social services such as clothing, welfare counseling, food distribution, and drug abuse treatment. Few centers offer preventive health care such as lead paint screening, early detection programs, and urban or rural community development in terms of economic self-sufficiency in basic areas such as housing and food. Three notable exceptions among neighborhood health centers are the Yeatman Health Center (St. Louis, Missouri) (Figs. 12-3 and 12-4), the Bolivar County Health Cooperative (Mound Bayou, Mississippi), and the Rodrigo Terronez Memorial Health Center (United Farmworkers, Delano, California).

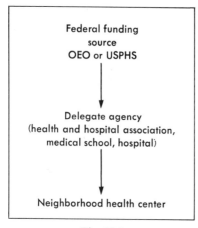

Fig. 12-1

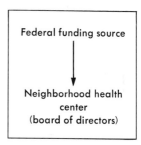

Fig. 12-2

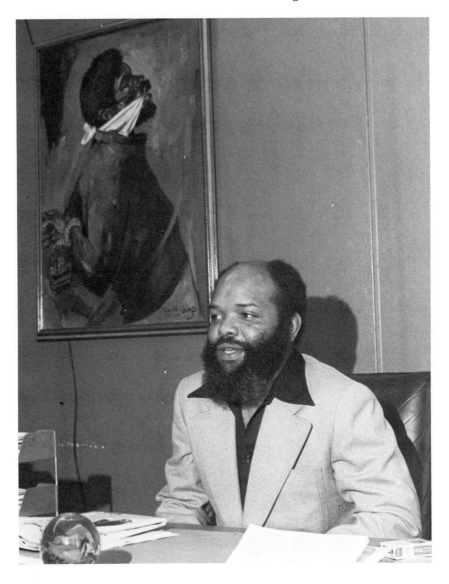

Fig. 12-3. *A. J. Henley, administrator of the Yeatman and Sarah Union Neighborhood Health Center in St. Louis, Missouri.*

Innovations

Perhaps the two most significant aspects of neighborhood health centers that distinguish them from more traditional health care organizations such as hospitals or group practices are (1) consumer participation in health care decision making and (2) the development of the health team and new medical career models. These two innovations will be discussed within the contexts of neighborhood health centers. During the past decade, the neighborhood health center has emerged as the major proving ground for the development and testing of these two concepts, which theoretically have the potential for changing the organization and production of medical work.

Consumer participation

"Maximum feasible participation" of the poor was a rallying cry of the War on

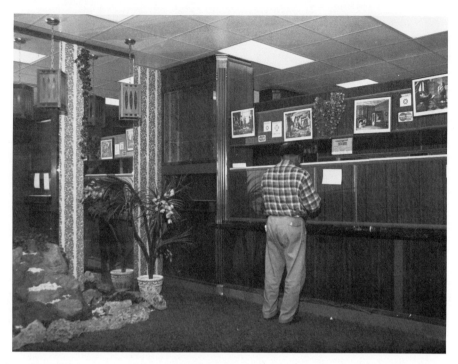

Fig. 12-4. *Filling a prescription: the Pharmacy with Soul in Yeatman and Sarah Union Neighborhood Health Center located in a low-income, inner-city neighborhood of St. Louis, Missouri.*

Poverty. This concept, although ambiguous and never clearly defined operationally, was applied to neighborhood health centers and became one of their major organizing principles. Funds for establishing centers were granted by OEO and USPHS only if the applicant had provided for the participation of neighborhood residents or potential consumers in the decision making at the centers. It is important to recognize the fact that consumer participation has its roots not in health care delivery but in the larger War on Poverty, a program which ostensibly sought to intervene in the "cycle of poverty" to improve the quality of life for the poor. Of equal importance is the recognition that the War on Poverty was conceived and mandated to a large extent by white middle-class American liberals (Moynihan, 1969).

In short, the poor became the recipients of a middle-class ideology of equalitarianism, and the neighborhood health center is one stage at which the drama unfolded.

Who participates in what fashion? The organization of the center's decision-making structure and the type of consumer participation extant determine to a great extent the character of the interaction between providers of medical care, that is, members of the medical establishment, and consumers, who are the poor in the case of health centers. Whether the actors on the scene will be antagonists or protagonists, whether the relationship between provider and consumer will be one of conflict or cooperation, and ultimately whether health care is organized to take the social, cultural, and economic needs of the community into consideration is a function of who participates and how they participate; in short, the form and content of participation in health care.

The organization of neighborhood health centers and consumer participation is not

Table 12-1. Stages of development of neighborhood health centers

Stages of development	Expectations		Role of consumers	Content of consumer action	Issues
	Providers	Consumers			
Formative	Delivery of health care services Medical education Career enhancement	Employment Upward social mobility	Narrowly advisory	Broad policy matters	Preventive vs. primary care Who participates? How are participants selected? Who works and how decided? Who is served? How is center organized and run?
Charisma testing	Delivery of health care services (primary) Evaluation Maintaining control and authority	Control of center decision making (e.g., hiring and firing administrative personnel)	Advisors on policy matters	Seek to control administrative decisions Conflict over administrative autonomy	Hiring and firing personnel Administration vs. policy Advisory vs. control Board training Racism
Routinization-purposive action	Control of administration and budget	Control of policy setting	Board of directors	Program development	Funding Professional turnover community relations Succession of board Quality of medical care

an event with static boundaries but must be seen and interpreted as a process. This is complex reality, and consumer participation varies according to the stage of development of the centers. Issues are linked to the form and content of participation as well. In an attempt to simplify matters we propose the following organizational model. We will draw heavily upon data from our study of neighborhood health centers to highlight and illustrate the model.

Centers go through at least three stages of organizational development: (1) formative, (2) charisma testing, and (3) routin-ization-purposive action (Table 12-1). There is a period or continuum of time that any given center will take in order to negotiate the first two stages (i.e., the duration of the stage).

Consumers and providers enter the scene with expectations concerning the objectives of the health center and their respective roles. Furthermore, the actors on the scene assume roles that can be described in terms of (1) forms of control and (2) the content of consumer action. Finally, issues emerge that can erupt into full-scale conflict between providers and consumers. The expectations, behaviors, content, and issues vary according to the stage of health center development.

FORMATIVE STAGE

Neighborhood health centers began with a broad model of what comprehensive care should include. This broad conception is what OEO and later USPHS had in mind when requests for proposals went out to potential provider groups such as medical schools and hospitals. If enough interest in designing and building a neighborhood health center was generated, then the interested party was encouraged to write a grant proposal for establishing a neighborhood health center within the broad federal guidelines.

Medical education and the delivery of primary health care services were the two major expectations or objectives of providers during the formative stage. The community was viewed as an extension of the medical school's laboratory facilities, where students could learn about the dynamics of poverty and acquire knowledge of those community processes, such as life-style, family structure, and nutrition, which are associated with sickness, health, and the physician-patient relationship. Certainly most provider grantees were interested as well in providing desperately needed health services to the poor.

As the first grants were written, the requirement that consumers were to be involved somehow in health center decision making emerged as a difficult mandate for providers. Expertise in medical science did not translate easily into the skills necessary to orchestrate a community organization for participation. In several instances, providers defined consumer participation as an unreasonable and meaningless device designed by OEO to placate militant communities. For the most part, however, providers considered consumer participation as a legitimate attempt to shift from peer accountability to community accountability and thought that the glaring deficiencies in the health system—self-serving health insti-

tutions, user alienation from services, unmet community health problems—could be overcome through vigorous consumer input. What they could not see, on the other hand, was the strategy and tactics for instituting this innovative concept.

As a result, three significant issues emerged in the formative stage of neighborhood health centers that affected profoundly the interaction between providers and consumers: (1) provider and consumer expectations for health care delivery, (2) the question of who participates and how are they selected, and (3) the role of consumers in health center decision making.

Expectations

During the formative stage, providers anticipate establishing high-quality primary care, and if money and manpower is available, preventive programs would be established to change social and physical characteristics of the environment, such as bad housing, rats, unemployment, and other factors associated with poverty and causing disease and illness.

On the other hand, consumers view the proposed neighborhood health center as an opportunity to obtain work and social programs, thereby pulling themselves out of a situation in which unemployment runs as high as 20% to 25% of the work force. We are reminded of the fact that health care relative to other matters of daily survival is a low priority for the poor by Dr. H. Jack Geiger, the former project director of the Tufts-Delta Comprehensive Health Center in Mound Bayou, Mississippi. Dr. Geiger reported that after opening the doors of the center and serving the health care needs of the community for a few weeks, he and the other staff members called a meeting, inviting consumers to attend and to provide the staff with feedback concerning the job they were doing. The local residents came to the meeting, and after thanking the medical staff for sharing their medical skills with the community, they proceeded to make the following statements, which Dr. Geiger has described as the most embarrassing of his professional career: "We deeply appreciate the medical care but for the love of God do you think you could spare some food"; "We think we would be healthier if we didn't sleep in housing where the rain comes through the roof and freezes on us"; "We think we would be healthier if people had work"; "We think we would be healthier if we didn't get our water out of the drainage ditch." As Dr. Geiger recounted it, the embarrassment stemmed from the fact that provider expectations were far off the mark, whereas the consumers had touched much closer to the heart of the original philosophy and strategy behind neighborhood health centers, which was to break the cycle of poverty by using health as a multiple entry point for changing those aspects of the social, political, economic, and physical environment that are damaging peoples' lives. It is important to note that Dr. Geiger moved quickly after this meeting to establish a farm cooperative, sanitation programs, and other social services to meet this challenge.

The important point here is that consumer and provider expectations of the health center are different at the formative stage, with consumers looking to the health center as an answer to the pressing exigencies of everyday survival, health care notwithstanding. On the other hand, providers view the center as an organization designed to deliver primary health care, and only as money is available will the center move seriously into areas of social change. This difference in basic orientation toward the program forms the basis for much of the conflict between providers and consumers that usually occurs in the charisma-testing stage.

Consumer participation

Who participates and how are they selected? As mentioned earlier, the issue of who participates and how they are selected is thrust on the providers by dint of federal guidelines, which strongly urge grantees to have an active consumer participation component at the health center. This is predicated on the assumption that organized consumers have more influence and power than unorganized consumers. Of course, the question of who participates and how one obtains their services becomes the key issue to be negotiated but not settled during the formative period.

Each health center and its adopted community evolves a different strategy for answering the "who participates?" question. Nevertheless, two approaches can be discussed and applied generally to developing centers. In our research, we have found that providers took one of the following approaches to the problem.

At some centers, they identify the potential consumer participants as those individuals who are actively involved in community service organizations. We call this the "community elite approach" for the simple reason that those individuals in the community with the highest status, greatest visibility in terms of public knowledge about them, and greatest vested interest in the community are either criminals or active members of several service organizations in the community. Happily it is rarely a case of the former.

The other method, which we call the "populist approach," is to develop consumer participation at the grass roots level. This usually means that providers devise a plan for involving those consumers who are not participating in community organizations but who manifest an interest in the development of their community in one way or another. Using this approach, one would attempt to contact community residents who are not actively engaged as members of community groups and organizations to ensure that at least some of the nonparticipants are represented among the health center consumer participants. Needless to say, the two approaches spell different consequences for the type and style of consumer participation at centers. Nevertheless, both assume that the term "consumer" refers to all community residents who are eligible for services at the center and who do not earn their income through any work in health care in contrast to "providers" who derive their major income from health care delivery and who are not eligible for treatment at the center.

How are consumers selected? The reply must be "with great difficulty." There are three widely used approaches for selecting what usually is between ten and twenty consumer participants from the ranks of interested community residents: elections, self-selection, and appointment. These have been used roughly equally in centers across the country.

Elections are costly and difficult to organize, and for these reasons, centers seldom hold their own elections to choose consumer participants. The usual pattern is for the center to hold its election concurrent with a larger election such as a Model City or OEO election in the community. Center candidates are placed on a single ballot with the candidates for the Model Cities or OEO boards, and what amounts to two elections are held as one.

One problem with elections stems from the fact that at best only 10% of the community votes. We have observed health center elections in communities where 1% to 2% turnout occurred. Obviously this raises the question of representativeness, and both consumers and providers have questioned the meaningfulness and utility of elections. Furthermore, instances of election fraud have occurred. For example, in one OEO–neighborhood health center election held in a large southern city, a fierce debate developed between a militant candidate for the health center board and a more conservative incumbent running for reelection to the board. The OEO election officials ruled that the militant was not a legitimate candidate, since she had not gone through the complex nominating procedures. In turn she argued that her neighbors in the housing project had elected her as a write-in candidate, and the small handful of votes she received was enough to push her to victory over the official candidate, given the 1% overall turnout. Later

this issue played a significant role in a major conflict between consumers and providers at the center.

Self-selection occurs when community residents, generally influential and active in organizations, identify themselves as representative of the community and succeed in convincing the administration at the center that they should be the consumer participants. Obviously self-proclaimed leadership can fall far short of the real thing, and the self-selected board may represent only a limited and narrow range of interests instead of pushing for issues and concerns that better fit the needs of the larger community served by the center.

With the appointment method of selecting consumer participants, usually the center administration runs an advertising campaign for board membership, screens applicants, and then selects those who meet certain criteria. A major problem with this approach stems from the tendency of members of groups or organizations to establish admission criteria that reflect their own values and attitudes. Humans strive to interact with those who possess similar values and attitudes (Homans, 1950), and health centers are no exception to this principle of organizational life. Thus we found that for centers utilizing the appointment approach, consumers selected tend to fit the provider conceptions of what consumer participants should value and be interested in accomplishing with the center. Once again the problem of community representation exists to plague center operations.

Role of consumers in health center decision making. During the formative stage, the role of consumers in decision making is ambiguous, vague, and therefore tentative. Frequently, at the level of expectations, providers have a reasonably clear sense of the objectives and program commitments of the center, whereas consumer participants have little knowledge of what it takes to manage a budget, how administration is possible, or what the limits are to comprehensive health care. What they do know about are the cultural, social, and economic dynamics of the community. However, in the press of staffing and health program development, consumers' expertise takes on secondary importance, and consequently the consumer lands on the fringes of the health center decision making.

By formal or occasionally informal agreement, the consumers usually agree with the providers to take on an advisory role, serving as sounding boards and critics for the providers, who then make the decisions. An advisory board member at one center put her role in perspective when she said, "The problem with being an advisor is that the man can take your advice or leave it, depending on what's good for the doctors. If he leaves it, there ain't much you can do about it except be cool."

And so it goes during the formative stage, with the consumer serving as advisor. Important decisions of great relevance to the community are made by providers occasionally with the informed advice of the advisory board, but often they inform the consumers of the decision after the fact. For example, the hiring of the project director and the directors of various medical and social services, hours that the center will be open, payment and billing procedures, and job classifications and requirements are but a few of the decisions that consumer participants play a minor role in.

Thus it is that the center begins to deliver health and social services, and for a period of time, providers and consumers coexist in an uneasy but relatively peaceful relationship with one another. The uneasiness is best illustrated in the words of a Chicano member of one center's advisory board in the southwestern United States. Standing alongside the dirt road in front of his adobe casa, I asked him why he agreed to be an advisor and not a decision-maker. He replied, somewhat amused at the bias in my question, "Do you know the difference between thinking and knowing?" I waited. Then he said, "A man thinks it's his child, a woman knows it's hers." And thus the honeymoon ends.

CHARISMA-TESTING STAGE

Once the doors are opened and services are delivered, the neighborhood health center enters a stage of development in which personal qualities and new ideas prevail and account for much of the success that the organization has in establishing its spheres of action and viability. Because of the important role that new ideas and personal qualities of the consumers and providers plays in establishing the center as a community institution, if not simply in protecting the center from being burned down or otherwise run out of the community, the concept "charisma" is applied to this stage of development. In this sense, the center is viewed as a social movement in which the charismatic stage plays best to large-scale efforts to acquire and to consolidate power on the basis of personal qualities and the saliency of new ideas (Weber, 1947).

During this stage, the administration becomes increasingly concerned with maintaining control over those decisions that relate to the everyday operations of the center such as hiring, firing, productivity rates, the way the staff relates to patients, and the quality of care provided. This concern grows as the consumer advisory board members seek to probe the basis for authority and the locus of control at the center. Typically consumers become disenchanted with their status as advisors, and they begin to seriously consider the possibility of assuming control over administrative decisions during the charisma stage. Frequently, one finds the classical case of an irresistible force meeting immovable objects, and predictably, the neighborhood health center becomes an arena where conflicts between providers and consumers erupt.

Health centers, like all complex organizations, must attend to four fundamental problems to provide service: setting goals, control, innovation and change, and intelligence (Wilensky, 1960). Wilensky defines intelligence as "the problem of gathering, processing, interpreting, and communicating the technical and political information needed in the decision-making process." He assigns great importance to intelligence as one of the major informing principles of organizational life and survival. The point is that during the charismatic stage, the central thrust of providers and consumers alike is toward control over administrative and policy decisions at the center. New ideas in the form of issues and strategies for action are developed around select individuals who are capable of generating great interest and support by means of personal characteristics; for example, a black leader who has demonstrated commitment to the movement by confronting the establishment at great personal risk may command the respect and allegiance of fellow health workers by dint of this charisma.

The major conflicts that occur during this stage emanate from the struggle over who shall control the administrative decisions at the center. For the most part, expectations and primary objectives of the administrator and department heads are to provide health services in the best manner possible, to evaluate these efforts, and to maintain administrative control over their domain with a view, possibly, of expanding their spheres of influence through the expansion of services or promotion to more powerful positions. Pitted against the dominance of providers are the consumer participants who draw on their community ties for assistance as they seek to change the nature of the situation to gain more control than their advisory status affords.

The conflicts can be serious, and the case we present is one in which the health center was picketed and the doors shut against patients for 3 days. One is reminded of the following important principles that underlie such conflict:

1. There is no one "true" position, but instead one finds multiple realities. What is real and at stake for the providers may not be seen as real and important by the consumers and vice versa. Nevertheless, the fact that both parties do not share the same

reality does not diminish the important effect on behavior.

2. Despite intentions to the contrary, no one on the staff at the center or on the consumer board can remain neutral during a conflict. Frequently, individuals are drawn into the struggle unwittingly either because one force sees them as part of the problem or as a source of power and influence.

3. There are manifest and latent issues, the manifest issues representing strategic means to achieve the latent issues or ends.

The following incident took place at a neighborhood health center in the South and illustrates the process of conflict in the charisma stage. When the incident occurred, one of us (R. M. H.) and two colleagues from Tufts University in Massachusetts had already completed two rounds of interviews at the center spaced over 2 months (New et al., 1973). When the incident erupted, the researchers immediately went to the center and spent a week interviewing all parties concerned.

The incident that led to the conflict involved eight black staff members (social worker, nurse, personnel director, assistant director of research, nurse coordinator, medical director, and two other physicians) who held a caucus to discuss their concerns about the health center's operation. Notes were taken and typed up, and copies were distributed to personnel throughout the center, including the administrator and director of the health center.

At a regular staff meeting a week later, the director asked the leader of "the Eight" to explain the grievances. This was the medical director, who refused, and the director immediately asked him to resign due to "insubordination." In an unrelated action the director had just suspended the personnel director who was a member of "the Eight." These actions touched off a strike by some of the staff, and the most active consumer participants joined the struggle. The demonstrators demanded that the medical director and the personnel director be reinstated and that the director of the center be removed. Since the center was under the fiscal control of the medical school (delegate agency), the administration of that institution held meetings and got involved as well. Other meetings were held in the neighborhood and center, and newspaper and television reporters eagerly joined in the action. Charges of racism were leveled at the director of the center (a white man) by the eight center health aids and consumer participants, most of whom were black. Other manifest issues included charges that the center administration was anticonsumer and that consumers did not play an important part in the decisions that were made. Furthermore, the concept of health care teams was severely criticized for allegedly reducing the quality of medical care, and the lack of communication between the center administration and staff was roundly cited as a cause of the trouble. Pickets were thrown up, and the center closed its doors for 3 days. It should be noted that these manifest issues are not unique to this particular center (Abrams and Snyder, 1968; Wise, 1968; Bakst, 1969; Davis and Tranquada, 1969; Hessler et al., 1970; Campbell, 1971; Banta and Fox, 1972; Hollister et al., 1974).

The "palace revolution," as one staff member called it, ended when the medical school administration fired the director of the center, a psychiatrist, who was given an academic job as professor in the medical school. On the surface, the causes of the conflict appear to be represented in the manifest issues. However, closer scrutiny reveals that latent issues, silent and hidden issues, were the culprits, and undergirding all was the absence of viable consumer participation, which created an enormous gap in the accountability of the center administration. The following is an analysis of the part that the latent issues played in the conflict.

Sponsorship of the health center

The health center was born in the dreams of a group of consumers. As the chairman of the consumer advisory board said:

Six years ago, before the health center was started, I was the president of the Coordinating Council of the southern part of the city. This was a civic group of leaders formed to consider community needs and we wanted to develop action programs to meet these needs. I set up a health committee, with (a nurse supervisor of a county health center) as my chairman, and they brought out the needs for mental health care. The government wanted a proposal, the health committee wrote it, sent it to Washington. They liked it so well that instead of having only a little mental health item, they said, "Let's get into comprehensive health." That is how the thing was born. The Coordinating Council set up a meeting with (the local poverty agency) about this. They told us to have a mass meeting at St. Paul's Church. The meeting was packed, and it was clear the community was with the Council (New et al., 1973:199).

According to the chairman and other advisory board members, all that they wanted was $13,000 to establish a halfway house for former mental patients and alcoholics. Instead of this modest but needed facility, a federal agency, working through the local medical society and the medical school, funded millions for a comprehensive health center. The consumers never saw the halfway house nor did they have control over the several million dollars per year budget, and their dream vanished. Whenever we met community persons, this was the same story told. In the rush to get the center started, little attention was paid to the citizens in the black area served by the center, and even less attention was paid to the role they would play in health center decision making. The stage was set, and the disenchantment with and lack of commitment to the center was programmed early, only to erupt during the charisma-testing stage of the center's existence.

Consumer participation

In an effort to make the center more accountable to the patients and the community in general, the consumers mounted challenge after challenge against the authority of the project director, and this striving for control was one of the most central and salient latent issues during the charisma-testing stage. The project director correctly identified the source of consumer disgruntlement when he mentioned; "Of course, our policy board had long since decided they had read "policy" as "control" and they realized they were not in control even with our bylaws which they had generated according to the guidelines.

The consumers were told by a representative from the federal granting agency in Washington, D.C. that only after it became a duly constituted corporation could it became a governing or control board. The bylaws, which had been rejected once before by the federal granting agency, were resubmitted and met with rejection again by the agency in Washington. The project director had the unpleasant task of carrying this bad news to the consumer advisory board, who through its increasing frustration thought he was manipulating them.

Since there were no acceptable bylaws, consumer participants found themselves caught in the plot of a *Catch 22* scenario. The advisory board agreed to have elections to obtain new and hopefully representative board members, but there were no official norms regarding the length of term of office nor the rules of succession for incumbent board members. Model City, OEO, and the health center elections were held simultaneously, and conflicts over eligibility and other voting procedures emerged. After the election, five irregularities appeared, all having to do with the health center. Four of the persons involved resigned from the advisory board but a fifth refused. She was a member of the old board and would not relinquish her seat. The matter was thrust into the hands of the project director of the center, and the issue remained unresolved but potent during the conflict. Throughout this debate, the advisory board members' views were not sought.

According to an earlier analysis of this conflict (New et al., 1973:204-205):

On the other hand, perhaps these seemingly inconsequential deliberations are really not so insignificant. Behind every innocuous act, the citizens, in their way, are testing the system for accountability. To a certain extent, the citizens did create a palace revolution, as a test, and they may have unhinged the establishment in this process. They did not feel they got anywhere in the earlier attempt to establish a half-way house for their own. Instead they felt the university took their idea and created another child in its own image. Substantive issues associated with the lack of neighborhood health center in part stimulate citizen participation and, in turn, growing participation and demands for accountability and control stimulate the development of substantive issues. To use an analogy, dominoes are repeatedly set up and knocked down and, with every collapse of the system, more dominoes are added to the stakes.

As shown by our example one outcome is clear. When direct accountability to consumers is lacking, struggles over control of decision making at centers will occur. Each locus of accountability constructs its own reality and priorities that may not coincide with the realities of others. The medical school perceives the center as a place for training students, the federal government views it as a vehicle for social change, the center administration considers it a primary health care organization, and the consumers see it as an opportunity for employment and ultimately as a test for the idea of whether participation could lead to control over health and other community institutions.

ROUTINIZATION-PURPOSIVE ACTION STAGE

The routinization-purposive action stage is where one finds what one project director called the "mature" centers. After all the battles have been fought and the center has survived the charisma-testing stage, the providers and consumers settle into relationships with relatively fixed and commonly held expectations. The big question of accountability and control by means of consumer participation has been resolved or at least suspended from active consideration, and the actors on the scene settle into routine and quiet roles.

The routinization of expectations and roles is the major identifying feature of this stage, and perhaps the most important feature is the settling of the question of accountability and who controls what.

For the most part, the providers and consumers agree to the following distinction between administrative control and policy control. The consumers are given authority to decide health center policy (e.g., which programs to have and which ones to eliminate), whereas providers retain authority over the nitty-gritty of daily center operations (i.e., the administrative arena).

This distinction of administration versus policy control is one hallmark of the routinization stage, and it depends to a great extent on one important structural feature of the consumer board: that the consumers reasonably become a governing board of directors during this stage by legally incorporating, educating themselves regarding the duties of a board, and then receiving the grant directly rather than having the money received and distributed by a delegate agency such as a medical school or a health and hospitals association. This structural feature stands as symbolic if not real evidence of the consumers' extended responsibilities and accountability. Furthermore, it saves money by avoiding the payment of overhead costs, which the delegate agency rakes off the top as a matter of course.

Accountability during the routinization stage has two dimensions: technical and social (Geiger, 1971). The providers assume control and responsibility for medically technical issues such as personnel qualifications, professional turnover (which is high at all stages), the quality of medical care, and fiscal viability. Social accountability becomes the domain of the consumers, who control issues involving relations between the center and community, planning for new programs and other innovations, and the succession of the consumer board. Health professionals are reluctant to become accountable to consumers as peers when questions of technical competence arise, and consumers seem reluctant to challenge this control of the technical sphere. This appears to be generally true of health centers that have reached the routinization stage.

Of course, we contend that technical and social aspects of health care delivery shade into one another. Most technical developments have social consequences, and to render providers accountable for the mechanics of producing health services while consumer participants are held responsible for the social side of these health services is not only extremely artificial but potentially explosive as well. At some point, perhaps during the routinization stage or perhaps in some future direction yet unknown, someone will lay aside the issues of economic survival, professional turnover, and community relations and once again question the relationship between neighborhood health centers and social change in the community. Can the center intervene in the political, economic, and social order and make people healthier or even prevent illness from occurring? Can consumers assume a more active stance and take more responsibility for technical decisions about their bodies and other aspects of their lives? Is health care a right to be enjoyed by all or a privilege for those who can pay or maneuver through the welfare bureaucracy? These and other similar questions could become the next issues to be fought as neighborhood health centers respond to the changing needs of the social order.

COMMUNITY HEALTH WORKERS

Neighborhood health centers were established ostensibly as a strategy for improving medical care for the poor in this country. One lesson learned about inner-city and rural areas of medical scarcity was that medical services must be available to be delivered. Inadequate or nonaccessible supplies of medical manpower would negate even the most innovative consumer-oriented delivery system. Thus of all the strategies for improving medical care for the poor, the substantial increase in new nonphysician medical manpower is possibly the most important innovation within the context of health centers. This is why a look at community health workers merits our attention as the second unique aspect of health centers.

Immediately on close scrutiny, a paradox emerges. Changes in medical manpower potentially is the best guarantee for achieving the goal of providing health care to the poor. However, manpower is the one area that is essentially blocked from significant change. The physician remains the producer of medical services by exercising primary responsibility for examining, diagnosing, and prescribing treatment for the patient. This is true in spite of the fact that there are currently approximately 2,500 AMA-approved training programs for allied health manpower in fifteen medical care fields and that the supply of this manpower is projected to increase from approximately 900,000 workers in 1971 to 1.3 million by 1980, a 67% gain (Pennell and Hoover, 1970). Although the nurse practitioner and similar medical professionals are assuming a great deal of responsibility and primary authority for patient care and cure, in general the push for new medical manpower has amounted to little more than a strategy for increasing the physician's supporting cast.

But what of community health workers? Why do they exist, what are their responsibilities, and does upward occupational mobility occur within the ranks of health workers?

The concept of community health workers as is currently known was developed within neighborhood health centers for two essential reasons. First, these workers represented a solution to the demands for jobs by community residents who live in areas where unemployment runs 15% to 20% of the work force. This coupled with the

lower salaries one would pay community health workers compared with health professionals made the concept attractive politically and economically. In short, it was a trade-off that the providers at the health center made with the community and consumers: jobs for healthy survival of the center.

Second, community health workers were trained and hired at the centers because they were familiar with the community, its cultural and political processes, and therefore they could serve as the liaison between the health center and the community. Public relations and a certain amount of "cooling the community out" were important reasons for the development of community health workers.

A good way to analyze the responsibilities shared by community health workers is to examine the training they receive. The remainder of this discussion is based on a national study of neighborhood health and community mental health centers, which provided much of the material for this chapter (Holton et al., 1972; New and Hessler, 1972).

One important function of being a health professional is to know something well and to convince others of this, thereby achieving relative autonomy in one's work. Extensive training is a direct route to achieving professional status in any given area of work. Training of community health workers was actively pursued in all the health centers studied, and such programs comprised all or most of the initial socialization process as the community resident was transformed into a health care worker.

Although many of these programs varied from relatively trivial first-aid courses to sophisticated medical and work habit training, a common factor or denominator emerged as a major impediment to professionalism for the community health worker: the nature of the special knowledge or competence of the paraprofessional relative to the physician. Training of health workers centered around medical care tasks that could be identified as supportive of the physician and his work. In no case was the health worker trained to perform well any medical care role that was essential to the physician maintaining control over the production of medical services. At several centers, especially the mental health centers, health workers were trained to perform limited segments of the physician's tradimedical roles. In none of these was the training extensive enough to ensure a high degree of competence. This placed the health workers in a compromising position relative to their autonomy from the physician. Mistakes at work were common, and physicians openly questioned the quality of the paraprofessionals' work, thereby effectively blocking any encroachment of their medical roles. For example, one of us (R. M. H.) was observing an intake interview at a comprehensive mental health center where paraprofessional workers did the initial interview with the prospective patient to make a diagnosis. During the course of the interview, it became apparent that the mental health worker was not asking the patient or family about alcohol problems, which, given later conversations with the patient's husband, turned out to be an important component of the presenting psychotic episode. As a result, the patient was labeled schizophrenic, and no mention of a drinking problem appeared in the intake record.

Community health workers are socialized for linkage rather than depth functions; that is, they are trained to serve as a liaison between the health care facility and the community rather than to control aspects of the production of medical care. Thus health worker training is technical but also peripheral to those skills which enable one to function with some measurable degree of autonomy as a medical care decision maker. This leads to a great deal of uncertainty in the minds of the workers as to who they are and what they can do. Decision redundancy prevails, and health workers often find themselves confronting a complex administrative chain of command in which physicians or other professionals involved simply go over the ground covered and essentially duplicate the task or decision making of the paraprofessional. Regarding the administrative hierarchy, one paraprofessional expressed her dissatisfaction with the health center's administrative structure, which she viewed as an impediment to her work, as follows:

You know, one thing that gets in the way of my doing my job is that there is such an extensive chain of command. There are so many commands and steps that you have to go through before you can do anything for a patient that it is really becoming a waste of time. We have a supervisor of neighborhood health agents called a field supervisor and this person should make the decision for our problems. Now you have to go to her first and then she has to go to the supervisor of social workers who has to go to the chief of the department who then has to go to the Medical Director and the decision comes back very slowly to say the least.

For her, the decision redundancy symbolized the professionals' unwillingness to accept and trust the health worker as an autonomous member of the health care delivery effort. Another health worker described her feelings:

We have an emergency food relief here at the center for patients who need food. The first thing I do is determine whether or not the patient needs the food program. This I do by going to the patient's home and talking with the patient and then making the decision. Now once I make the decision there are the things I have to go through. I have to go to the doctor at the health center first and the doctor makes a determination on a consultation form. I take the form to the dietetic department and they have to call the patient in and question the patient to the fullest extent. Now here is where I mean they are not taking my judgment. From there, it goes to the administration who then passes or rejects the application. Eventually I hear from my field supervisor as to whether or not the patient got the food. Now several times my judgment has been reversed. So now I try to ask outside agencies who give food before I approach the center. If a person is hungry you don't have the time to play these kinds of games, especially when children are involved. They (the health center) say this is the way that it has to be done. But I never got a reason for the policy. You know, a person (patient) has to choke down his pride and I have to tell the patient I'm sorry but we don't have the funds when deep down inside I know that it is only $15 and I know we have the money.

In addition to the serious morale problems and strains created between community health workers and health professionals, the training issues and attendant decision redundancy have placed workers at simultaneous risk, accountable correlatively to their community peers and to the professionals at the health centers. Their plight is one of marginality in both sectors, since their employment within the medical establishment mitigates in part claims of unswerving loyalty to community issues while at the same time the door to professional status and autonomy is blocked.

Finally, we turn to the question of upward occupational mobility. The concept of new health careers emanated from the 1967 New Careers Amendment to the Economic Opportunity Act, which provided for training and employment of the poor and undereducated in health and other human development work. For the indigenous community health worker, this concept included full-time work, release time for educational training, on-the-job education, and career ladders for occupational advancement. Most importantly, the career ladder concept has become the major thrust for new sources of health care manpower (Riessmen, 1969). Smith (1973) has hailed the career ladder concept "as a means of upgrading indigenous health workers to paraprofessional and professional status," calling it "one of the most innovative features of the new careers program."

Within the contexts of community physical and mental health centers, the notion that community health workers move up a career ladder falls within the ethos of Horatio Alger. Indeed a few climb their way into specially created jobs unique to the comprehensive health setting. For example, in a neighborhood health center serving blacks in one city in the South, the administration provided occupational mobility by creating the jobs of team manager and team director. However, this is an uncommon strategy of limited efficacy.

In most of the centers studied, career ladders were nonexistent for the community health workers. The major reason for this blocked occupational mobility rests in the fact that there are no systems in community health for creating and maintaining an expanding paraprofessional competence that is compelling to the other organizations which comprise the health care network. A lack of fit and coordination between the community health worker system and the present health care system exists. Hospitals, group practices, extended care facilities, and other settings must be open to the paraprofessional in the sense of providing the occupational rungs on the career ladder. To create a viable job hierarchy within the ranks of health workers, one must see to it that an appropriate job market exists outside of the health centers per se, and the absence of such a market has effectively prevented these workers from moving out of the health centers into related health care roles. This blocked mobility has had profound impact. Without hierarchial occupational levels within a given occupation, a health facility is neither able to weed out the ineffective workers, nor can it provide sufficient job turnover to increase the technical competence and effectiveness of workers and also to create new jobs for the community in an ongoing fashion. Furthermore, health workers view their situation from the perspective of one on the bottom with a dead end looming ahead. Some place the blame on the physician whom they view as an active hinderance. As a neighborhood health agent working in a community-controlled neighborhood health center located in a black ghetto on the West Coast expressed it:

The professionals orient us to get along with them. I strongly feel that professionals should be oriented to adjust to us. When the center first opened there was one doctor who said at each meeting (staff) "What do you say your role is?" This was his way of telling us that he didn't think that we had a valuable role to perform. Now, some neighborhood health agents are shy and I am not one of them, but the professionals try to make neighborhood health agents feel like they are in a bracket all by themselves. If there is any learning to be done, it has to be done on both sides. There was never a thing as neighborhood health agents before and so how do the professionals know how to relate to a neighborhood health agent? You know I went to a conference in Denver and I learned that some agents are not allowed to talk to the doctor. Well this is just one example of our problem here.

Another health agent at the same center identified the lack of formal training consonant with the existing health care structure as the prime reason for her inability to move into a health care role outside of the center:

On the new career program, this is all fine. But I don't have a degree, so if I left here I may have to go and work in the government. Maybe I will go back to National Cash Register business machines. . . .

On our new career program, I don't really feel secure. If something happens, you have to try and get a job. It creates a problem. If you have a degree, then that makes a difference. The main thing is the stress that it creates. You should at least get an associates degree in college. Otherwise, it is in vain. It's just like a person who is qualified to do things but you are confined to an institution.

There should be a stipulation that after a few years in the new career, you should be able to go to a college. As it is now, if you happen to drop out, then its damaging to the new career program and it's damaging to the individual. If he were on welfare and went into new career, and then he had to go back to welfare, that would really be discouraging and damaging.

Finally, an administrator of an East Coast neighborhood health center, which serves an ethnically mixed population, described her training program as one that produced medical care freaks who were unequipped to move into more traditional

medical care roles because of the innovative nature of their medical care skills. According to this administrator, both professionals and nonprofessionals were victims of this process:

One of our innovations is the training of the aides (paraprofessionals) who are getting pretty professional, but sometimes I wonder whether we should let them stay too long. On the other hand, where are they going to go? They can't fit into the traditional hospital structure because it violates everything we've taught them. They're freaks, you know, we raised freaks. We made freaks of the nurses and the neighborhood health aides. The nurses who come to work in the health center program can't go back to the hospitals. They just can't stand it. They can't go into traditional agencies because they are too outspoken and too analytical. They say what they think and they expect people to respond to what they say.

Thus they are prisoners of their positions, and job turnover for community health workers is extremely low as a consequence. Furthermore, these structural constraints are exacerbated by the fact that most community health workers seem to be highly enthusiastic about their work and consequently reluctant to leave the centers, even given the lure of upward occupational mobility in a health career outside of the health center. Perhaps as a monument to one of the successes of the neighborhood health center program, the dedication of community health workers toward their health care roles, their communities, and patients emerged as one of the major themes in our study. For a majority of workers, being a health care worker carried with it a degree of drama not to be found in other jobs within the community. The community accords prestige and status to one who is associated, albeit tangentially, with the mysteries and enormous privileges inherent in the everyday work of nurses, physicians, and other health care professionals. This excitement and drama in work was expressed well by a health worker employed in a neighborhood health center. He saw the community-linked prestige of his work reflected in his son:

> My five-year-old boy says, "My dad works in the health center." He really gets a big thrill knowing that I work at the health center. Most people don't try to knock it. It makes me feel good.

He also mentioned the excitement derived from rubbing shoulders with nurses and physicians and sharing some of the mysteries that are medicine's alone:

> This training is beautiful. They teach you the body structure, psychology, how to interview, also how to talk over the telephone. We are conditioned to help and comfort people. Some mornings we have phonics, English. Out in the stations we also learn a lot. Now, I am on Surgery South. I fill out the 103 forms. I give patients information on when the doctor is coming in. Sometimes I go on house calls. I pick up records or x-rays. I also learn a little bit about the doctors.
> Yesterday, I really worked hard. I was running back and forth all day. When they rotate us around the stations, that helps us a lot. We get to meet the chart nurses and we also see all the memos that are sent around. You'd be surprised how fast people get to know you. I think the most interesting jobs the ladies have here is being a medical stenographer. They listen to the tapes of what the doctors say. That would be interesting. Its a real big job.

Dedication to the job was best reflected by two comprehensive mental health workers who worked for 1 and 2 months, respectively, without pay as a result of problems with the federal funding agency. During these financial crises, the professional staff remained off the job until it was determined that salaries would resume. The mental health workers at the two centers mentioned these examples to us as symbolic of their dedication to the patients and the professionals' dedication to dollars. Although there appears to be an element of sanctimonious posturing contained here, suffice it to say that even when they are payed, the salaries that community health workers command are slightly above the poverty level.

CONCLUSION: STRATEGIES FOR CHANGE

We have taken a thorough look at two of the most innovative aspects of neighborhood health centers. Although it is reasonable to accuse the neighborhood health center movement of being traditional medicine packaged as a medical care outpost (New and Hessler, 1972) and thereby failing to really change the balance of power in favor of consumers or failing to create new manpower strategies, we may be too harsh by expecting too much of the concept. As Boswell concluded long ago, it is not a question of how well a dog walks on his hind legs but that he walks at all that counts.

It must be remembered that the neighborhood health center programs were virtually token ventures in light of the enormous expenditure in time, manpower, and dollars for health care organization and delivery in the United States. Expecting them to change the basic thrust of health care in terms of consumer participation in decision making about matters that affect the health care they receive is unreasonable and unlikely.

Some changes have occurred as a result of neighborhood health centers, and these are worth noting, since they involve the two innovations that we discussed, consumer participation and community health workers.

First, consumer participation has unquestionably altered the thinking of increasing numbers of the public, who are beginning to take an active role in solving their health care problems. Consumers are beginning to ask questions of physicians about medical decisions that previously were accepted on what could be called "blind faith." There is growing unrest with the notion that medical treatment must originate with a physician, and consumers are actively seeking to educate themselves medically to do self-examination, diagnosis, and even treatment. For example, women's rights groups have produced manuals on self-examination and diagnosis for breast and cervical cancer, and they have raised the consciousness of consumers concerning the problems of sexism and racism in medicine. It is our contention that consumer participation at health centers provided a great stimulus and model for much of the consumer movement in health care which is occurring today. In fact, many of the currently active consumer health rights groups can be traced to the National Consumer Conferences held in Berkeley and San Antonio in 1970 and 1971 for neighborhood health center consumer groups.

Finally, as community health workers increase in members and become organized, their roles in medical care will challenge the established hierarchy of medicine in the United States. True that within the context of neighborhood health centers the community health worker is an occupation of not quite a community person and not quite a health professional; nevertheless the seed has been planted for changes in health manpower. If health care is to be made available to all as a right on the order of public education, then change must occur primarily in that sector of the system in which control is vested in the production of medical care services. The community health worker program has provided a model for the creation of a new occupational hierarchy in which health workers and other health professionals can move from under the direct aegis of the physician and actually produce diagnoses and treatments. The pediatric nurse practitioner and emergency medical technician programs are examples of the beginnings of this movement, and some of its impetus can be traced to neighborhood health centers and their community health workers.

Neighborhood health centers will continue to contribute to the development and production of vitally needed health services in spite of the serious shortcomings and issues discussed in this chapter.

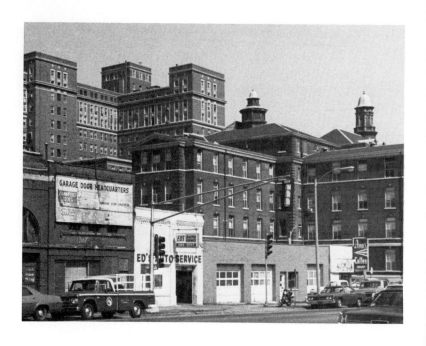

CHAPTER 13

The health care system

There is no health care system in the United States. . . . It is a non-system.

Medical Committee for Human Rights (1966)

If you think there is no system, just try and change it.

John Knowles (1969)

Square doctors are usually good bod mechanics. . . . But somebody who's been through square doctor's school, it's really hard for him to learn anything about healing or to put enough holiness and enough value in the human body to really let it come on and do its thing.

Stephen and the Farm (1974)

The way in which health care is organized differs from one nation to another. Every nation, in fact, organizes its health services in a different way. In this chapter, we will explore some of the dimensions of these differences and try to identify at least some of the sources. Given that there are a multitude of nations, it is obvious that we will not be able to discuss all the alternative arrangements, nor, we suspect, would

the student be able to tolerate such an effort even if it were possible. Instead we will refer to a limited number of countries that have distinctive differences which illustrate some types of solutions to problems in the delivery of health services.

Before beginning this task, one must be clear about our meaning when we use the term "system" with respect to health services, and we will have to address the issue noted in the quotations at the head of this chapter as to whether there is a system at all. This aside, some sources of national differences will then be identified. Anticipating our argument, two of these sources, economy and ideology, will be singled out, and some ways in which they influence health systems will be presented in an abstract form. The next two sections of the chapter will apply these formal propositions to the concrete organization of health care services in the United States, the United Kingdom, Sweden, the Soviet Union, the Peoples' Republic of China, and Cuba.

THE CONCEPT OF SYSTEM

One of the holdovers from the organic tradition in sociology discussed in Chapter 1 is the concept of system. Societies from this perspective are seen as analogous to biological organisms. Although the notion of societies as a form of organism has been abandoned by almost all sociologists, some concepts from that tradition are incorporated into the modern notion of social systems.

To posit the existence of a social system (and we should be clear that to do so is a conceptual act rather than an empirical observation) usually involves two ideas: that parts of the society can be identified and that these parts go together (or are integrated) so as to form a more-or-less unified whole (Rose, 1971; Wilson, 1971). From this perspective, societies may be seen as composed of institutions such as the economy, politics, the family, and others, all of which are related in some distinctive pattern to constitute "the society" (Parsons, 1951).

Such a model has the distinct advantage of focusing attention on the question of how parts "hang together"; it leads to a search for the components of any given group, society, or organization and allows for the description of how the unit in question maintains itself over time. This produces an aspect of the true state of affairs. At the same time, however, it leads the focus of attention away from the fact that members of any group, organization, or society are often in conflict with one another. There may be significant differences of not only opinion but also action, leading to a fragmentation rather than a unification of human experience and effort. Whether it is true that conflicts are a source of unification (equilibrium or integration) or whether integration exists in spite of conflict has not been resolved. In fact, the existence of a system is possibly not demonstrable.

In this book, we take an agnostic position on the existence of a system, if by this we mean an integration of parts analogous to that implied by the biological concept of homeostasis. What we can observe is that different large aggregates of people have tended to solve problems in different ways, and the way in which they solve one type of problem (e.g., health care delivery) tends to correspond to the ways in which they solve others (e.g., the allocation of other goods and services, family organization).

HEALTH CARE: SYSTEM OR NONSYSTEM?

In recent years, several individuals have referred to health care in the United States as a "nonsystem" (Glasser, 1972; Reuther, 1972). By this they mean to call attention to certain features of health service delivery that fall short of those considered optimum. These persons have correctly noted that in the United States there is no national program of health insurance and that many people do not have the financial resources to afford medical care, that we place the burden on the sick person to select the right physician from a confusing array of specialists, that our insurance companies often artificially inflate the rates of hospitalization because they will not pay for simple procedures outside the hospital, that patients often get lost by "falling through the cracks" when being referred from one service provider to another, and that each provider maintains his own records and vital information about the patient is often not communicated from one to the other. In short, health care services are fragmented and disjointed; they are provided at increasingly higher costs; and there are manpower shortages, partly because of the wasteful way in which services are currently organized (Corey et al., 1972; Glasser, 1972).

Others such as John Knowles, former Director of the Massachusetts General Hospital and current President of the Rockefeller Foundation, have focused, also correctly, on the resistance of health care providers to changes in their work environment. The legislative proposals for health insurance for the aged in the mid-1960s, for example, faced well-organized opposition from the AMA (Harris, 1966). The attempt of the Kaiser Foundation to establish prepaid group practice was fought in the courts for a period of twenty-five years.[1] From this perspective there is a system of medical care that is organized and committed to maintaining the status quo, and those who believe that it is a "nonsystem" are challenged to "try and change it."

Whether health care is considered a system or nonsystem depends on one's perspective. The proponents of each view are looking at different factors. Those who argue for "nonsystem" tend to see health care delivery from a consumer viewpoint. From this perspective, health services are chaotic, disorganized, fragmented, and expensive, and the consumer in the United States has little to no voice in deciding the conditions under which what kinds of services will be offered. In fact, all recent proposals and policies for changing the organization of health services and financing in the United States have kept the control of resources in the hands of the providers (Navarro, 1974). At the same time, the providers are well organized to protect their interests with respect to both economic rewards and the maintenance of their autonomy in setting the conditions of their work.

Although we would expect that in most countries providers are organized to protect their interests, we also expect that great variation exists in the extent to which they see their interests as including satisfying public (consumer) needs. There will also be great variation in the extent to which the consumers are organized, the extent of their voice in the delivery of health services, and the extent to which they are *part* of the system. Thus as we examine the systems in various countries, consumer involvement will be a key issue.

SOURCES OF NATIONAL DIFFERENCES IN HEALTH CARE SYSTEMS

Sources of national differences in health care systems can be identified in many ways. Nations differ in geographical size, in the size and distribution of their populations, and in the composition of their populations with reference to age, sex, marital status, and other characteristics. Such differences are *ecological,* since they involve the relationships between populations and environments, both physical and social (Hawley, 1950). Another way of approaching the problem is in terms of the *social organization* of the society as a whole. Ethnic composition of the populations, the pattern of social stratification, and institutional arrangements with respect to government, family organization, education, and other entities influence the organization of health services. Another way is in terms of the *economic structure* of the society, including the available technology, the characteristic ways of financing goods and services, and patterns of expenditures. Finally (in the sense that we are limiting our focus in this chapter, not that we have exhausted the possibilities), nations differ *ideologically* with reference to political, religious, and health values.

In the analysis later in the chapter we will concentrate on the last two sources: the economic and ideological. Ecological and social dimensions will be considered as needed and much less systematically.

Before turning to the analysis, however, we must briefly delineate a few ways in which each of these dimensions can influence health services.

Ecological sources

Both the pattern of disease and the organization of health services are influenced by characteristics of the population and the ways in which the population relate to the environment.

In Chapter 3, we noted several effects of personal characteristics on the distribution of disease. Acute disease was more common among young people, and chronic disease was more common among the old. Women had more disease than men. Rural residents were more likely than urban residents to have chronic disease than whites. High socioeconomic status was associated with high rates of acute disease and low rates of chronic disease.

Viewed from another perspective, these same findings apply to the patterning of health care at the national level. A country with a high birth rate and a low death rate will have a high proportion of young people as compared with one in which both the birth and death rates are either high or low.[2] Such a population will have more acute disease and less chronic disease. The health care system will necessarily be more oriented toward short-term care. A predominantly rural country will have to provide for relatively more long-term care, whereas an urban one will have to have an organization capable of handling short-term cases (holding constant, of course, the differences in age and sex distributions of the population).

It is not only the population that is at issue but also the way in which it relates to the environment, particularly through land use. To some extent the organization of health services depends on the distribution of the population over a land area and the modalities by which resources are exploited.

Some types of services such as specialized hospitals and technological apparatus, which are expensive and used by relatively few people, require a large population base within a small area. Agrarian societies, in which the vast majority of the population is rural and relatively evenly distributed over a large land area, cannot economically support some types of services that are feasible in urban societies. Highly specialized physicians such as neurosurgeons must locate in an area with a large enough population to ensure that there will be enough patients to keep them busy. Since relatively few people will have reason to use such services, they tend to be found only in urban areas.[3] In countries such as the United States and the United Kingdom, the population is highly urban, and there are a large number of specialists in medicine, as well as a system of large hospitals capable of carrying out a number of esoteric diagnostic and therapeutic procedures. A more rural country such as China relies more heavily on generalists who can locate in smaller population units because their services are used by a large number of people.

Population density and concentration are also related to technology, but these are discussed later in the section on economic sources of national differences in health care systems.

Within urban areas, the more highly specialized services tend to be more centrally located, since this is the point of maximum access, that is, the easiest place for all people to get to generally. This point is the shortest distance measured in terms of time and cost from all other places in the community. Hence large hospitals, specialized medical services, and other facilities that serve the whole community tend to be centrally located in the business district of the cities, whereas less specialized services tend to be more evenly distributed within the urban area.

It is only when the technological base allows for a high degree of specialization that such factors tend to be taken into account in the organization of services. This kind of calculus is more characteristic of urban than of agrarian societies.

How a population exploits natural resources also affects health care. The reliance of industrialized societies on large amounts of energy not only has led to the prospect of long-term shortages when the energy sources are nonrenewable, but also the resulting pollution of the natural environment has become a threat to life. Many modern chronic diseases are seemingly the result of environmental pollution, requiring a larger amount of energy to be expended in health care services. Much of this problem is due to a short-sighted ideology that supports waste and will be discussed later in the chapter.

Social sources

The organization of health services depends on the ways in which aspects of the society are organized, including the economic structure, the presence of ethnic populations, the organization of the family, and the political structure. Since some of these topics are covered later in the chapter, this section will deal with stratification and the family briefly to illustrate some key dimensions.

Stratification systems can vary in both degree and kind. Although some form of social differentiation and ranking can be found in almost every society, the basis on which people are ranked varies in almost every society. In most industrialized countries, the basis is power or income (which are usually highly correlated). In more "primitive" societies, other criteria are used. The Lenape, for example, differentiated between visionaries (who had powers and protections granted by the spirits, or *manitu,* and hence could perform functions denied to others such as name giving and healing) and those who were *a-sohn,* or "empty" (Westlager, 1973).

By any given criteria, societies differ in the degree to which they are stratified. In the United States, for example, there is a steep stratification structure based on income. Most people have modest incomes, with the wealthiest having many times that of the poorest. Reports of visitors to the People's Republic of China claim that there the income structure is relatively flat, with the wealthiest making little more money than the vast majority at the bottom of the structure. In addition, although poorer in material possessions than their American counterparts, the Chinese are not denied the essentials of life, such as health care, on the basis of income. The implications of poverty are different in the two societies (Sidel and Sidel, 1973; New, personal communication, 1976). Much of the reason for these differences is ideological.

The nature of the family structure typical of any given society, particularly with reference to the position of women, affects both the number of hospitals in that society and the organization of the hospitals (Glaser, 1970). In those societies in which there are extended families and women are sheltered, there tend to be few hospitals because a work force of nurses is essential, and such a structure depresses the potential work force. Also such societies tend to have a tradition in which families take care of the sick at home.

In societies in which there are nuclear families, a larger work force is required for any given hospital. In Greece, for example, when a patient is admitted to the hospital, the whole family moves in with him. The housekeeping chores are done by the family members, who also prepare the meals. Such a system requires fewer nurses and a smaller staff in housekeeping and food service (Friedl, 1958).

Glaser also found that the nature of hospitals is affected by the interaction of social class and family structure. For example, in societies in which upper-class women are sheltered and lower- or working-class women are not, the hospital work force is less skilled, and hospitals tend to care for lower-class people. Under these circumstances, upper-class people tend to avoid hospitalization.

Economic sources

The term "economics" is derived from two Greek words: *oikos,* meaning living unit, and *nomos,* meaning management. Economics deals with the management or allocation of scarce resources that people value. For most of us, the term evokes images of the business world, of General Motors and the stock market. Seldom do we consider economics as applied to health services, the second largest industry in the United States.

Given the conflict and indecision associated with governmental economic policy, it should come as no surprise that there is dissent among economists concerning the basic theoretical assumptions underlying the view of the individual in the economic system. Furthermore, it is important to understand that two major theoretical assumptions of economics commonly applied to the business world may in fact lead us astray in considering the economic structure of health care. These assumptions are (1) the concept of profit maximization as it explains organization behavior, and (2) the concept of consumer sovereignty, in which it is supposed that the producer is governed by neutral and technical cost functions and functionally accommodates to the consumer's demand function. These assumptions are not helpful in understanding the impact of economics on health services.

THE COST OF HEALTH CARE

In 1974 health care in the United States cost over $100 billion, fully 7.7% of the gross national product. To get an idea of the magnitude of the increase in costs for health services over the past thirty years, the percentage of the gross national product spent on health care was only 4% in 1940 and 5% in 1960. The reasons behind this great increase in the cost of health care are somewhat of a mystery. However, the primary reason appears to be a rapid increase in the unit cost (price) of hospital care, spurred on by rising demand and an increase in the government's share of payments for services provided.

Demand rises with family income. The growth of health insurance has drastically increased demand for hospital care. Although the net cost to the consumer of hospital care has barely changed in twenty years, insurance has gone from paying only 37% of consumers' expenditures for hos-

pital care in 1950 (when average cost per patient day was $16) to 82% in 1972 (when the average cost per patient-day was $103) (Feldstein, 1973).

The degree to which a government is involved in paying the bill for health services, coupled with the extensiveness of subscription to third-party insurance plans, will have a telling effect on cost. The greater this involvement the higher the cost for medical services.

For example, the United States federal government in 1974 paid for more than 40% of health care costs as compared to 20% in 1950. Medicaid and Medicare represent the major source of this increased governmental involvement. This, coupled with prepaid insurance, is a stimulus to hospitals and other providers to produce services that are costlier and more extensive than consumers actually want or need. In short, the impersonalization of payment procedures is a major source of increasing costs.

Technology

The economic order, particularly the growth or decline of economies, will define the level of resources within which national goals, including health care goals, must be achieved. For an analysis of health care systems, it is vitally important to point out the interdependence of economics and technology. In all countries, economic growth has been as much determined by new technology as by the investment of capital. The growth and diffusion of technology expands the goods and services available to people and thereby stimulates the economy (Teich, 1972). The economic order in turn stimulates or retards the growth of technology, depending of course on whether the economy is growth oriented, in a stable state, or in decline.

Theoretically one side of technology encompasses the argument that technological developments lead to economies of scale, greater efficiency in terms of cost per unit produced, and improvement in the quality of life by creating new opportunities for fulfilling people's needs. A classical example of this is Field's study of changes in the health care system in which he demonstrates that advances in biomedical technology have made hitherto unthinkable areas available, thereby providing the necessary conditions for health care to be considered a right rather than a privilege (Field, 1967).

However, another side of technology is less pleasant. These are the costs of technology, some of them well known at this time. In health systems, technology is related to the increasing scarcity of the general practitioner in certain industrial countries, the acceleration of the power of differentation of medical personnel, and the concentration of medical services. These have left vast populations with inadequate care, unmet needs, and a growing problem of quality care and accountability. Furthermore, as the medical buffet expands its offerings, the patient tends to become less important as a person. A high level of consumption is made an evil in itself (Duesenberry, 1949).

Medical care systems internationally are characterized by an increasing use of and dependence on technology. In some countries such as China and Cuba, technological advances in the forms of machines, processes, and techniques are not linked to corporate profiteering. Such is not the case in the United States where medical technology is big and profitable business for a few extremely large and powerful corporations. In fact, because producers of medical technology form monopolies in the sense of exerting common control over the allocation of resources, the market, and prices (Robinson, 1933), health technology producers have been called "the 'medical-industrial complex,' the business of manufacturing and selling the varied equipment, from bandages to two-million volt cobalt machines, that doctors and hospitals use" (Meyers, 1970). Corporations such as Zenith, Phillips' Petroleum, Motorola, IBM, Monsanto, Litton Industries, Bigelow-Sanford, and even Phillip Morris (sutures and surgical knives) have moved decisively to capture the health dollar. The best example of the enormous growth experienced by a health care business is the American Hospital Supply Corporation. As Meyers (1970) points out, 45% of its sales involved its own manufactured products, varying from rubber gloves to oxygen preservation machines, which cost over $15,000. Sales rose from $219 million in 1964 to $387 million in 1968, and earnings more than doubled during the same period, going from 33 to 67 cents a share. Unlikely consortiums have emerged as technology is pushed to the limits of human knowledge. The Lockheed Space and Missile Center, National Aeronautics and Space Administration (NASA), and United States Department of Health, Education, and Welfare have combined forces to apply exotic medical technology developed for outer space to rural health care systems (Anderson, 1971; Garrett, 1972; Carlton and Hessler, 1973).

United States hospitals have been the scene for the most rapid changes in and uses of medical technology (Feldstein, 1973). For example, manufacturers of surgical dressings and instruments profit from sales of over $500 million. Adhesive tapes alone bring in $163 million, cotton balls $30 million, and surgical instruments cost over $120 million a year (Goddard, 1973). Anesthetics, solutions, syringes, laboratory ware, stethoscopes, x-ray film, and supplies are expected to hit sales of $4.2 billion in 1980 and are currently bringing the manufacturers $3 billion a year in sales. Electronic hospital equipment, including patient monitoring devices, organ preservation machines, and automated laboratory equipment, may reach sales of several billions of dollars by 1980. Sales of prosthetic and corrective devices may hit $890 million by 1980. Many of these increases are due to the enormous proliferation of technology both in terms of new devices and multiple variations of a given model, such as gauze with or without lubricants or pacemakers with chemical or plutonium energy sources.

Consumers, either on their own or covered by a third-party payment scheme, pay the bills for medical technology. Hospitals and physicians make the decisions to employ or not to employ the technologies but do not gain financially from the technology directly. Costs are passed on to the consumer through the hospital's or physician's bill.

Evidence suggests that the growth of medical-industrial technology has had a negative impact on various sectors of the health area system. These effects will be discussed later in the chapter, as will how the use of medical technology in the United States has decreased productivity and other facets of economic efficiency (Feldstein, 1973) and have created moral and ethical dilemmas for health professionals and patients.

Ideology

The term "ideology" has become one of those buzz words that through abuse and overuse has lost much of its explanatory utility. This is a problem because a careful analysis of ideology is extremely important for understanding health care systems. Ideology in fact is a major source of the organizational form that a national health care system takes. Furthermore, the organizational structure of the health care system influences the ideological stance of a country or group of individuals, as the case may be.

The concept of ideology was born sometime during the period beginning with Galileo (1564-1642) and ending with Leibniz (1446-1716) called the "Age of Reason." This period marked the decline of medieval religious systems of thought based on faith and the rise of science, particularly physical scientific thought. Bacon, Descartes, Spinoza, and other philosophers of the period introduced rigorous mathematical thinking into the pursuit of truth to eliminate personal vested interests and other human biases.

The term "ideology" was first used by a French philosopher, Destutt de Tracy, during the late part of the eighteenth century.

For de Tracy, ideology was the science of ideas in which empirical objective truth could be discovered by boiling down ideas into their empirical referents. In short, ideas determine reality.

Karl Marx turned the concept of ideology completely around. Instead of ideology representing the pared-down, objective representation of the empirical world, Marx used the concept to mean idealism, that philosophy first expressed by Plato which argues that ideas per se explain natural processes and embody reality. For Marx, who held that reality determined ideas rather than the converse, ideology became false consciousness which served the function of covering up the vested economic interests of groups. However, one would not know this by a casual reading of the ideology, since it is designed to hide vested interests by appearing to be universal, general representations of reality or the truth, according to Marx. Therefore Marx defined ideology as an attempt by a vested-interest group to claim universal applicability of some general truth, such as, the right to health care, which in reality masks the objective, social class interests behind the idea. In his "18th Brumaire," Marx urges the researcher to look behind ideology for the objective interests represented.

Karl Mannheim (1936), in line with the thinking of Max Weber, viewed society as a network of intersubjectively meaningful actions of individuals. How well humans adapted to the social and physical environment is a function of knowledge, according to Mannheim. Knowledge is class based because the social order is structured according to social classes.

Mannheim defined ideology as that type of knowledge which serves to defend the vested interests of the political and economic classes of the society. He distinguished between two types of ideology in terms of the functions they serve: "ideologies," which are ideas that defend and preserve matters as they are; and "utopias," which are ideas that support the interests of the downtrodden and the underdog and that seek to change the economic, political, or social organization of society to improve life for the disadvantaged. Mannheim refined the concept of ideology further by distinguishing between "total ideologies" (all-inclusive, global interests claiming utility for all facets of life and social organizations), and "particular ideologies" (ideas of a specific group such as nurses with limited vested interests). Finally, the agents of ideology, those who define and pursue the ideas, are important in Mannheim's thinking about ideology. For Mannheim, the elites of society (political, technical, religious, managerial, intellectual, moral, artistic) are the principal agents of ideology, and the task of achieving some degree of order in society depends on the skill of the elites in developing ideas that reduce the tensions betweten laissez-faire capitalism and totalitarian control of society.

The functions of ideology are complex and are as follows:

1. *To build and maintain the power and prestige of an individual or group.* For example, physicians' commitment to serving mankind masks another value of professionalism whereby physicians assert that freedom to control the level and direction of their work is absolutely necessary for the effective practice of medicine.

2. *To retard social change.* If the vested class interests are maintained by ideology, then ideology becomes a tool or strategy for implementing the status quo.

3. *To gain adherents or a constituency for the ideologue.* For example, pharmaceutical companies claim dedication to improving people's health by improving the quality of drugs. The industry hopes that this idea will gain the approval of the public, which would limit pressure on the political regulatory bodies designed to control the production of drugs.

Ideology interacts within health care systems by taking the form of political, religious, and health ideas. In some societies, all three facets of ideology are bound together in one package within the health care system. For example, the Cuban health care system under Castro has adopted the political and economic ideology of the larger society. The attempt to eliminate social class within educational institutions affects admissions to the three medical schools and other medical training programs. One result is that health personnel come from all sectors of Cuban society. To develop the idea that there should be no economic elitism born of occupational prestige hierarchies, Cuban physicians are required to spend some time at manual labor in the fields alongside peasants (John et al., 1971). In turn, this is related to the health ideology, which precludes elitism and status differentials in the health professional-patient relationship. In Cuba health care is defined as a basic human right rather than a special privilege.

Religious ideology is seldom a manifest, formal part of the health care system. Religious beliefs enter the health care system by way of patients and practitioners who may subscribe to specific religious dogmas. These are related to medical beliefs and practice either directly or tangently. For example, from Chapter 6, one will recall that certain cultural and religious beliefs direct health content and are applied to health and illness behaviors. In many Native-American tribes, health is the measure of the degree to which the individual is connected with the spirits in nature and other people. Similarly, a physician who for religious reasons believes that abortion is wrong will engage in health practices consistent with those beliefs.

DIMENSIONS OF DIFFERENCES IN NATIONAL HEALTH CARE SYSTEMS

Nations differ in a number of ways in their health care systems, including modes of organization, characteristics of the persons who become health professionals, relationships between health workers, the range of services provided, the quality of service, and the accountability of the health care system to consumers and the public at large.

In a study of hospitals, Glaser (1970) identified a large number of differences when sixteen countries were compared. The major differences, which were discussed in Chapter 11, are the following:

1. Inputs into hospitals, including recruitment of employees, investments in buildings and technology, the utilization of ambulatory services, utilization of inpatient services, time or referral, and regional distribution
2. Organization of the individual hospital, including its size, number of departments, and number of personnel
3. Authority within the hospital
4. Performance of employees
5. Relations among hospitals
6. Output of hospitals, including rate of recovery at discharge, rate of relapse after discharge, type of treatment by clinical specialty, and consensus about goals and rate of success

Hospitals are only a part of the picture, perhaps a minor one. The student will recall that a minority of illnesses are treated by health professionals, and a minority of these are treated in hospitals. We must be concerned with a much broader range of services. The extent to which hospitals dominate a system of health care delivery is itself important. Given the realities of economic life, a heavy investment in any one sector usually means that another is being shortchanged.

Organizational forms

At the national level, health care systems differ in the degree to which they are financed by the government or private means. In the first case, the health care system is more influenced by the political process of the country (which may differ widely in its responsiveness to public needs), and in the second instance, it will be more influenced by the market economy. This difference can influence accountability, flexibility in adaptation to local differences, the availability of services needed by only a small portion of the population, and the degree to which alternatives can be explored.

Nations also differ in the degree to which they emphasize large-scale or small-scale organizations, including the relative emphasis placed on hospitals, the size of hospitals, the thin distribution of resources over a wide area, or the concentration of services in a few places. In general, an emphasis on primary care and preventive medicine is associated with a system in which personnel are widely dispersed and there are few concentrations of large numbers of specialized people. Systems that emphasize secondary care tend to develop large-scale organizations, which are centralized in a few locations.

Closely related to scale of organization, nations differ in the extent to which they focus on technological innovation for solving health care problems versus the emphasis on providing personal services. In the first case, the best service will be much more sophisticated but available to a smaller proportion of the populations, and in the second, the average care will be of higher quality, but the best will be somewhat lower.

Health professionals

Different nations have different patterns in the nature of their health professionals. Some emphasize the highest skilled occupations, which require long years of training; others place more emphasis on lower levels of skill. There are differences for any given occupation in the nature of work, the kinds of activities occupants are expected to do, and the degree of their authority. Some countries have unique occupational roles that are not found in other countries, usually designed to meet specific needs of that country in ways that traditional occupations cannot.

For those occupations common to all countries, there are differences in the kinds of people recruited to work in those occupations. In some countries, for example, nurses are recruited from the working classes, whereas in others they come from middle-class backgrounds. In some instances, particular groups of people have traditionally filled certain positions; in others the filling of positions is competitive. How people are recruited influences the image of the health professions and the kinds of people likely to make use of the particular services (Glaser, 1970).

The development of a profession of nursing requires a relatively emancipated group of women who are free to work outside the home, an ideology of service to others, and an economic structure that can support organizations on the scale of hospitals (Glaser, 1970).

Another way in which countries differ is in the kinds of relationships among health occupations that could be considered typical. In some instances, all health occupations are relatively equal, each having an area of special expertise or all having significant overlap. Here decision making is a matter of negotiating a plan of action in each case. In other countries, certain occupations are always above others and have the right to overrule decisions. In this case the relationships are relatively authoritarian.

Services provided

A vast range of services are available in some countries. These range from primary care to several levels of specialization within medicine, including some extremely esoteric procedures suitable for only a small number of people each year. Outside of medicine, a vast range of occupations may be available either to support basic medical functions (e.g., laboratory technicians), to augment them by providing additional services outside the normal scope of medicine (e.g., nursing), or to provide a range of services that relate to health but are not considered as traditional members of the health care fields (e.g., learning disabilities specialists).

The inclusion or exclusion of any type of service is an economic and political choice. Given that resources are finite, the inclusion of any particular service means a reduction of the resources available for another. Each country is forced by necessity to make choices that will alter the organization of its system of medical care. Money spent for experimentation with open heart surgery, for example, is money not available for primary care (Fox and Swazey, 1974). Money spent on medical care is money not spent on education. Thus what is provided is not just a matter of relative sophistication but of the choices made in each country.

Quality and accountability

Nations differ in the technical quality of the services that they offer and in the degree to which they are accountable to those they treat.

It is useful to distinguish the quality of the *best* services available in the country and the quality of the *average* services. The two do not necessarily go together. As noted in Chapter 3, according to one indicator of the quality of medical service, the infant mortality rate, the United States does rather poorly. However, at the same time, few would deny that the best medicine in the United States, that delivered by the Mayo Clinic in Rochester, Minnesota, for example, is the best to be found anywhere in the world.

State-of-the-art medicine is enormously expensive. A nation that elects to provide it, with only a few exceptions, also elects to provide poor quality average care. That is, a choice is made between providing the best for a few and providing good care for the many.

Nations must also make choices dealing with the issue of accountability. Medical care absorbs a large portion of the gross national product of almost every country (in Western societies only the military and education are in serious competition). Consciously or unconsciously, decisions must be made regarding to whom the providers must answer. In some instances, providers enjoy almost total autonomy, in which case the health care system tends to organize for the convenience of the health professionals. In other cases, professionals are held to account by a national government, communities, organized groups of consumers, or some mixture of these. The choices made will affect the way in which services are provided and conditions under which they are available.

In the following discussion we will illustrate with case examples some national differences in health care systems. Special attention will be given to the influence of the economy and ideology on the forms of medical organization, the nature of the health professions, the services provided, and the quality and accountability of that service.

IMPACT OF THE ECONOMY ON HEALTH CARE ORGANIZATION

In all countries, the health care system is linked to the entire economic and political structure. The evolution of health care, the type of health system that develops, and the issues or problems that emerge parallel the economic organization of a society. In short, the action in the larger economic system is reflected in the health care system.

The economic structure of a society affects the health care system at two levels: (1) the more general level of organization, including the organization of services, the medical professions, and the industrial sector; and (2) the more specific interaction that occurs between health care personnel and patients, including the health-seeking behaviors of consumers. Since the patient-health provider interaction has been discussed in Chapters 5 and 10, this section will focus on the impact of economic organization on the more general level of health care organization.

A good place to begin an analysis of the impact of the economy on health care organization is to examine the dominant form of economic organization in a society, particularly the form of the market structure. In the People's Republic of China, for example, the market structure is collectivistic. Economic policy is formulated and administered by a centralized bureaucracy, but the functioning and implementation of programs is highly decentralized in the

sense that these decisions are left up to local political entities such as individual communes or even smaller units. In the United States and other societies with capitalistic forms of economic organization, the market structure is characterized by competition and monopolistic control. Where technology is growing rapidly, monopolistic control of the market increases. In health care, as well as in agriculture and other sectors, the monopolistic control takes the form of large-scale corporate mergers of producers in which economic policy, administration, and implementation are highly centralized. In the capitalist system, increasingly complex technology and ever-larger scales of organization diminish the likelihood that small, independent producers can survive and compete with the corporate giants. This holds true for all sectors of the economy, including the health care system. One only needs to analyze the fate of the declining autonomy of the private practitioner engaged in solo, fee-for-service practice in the United States to substantiate this point.

For ideological reasons, which are discussed in a later section, the economic organization of medical care in the United States falls outside of public regulation and control. The medical system, particularly the economic aspect that relates to the production of services, is vested with the providers of care. As Navarro (1974) points out, the provider exerts major influence over the health care market by controlling the distribution of resources and the patterns of consumption. For example, studies have shown that fee-for-service payment systems of medical care have higher utilization rates than prepaid systems in which physicians are salaried or costs are fixed on a capital basis (Bunker, 1970; Perrott, 1971). According to Navarro (1974), "All these studies would seem to indicate that the 'invisible hand' of the market is increasingly visible, and the hand looks more like the provider's than the consumer's."

The economic order, particularly provider sovereignty, and the attendant growth of the medical-industrial complex have affected the medical care system in the United States in many ways. For the remainder of this section, we shall focus on the following impacts: (1) the distribution of health care resources, particularly medical services and personnel; and (2) the types of services produced.

Distribution of medical resources

The greatest inequalities in terms of the availability of medical resources occur in societies that have provider sovereignty and a capitalistic-monopolistic economy. These societies have pronounced maldistributions of medical manpower, for example, with the highest density of physicians found in those areas with the highest median income. For example, the United States has an acute and growing maldistribution of physicians, particularly in inner-city and rural areas of the country. Physician-to-population ratios are highest for the wealthier, more populous regions of the country, primarily the suburbs, whereas the lower income inner-city and rural areas have the lowest ratios, some being without any physicians (American Medical Association, 1971). United States physicians have been concentrating in the wealthier, larger communities at a much faster rate than the population increase for these areas would warrant, indicating the seriousness of the maldistribution in rural areas (Hobbs, 1974).

In the United Kingdom, the distribution of physicians is controlled by the National Health Service. In that country, the maldistribution is different from that in the United States. The rural areas (which, it should be cautioned, are much less rural than in the United States) have been oversupplied with physicians. The National Health Service implemented a system in which areas of the country were classified into one of four categories: *closed,* in which no physician could set up a new practice; *restricted,* in which a new practice could be opened only to replace one that has closed; *open,* in which new practices could be opened irrespective of what other physi-

cians did; and *designated,* in which the government pays special subsidies to encourage the opening of new practices. Since that time, the maldistribution of physicians relative to population has been decreased by 20%. Within the constraints of the classification, physicians are left free to practice where they choose. The system is basically one of incentives (Butler and Taylor, 1973).

In societies in which the economic aspects of the health care system are controlled by the public sector, the maldistribution problems are much less serious. For example, in the Soviet Union's *zemstvos,* the local governmental districts, feldsher-midwife stations are located on collective farms or in villages throughout the rural areas. The feldsher performs primary and preventive care functions independent of physician control, although there are some regularly scheduled visits to the feldsher stations by physicians (Sidel, 1968). A network of rural hospitals, organized along the line of ambulatory medical stations with one or two physicians on board, are spread through the rural areas. Each of these stations serves approximately 4,000 people (Sidel, 1968). In Cuba comprehensive community health centers, called "polyclinics" provide clinical, environmental, community health, and social services to a specifically defined area and population (Danielson, 1974). The polyclinic is under the leadership of a physician-director, and it serves 25,000 to 30,000 persons in urban areas and as few as 7,000 to 8,000 in rural areas. The task of the polyclinic, in addition to providing services, is to serve as a referral source for the regional hospitals where secondary specialist services are available. The full-time staff of the polyclinic includes primary care specialists such as internists, pediatricians, obstetricians-gynecologists, and dentists, as well as nurses and other medical workers. A new plan is presently being implemented that will change the organization of work in the area polyclinics. Under the new plan, physician-nurse teams will be assigned to specific sectors within the health

Table 13-1. Health services offered and personnel categories for Cuban area polyclinic, 1971*

Personnel categories	Personnel norms
Director	1 full time/polyclinic
Internist	4 hours/day/15,000 population
Pediatrician	4 hours/day/3,000 children, ages 0-14
Obstetrician-gynecologist	4 hours/day/20,000 women
Dentist	8 hours/day/7,000 population
Dental assistant	1 full time15/dentist hours
Nurse	1 full time/polyclinic
Auxiliary nurse	1/sector (3,000-5,000 population)
Administrator	1 full time/polyclinic
Statistical clerk	1 full time/polyclinic
Laboratory technician	8 hours/day/15,000 population
Auxiliary technical sanitarian	1 full time/two sectors
Assistant technical sanitarian	1 full time/2,000 population

*From Danielson, R. The Cuban health area and polyclinic. *Inquiry*, 1975, **12**, supp., June, 86-102. Based on data from Navarro, V. Health, health services, and health planning in Cuba. *International Journal of Health Services*, 1972, **2**, 409-410.

area (the geographical base of the polyclinic), and polyclinic physicians will no longer divide their time with hospital duties; rather they will perform home visits and health education (Danielson, 1976). The services offered and the personnel norms of Cuban medical care can be seen in Table 13-1 (Navarro, 1972).

Similarly, the distribution of health care resources in the People's Republic of China is more equitably managed than in the United States. Geographical and administrative decentralization of the political and economic structure of Chinese society serves as the context for the health care system. Health services are organized according to population density and the hierarchy of local governmental units. For example, urban areas are administered by municipal governments, a number of districts with their own separate administrative branch (covering 250,000 to 500,000 people), street committees within the district (administering to 50,000 to 100,000 people), a network of neighborhood committees (2,000 to 12,000 people), and factory administrations. China's rural health care is administered by communes of which there may be several within a district. Each commune, usually comprising several villages and a

large geographical area, is administered by brigades and production teams. For example, the August 1st commune has fifteen brigades and seventy-three production teams, serving a rural population of 20,600 persons (New, 1974). Health care services are distributed and administered according to the political structures established within the rural districts and urban municipalities.

According to observers' reports (Rozenfeld, 1963; Sidel, 1968), the Soviet Union has attempted to attain equity in the distribution of health care across class and geographical lines in the society. The production of medical services, although organized differently for rural and urban areas, is controlled not by physicians but by the state. Because the Soviet Union also experienced great difficulty in finding adequate numbers of willing physicians to practice in medically underserved areas, particularly after the abolition of serfdom by Alexander II in 1861, "middle medical workers" were introduced. These workers include feldshers who constitute the bulk of middle workers. In rural areas, feldshers, trained as generalists and midwives, work in a feldsher-midwife medical station located in a village or collective farm.

The rural felshers work independently of

physicians, aside from regular visits to the feldsher stations by physicians stationed at rural ambulatory stations serving approximately 4,000. Patients will see only a feldsher for primary and preventive services unless the medical problem is beyond the feldsher's capabilities, in which case she (feldshers, as well as physicians, are predominantly female occupations in Soviet Union) is required to refer the case to a physician-manned ambulatory station. The urban feldsher works at a polyclinic or possibly a hospital under the direct supervision of a physician. Medical care facilities and personnel are located in principle according to the size and scope of the population rather than the financial attractiveness of certain areas. Unlike the free enterprise economic models, Soviet medical services and personnel are controlled by the state in terms of numbers produced and where one practices medicine.

Types of services produced

The product mix of all societies occurs in large measure, as a result of economic organization. This is true of the service sector of a society as well, and the type of health service produced in large measure is due to the predominant form that the economic order takes in a given society.

Regardless of the type of economy extant, all societies develop some form of primary medical services, and some establish preventive services. Capitalistic and socialistic societies alike will produce these two basic medical services to meet the universal demand for a minimal level of primary and preventive health services.

However, the mix or types of services produced in a society is related to the economic structure of that society. We have taken a glimpse at several societies and have seen that their health care systems are formed by economic currents such as the degree of corporate action, private initiative, enlightened despotism, and so forth. These same economic forces affect the decisions of health planners in a society to emphasize certain types of primary services,

for example, as opposed to prevention of environmental problems associated with acute and chronic health problems.

The relationship between economic structure and types or mix of health services is evident in the case of the United States. For simplicity instead of considering the entire health care system as a unit of analysis, one can focus on hospitals as a component of the United States medical care system in which service mix relates to the monopolistic-capitalistic economic order. Furthermore, this focus has the advantage of building on the student's knowledge of hospital organization in United States society as presented in Chapter 11. In this sense, the hospital can serve as an analytical tool for understanding the processes of the larger health care system of which it is a part.

Hospital services in the United States tend to become more complicated dramatically over time. In short, hospitals tend to become larger, with greater bed capacities and higher ratios of full-time employees to patients served. The scope of services and facilities offered grows, and the technology associated with the services becomes increasingly specialized and complex.

The United States economic system, in spite of increasing federal control, is predicated on provider sovereignty in which the enterprise of deciding what gets produced, when, how much, with what quality, and with what accountability is vested with the providers of medical care. It is altogether too simplistic to argue that profit seeking by providers is the predominant economic force which motivates the behavior of hospitals and other institutions producing services in the health care system. In fact as explained shortly, the complexing of organization precludes reaping great profits because economy of scale operates to raise costs excessively. This is not to deny that excessive profits exist. For example, evidence on the drug industry has shown that the profit motive is a major driving force. In fact, it is important to recognize that the net revenue of the hospital and the income of the staff are important motivating forces as well. However, the mix of health care services is not explained well by the profit motive. A much more important factor, a variable much overlooked in theories of organizational behavior, is prestige. In corporate-monopolistic economic systems, the prestige of organizations—the reputation, status, and good name—is a critically important dimension of the ability to compete and survive. Under these circumstances, **management** might make decisions to deliver services that would be inconsistent with profit maximization but that would build the prestige of management through various ways, such as having a high-powered staff with international reputations or the most expensive heart-lung machine (Alchian and Kessel, 1962). Organizational theorists have argued that the power and professional satisfaction of decision makers are dependent on the prestige of the organizations with which the decision makers are associated (Thompson, 1961; Barnard, 1968). Finally, as Lee (1971) points out, hospitals strive to acquire inputs without adequate regard for the manner in which the inputs will be used to actually produce services. This means that hospitals use more resources than required to produce a given mix of services, or they may use a greater quantity or quality of services than necessary to accomplish a given task. Again the economic structure of third-party payment (impersonalization) and the lack of citizen participation in economic decision making (public ignorance about economic organization) facilitate this drive for status among hospitals. Lee calls this process "status gap minimization" or "conspicuous production," in which the mix of hospital services and facilities defines the status group to which a hospital belongs. Ultimately the mix of services produced is used as status symbols, and hospitals compete with one another by means of the acquisition of services and facilities. Consequently, the total expenditure of hospitals for services and facilities and its prices may in-

crease without any change in productivity or output (Lee, 1971). This results in an overabundance of highly trained employees who perform tasks suitable for persons with less training. Or the hospital uses equipment too sophisticated or overduplicated for the task at hand. In brief, the hospital engages in creative waste to maximize status.

As the product mix increases in scope and complexity, the following occur as a consequence: (1) the number of patients treated (hospital admissions and total patient days) goes up, (2) the mean number of patient days goes up, (3) the average length of stay in the hospital goes up, (4) occupancy rates increase, and (5) labor and capital per unit of labor goes up (Berry, 1973). With apologies to Parkinson, sickness expands to fill the available beds.

This process serves as an example of how the economic structure of the United States affects the organization and delivery of health services, particularly regarding the types of services produced. In the People's Republic of China or Cuba, where the economy is tightly controlled by a highly centralized governmental structure, the types of medical services produced reflect the production priorities of the state. Types of services appear to correspond closely to production goals in the sense that health and environmental problems affecting the work force are assigned high priorities for eradication. Conspicuous production and status maximization within health care institutions are minimized. One finds much greater coordination of decision making regarding the types of services produced, and reports of observers suggest that duplication of services is minimal in contrast to the United States with its competitive economic structure.

In the Scandinavian countries, creative waste is controlled by a welfare state apparatus. The control of the medical care system (although not of medical practice) is centralized in the governments, which place a premium on rationalization and efficiency. Sweden, for example, is di-

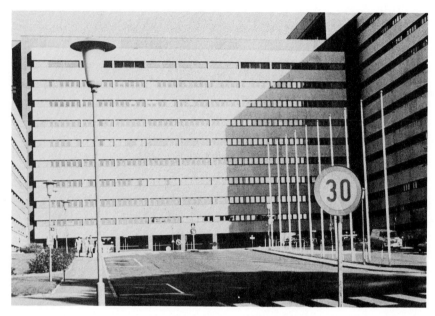

Fig. 13-1. *The Central Block Hospital in Lund, Sweden, one of seven regional hospitals in the country.*

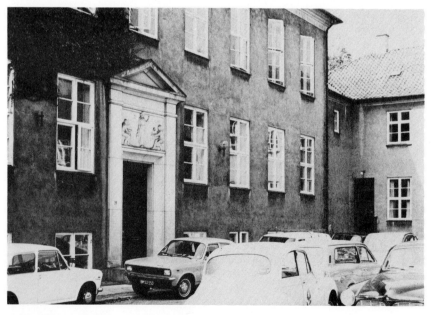

Fig. 13-2. *The Institute of Social Medicine in Copenhagen, Denmark, has responsibility for studying improvements in the delivery of health services.*

vided into seven regions, each of which has a "central block" hospital (Figs. 13-1 and 13-2). This hospital serves the general medical care needs of the region, including those specialty services that are required by large numbers of people. Each hospital, for example, has medical and surgical services, an intensive care unit, pediatrics, obstetrics and gynecology, cardiology, and other commonly used specialty services. Better than 95% of the needs of the population can be adequately met in such a facility.

Each hospital is surrounded by a large number of specialty clinics, each serving a national population and each existing in only one region. Of the approximately forty clinics surrounding the central block hospital at Lund in the southern part of Sweden, for example, one clinic is devoted to a surgical procedure in the treatment of arthritis. The demand for this surgery, which is appropriate for only a minority of arthritics, is approximately a hundred operations each year for the entire country. Should a patient in the extreme northern part of the country need this procedure, he is flown to Lund with the family and treated at the clinic. This has the advantage of avoiding duplication of services and ensures that somewhere in the country there is a skilled team with adequate experience in the procedure. Hence the success rate is higher than when surgeons do the operation only rarely and operating room teams are less highly trained in the particular surgery.

Although what is gained in this kind of system in efficiency may entail a sacrifice in the personal care with which a service is delivered and in freedom of choice on the part of the patient, casual interviews with Swedish patients by one of us (A. C. T.) in 1972 failed to reveal any dissatisfaction. It is possible that the Swedish people have an ideology favoring efficiency to a greater degree than other peoples and that such a system would not transfer easily to other countries for this reason.

IMPACT OF IDEOLOGY ON HEALTH CARE ORGANIZATION

Developments in health care organization rest on ideological bases. Recalling the Marxian conception of ideology, the reality of the political and social organization of society determines ideologies that reflect the needs of particular vested-interest groups. Because the vested-interest groups, for example, in health education or religion, claim universal applicability of some ideology (e.g., the equitable distribution of health services for all people) and because ideologies mask the vested interests behind the particular idea, according to Marx, it is imperative to assess the role that ideology plays as it in turn affects the organization of the health care systems. Although there are many functions of ideology in this regard, we will examine the following impacts: ideology as it forces the reexamination of assumptions underlying the social organization of the health care system and ideology as it is put into practice in medical care.

Ideology and reexamination

Ideology is used by vested-interest groups to call into question basic tenets that may appear immutable or be taken for granted by the members of society. New (1974) pointed out that political ideology has forced medical care planners in the People's Republic of China to critically examine hitherto accepted dogma. For example, the ideology of equal access to health services for all people in China has led to a recognition that the medical manpower shortage is due to an uncritical acceptance of the principle of educating only a few who then form an officially qualified elite who carry out their medical specialties. Similarly, why is it so important to prove the worth of medicines and treatments before adopting certain procedures? Is rigid adherence and attention to licensing procedures really necessary? With the political and economic ideology of equity in the distribution of goods and services throughout rural and urban China, health care planners have reevaluated these assumptions, a necessary step if they are to accomplish the changes necessary to meet their goals.

In Cuba the ideology of equity in the distribution of health services led to a reexamination of the premise that specialized health services ought to be developed at urban medical centers. Instead Cuban health planners established a health care system at the rural periphery of the society and worked the urban medical centers in as part of a referral network.

In the United States the emerging ideology of equity in the distribution of medical resources to rural and inner-city areas, chronically underserved, has led to a reevaluation of the belief that the physician must be the sole producer of medical care services. The rapid increase in the number and types of nonphysician health workers such as physician assistants, community health workers, and others is correlated with an equally rapid rethinking of the amount of supervision and control to be exerted over these workers by physicians. Whereas in the 1950s it would have been inconceivable to argue for nonphysician health personnel doing diagnostic and treatment work, currently this is a reality in some rural areas, and this concept of autonomy is gaining approval from ever-wider segments of the society.

Ideology put into practice

The dominant ideological positions of a society are reflected in the organization and delivery of personal health services. Health services' organization is embedded in a sociopolitical context, and the manner in which health services are delivered to the populace is in response to the dominant ideological forces in the society rather than as a result of formal, rational planning in any controlled, bureaucratic context. Crozier (1964) observed that organizational goals may be developed in a rational fashion, whereby one systematically seeks to maximize gains and minimize losses. How-

ever, such goals are limited or constrained by the sociopolitical environment of which the organization is a part. This includes the predominant ideological structure as an important yet much ignored influence.

In the United States the free enterprise ideology of economic individualism and self-determination has led to a health care system in which physicians are mostly in private practice, general hospitals are owned for the most part by nonprofit corporations in the private sector, and slightly more than a third of the cost for medical services is paid by various levels of government. In the main, health services are relatively diffusely organized with multiple levels of ownership, control, and financing. Individual striving places emphasis on the specialized and more exotic domains of medicine, in which personal reputations and self-development can occur with maximum probability.

The People's Republic of China presents a different picture. The predominant ideology places the common good of the society above any individual interests. Even in sports, the good of the people is considered to be a legitimate pursuit, and an athlete does not strive for individual acclaim or glory (*Sports Illustrated,* 1973). Individualism and self-determinism are viewed as sins against the state (Sidel, 1973). As such, there is no private sector as we know it in the health care system, and ownership and control over the means of producing health services are vested entirely with the various levels of government. Indeed the extent to which the ideology of the common good over individual needs is used to derive organizational principles for the health system and is put into the practice of medicine is vividly portrayed within the People's Republic of China's medical care system. For example, Gibson (1972) analyzed the *Peking Review* over the period June to November, 1969. The *Review* is published weekly in Peking and is a major source of information on the role ideology plays in the practice of medicine. One article cited by Gibson,

"Using Materialistic Dialectic to Cure Common Diseases," shows how ideology is used as a guide for establishing treatment methodologies. The Chinese physician who authored the article expressed his frustration with foreign texts on neurology, which focused "only with difficult theories and rare diseases" and said "very little . . . about common diseases and ailments which we often meet in practical work." As this physician wrote, according to Gibson (1972:70):

It was just at this time that the great leader Chairman Mao issued the brilliant call: *In medical and health work, put the stress on the rural areas,* pointing out the orientation of our advance as medical workers. In line with Chairman Mao's instruction, instead of staying in the hospital, we organized ourselves into medical teams and went to the P.L.A. units and the villages. What we encountered there were still common diseases. It is counter to Chairman Mao's proletarian line in medical and health work to neglect the study of these diseases and the improvement of their treatment, and to assign a huge staff and a large quantity of material to the research of difficult and rare diseases. In keeping with Chairman Mao's teachings, we resolve to launch attacks on common diseases and discover new methods of treatment.

Gibson goes on to show that ideology is applied to diagnosis and therapy, as an explanation of previous health care failures, as a channel or vehicle for expressing patient gratitude, and as sensitivity training for health workers.

New (1974), writing on medical care in the People's Republic of China, observes that the application of the ideology of the common good has resulted in the virtual absence of formal degrees, standard licensing procedures, or requirements throughout the education system, including medicine. Factory workers do some teaching at Peking University, and particular regions of the country establish their own training programs for barefoot doctors, depending on the particular medical problems the regions are faced with. According to New, this lack of formal requirements allows for great flexibility in the practice of medicine. Because Shen Yang has a school of public health, barefoot doctors receive two years of training. Other areas with less capability offer less extensive training programs.

Furthermore, New points out that the ideology of the common good also affects the manner in which health insurance is implemented in China. Local autonomy is emphasized, and many communes and neighborhood areas have health insurance schemes whereby the amount paid by individuals varies according to the financial resources of the commune.

NOTES

1. This is from a personal conversation in April, 1970, between the one of us (A. C. T.) and Dr. Edward Saward, the founder of the Kaiser-Permanente Health Plan. For a brief description of the Kaiser-Permanente program in relation to its attempt to address key issues in the delivery of health services, refer to Saward et al (1968).

2. This is not the place to describe the complexities of population composition. The interested student is referred to any one of several good population textbooks, including Stockwell (1968), Thompson (1953), and Petersen (1969).

3. Some countries such as Sweden have provided for some superspecialized services on a national level. They have some clinics that are the sole places in the country for certain procedures, and patients are flown in when the services are needed. Such a system requires a national system of health care with public financing.

PART FIVE

SOME URGENT ISSUES

In the Introduction and several times throughout the text, we have mentioned that the sociological study of health and health care relates to important issues in ethics. Furthermore, we have indicated that serious problems exist in the organization of health services.

In this final section each of these issues is highlighted. In Chapter 14 we bring together the various strands of ethical concerns and focus on them explicitly. Because of its focus on the application of knowledge and technology, medicine highlights many general ethical concerns. Giving special emphasis to the issues of abortion and human experimentation, the ways in which medicine has dealt with the problems and the key issues raised are explored. This is one instance in which the study of medicine has implications beyond the subject matter. The issues may not be as well defined with respect to other spheres of human activity, but they are nonetheless there.

In Chapter 15 we finally bite the hand that feeds us. There we attempt to list many deficiencies of medical practice and the organization of health services. This is done by treating American medicine as a hypothetical patient being admitted to Sociology Hospital. In the form of a standard admission workup, we review the patient's complaints, the objective laboratory findings, and the signs and symptoms of disorder. A differential diagnosis is presented along with a preliminary treatment plan.

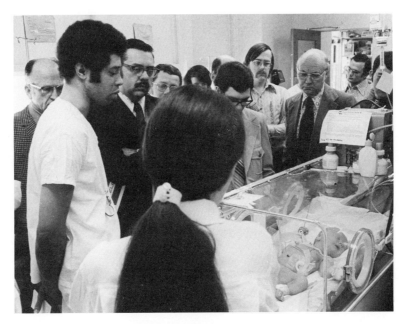

CHAPTER 14

Medical ethics

In 1958 researchers in the newborn unit at Los Angeles County Hospital conducted an experiment to see if prophylactic antibiotic treatment would reduce the high mortality rate of premature infants. All of the infants came from the same socioeconomic group—generally poor, uneducated Americans. The experiment set up four treatment groups: One group received no antibiotics; one group received penicillin and streptomycin; one group received chloramphenicol; one group received chloramphenicol, penicillin, and streptomycin. . . . The parents did not give what would today be called "informed consent." A "blanket permission" form was signed upon the mother's admission to the hospital. . . . The extent of knowledge about chloramphenicol at the time of the experiment was this. . . . There were numerous reports of bone marrow depression and deaths associated with the use of the drug. . . . There were no studies of the drug on newborn animals. Human infants were the first newborns to receive the drug."

Geoffrey Cowan, in the Congressional Record (Oct. 10, 1972)

Medical ethics is one of the most fascinating topics with which a medical sociologist or health practitioner could be concerned. Everyone currently alive invariably will confront some health care decision, either personal or concerning a significant other, in which difficult and even unresolvable ethical issues will emerge. This chapter is an attempt to raise some of these issues and to relate them to various aspects of the social order where genesis and resolution coexist. Because the topic of medical ethics is so vast, we have decided to simplify matters somewhat by hinging the discussion of ethics on the general topic of human experimentation in medicine. Toward this end, we will attempt to analyze the societal forces that shape and even

301

determine to a large extent the substance and process of the emergence of medical ethical problems in medicine. We will draw on some of the material discussed in the earlier chapters of this book. For example, the concept of stratification is relevant because position in the structure of hierarchical opportunities is related to the power that groups or classes of people have to decide whether a medical procedure should occur. Also the medical model, ideology, and the role of authority within the context of increasingly complex technology are important for determining the extent to which patients and their families feel free or coerced to make difficult medical decisions such as the management of pain and the treatment course for the terminally ill.

CULTURE AND THE CONCEPT OF LIFE

Basic to all the ethical issues that exist in medicine is the way in which life is defined as a concept by a specific culture. Basic cultural conceptions such as "life" form the basis for consensus among the people of a society. This consensus determines the extent to which people will follow or obey codified norms such as laws or codes of ethics. If the fundamental cultural consensus is in disharmony with a law or code of ethics, then moral and ethical issues will arise. This disharmony can occur as a result of planned intervention such as when a law is passed consciously by practitioners in opposition to a cultural conception (e.g., busing legislation or abortion rulings), or the disharmony can result from technological and ideological forces beyond the control of health practitioners and patients (e.g., machinery and legislation that encourages heroic measures to keep a patient "alive" long beyond the point at which death would have occurred unencumbered by technology).

Regardless, such basic conceptions are ideals or approximations for which people of a culture never achieve but only strive. The concept of life and other cultural concepts are relevant but are never absolutely applied because people are continually exploring and working out what these concepts mean and how they are to guide human action.

In Western cultures, life is conceptualized as something sacred. Frequently, people's deeds do not reflect the value placed on life, as seen in the Vietnam war, for example, or the absence of health services for large segments of poor people in the United States. Nevertheless, life is revered and valued above all other values in Western cultures. The high value placed on life is rooted in two dimensions of the culture: the sacred and the profane. The sacred or religious basis for the value of life is based on the general precept that life is a gift from God. As such, life does not depend on something within mankind for its value but derives its great importance from the Creator who transcends mere mortals. On the other hand, for those who do not believe in God, life may be defined as all important because of the nature of life itself within the natural order of things. Life is considered "sacred" because it is life (Shils, 1968), and its value depends on the infinite worth of every individual (Kant, 1949).

CULTURE AND CONCEPTS OF MORALITY

Another highly important principle that is fundamental to ethical issues in medicine is rooted in the concepts of morality which a culture adheres to. Western society contains two basic concepts of morality that are in opposition to one another. One concept, the "greatest good" concept, focuses on behavior and thought and seeks to maximize the potential in everyone by minimizing pain and suffering. The other concept of morality is proscriptive, since it attempts to define behaviors and thoughts that are abnormal or indecent. For example, euthanasia emanates from the first conception and antiabortion efforts from the second. Each of these concepts of morality takes one along different decision paths, and if one should attempt to approach an ethical issue using both concepts simultaneously, the contradictions inherent in the two concepts emerge.

If one considers the Western concepts of life with its two dimensions and morality with its two dimensions, one can begin to understand how it is that the ethical problems currently facing medicine are possible. For example, the concept of life that is dependent on believing in God is absolute to the extent that it provides a seemingly unshakable stance in support of life. From this perspective, it is difficult to justify any medical action that will allow life to end. However, the ground seems less solid when the greatest good concept of morality is thrust before it, and troublesome issues suddenly became possible in cases in which previously absolutism had ruled them out. An example is the Karen Quinlan case in which, on the basis of the theological concept of life, there is no question but that she continue to be supported by the respirator and hyperalimentation. Because her life is considered a gift from God, it is seen as inviolable from herself or others. At the same time, her parents responded to the greatest good concept of morality and from this perspective argued for a termination of the mechanical life-support system to alleviate Karen's vegetative and possibly painful state of existence. This course of action is in conflict with the theological conception of the sanctity of life.

On the other hand, the conception of life for life's sake admits the possibility that individual merits, be they genetic identification, malformations, psychological stress, or a decline in the quality of an individual life, can be used to decide whether life is allowed to exist. Since the sanctity of life does not transcend individual lives but instead is rooted there, decisions affecting life are dependent on the issues surrounding individual lives.

CULTURE AND THE ROLE OF TECHNOLOGY

The technology of a culture is the third major principle or force that determines the evolution of ethical issues in medicine. In simpler times, when complex machinery and techniques were not available, it was impossible to draw amniotic fluid from a womb to examine the genetic structure of a fetus, and the failure of major body organs usually meant that the sick person would die. Today medical technology has made it possible not only to know genetic structures but also to transfer genetic information from one organism to another. Positive pressure respirators, kidney dialysis units, microsurgery, and on and on through a long list of technological developments have made it not only possible but even mandatory that people be kept alive long beyond the point of "natural" death.

The advances of technological science have precluded any possibility of falling back on absolutes in meeting the ethical dilemmas faced by health practitioners and patients. The irony is that the sheer brilliance of medical machinery and know-how has cast long shadows of uncertainty in areas which previously were clear and unambiguous. We are no longer certain of when death occurs, whereas in simpler times, cessation of breathing and rigor mortis served as undeniable and absolute criteria.

The structure of medical technology within a culture is determined and supported by biomedical research. The research orientation of a culture and the formal procedures by which research is funded and monitored is a particularly significant source of technological growth and medical ethical problems, as discussed later in the chapter. The magnitude of this impact by research can be seen indirectly when one considers that the budget for the United States National Institutes of Health (NIH) rose from around $2.5 million dollars in 1945 to 1.5 billion in 1970 when NIH awarded biomedical research grants to more than 3,000 projects (Frankel, 1972). Much of this research has a direct bearing on the ethics of human experimentation because of the research procedures and the application of findings to the practice of medicine.

ETHICAL ISSUES AND HUMAN EXPERIMENTATION

The basic cultural conceptions of life and morality are historical concepts because they evolve over the course of a culture's existence. For this reason, it is important to consider the historical development of the ethics of human experimentation because the ethical concerns about medical experimentation are as old as the discipline of medicine and the cultural conceptions of life and morality. For example, the ancient Egyptians left records from 2500 BC that portray clearly the concerns of medical practitioners about the uncertainties of medical treatments which were viewed as inherently experimental. We will focus on more recent times to illustrate the historical evolution of ethical concerns surrounding human experimentation in medicine.

The first recorded United States' study involving a public epidemiological experiment occurred in 1721 when Zabdiel Boylston of Boston (1726), a medical practitioner with no medical degree, undertook the first smallpox inoculation trials. A number of persons, including his child, were given live smallpox virus, and Boylston kept careful written documentation, including the names of those inoculated and the outcomes. Interestingly it appears that approximately 2% of those receiving the inoculations died as opposed to a 15% mortality among those contracting smallpox without inoculation. The risks of inoculation were tremendous given the fact that Boylston had not a clue as to how the process of immunities worked, nor had inoculation trials been conducted on lower animals prior to humans receiving them.

Ethical concerns about human experimentation were published by the nineteenth century French philosopher of science and research, Claude Bernard, and an American researcher, William Beaumont, in 1833 (Beecher, 1970). Beaumont raised issues of informed consent and the necessity to weigh the risks to the subjects against the potential gains for science.

More recently, Nazi Germany brought into sharp focus many of the major ethical issues involving biomedical research on human subjects. In one of the most heinous natural experiments of the Nazi era, the lesson that there are no ethical absolutes emerges forcefully. In Warsaw the Germans forced over a million Jews into a ghetto that could support only 50,000 to 60,000 people. The experiment in this case was to ascertain the effect of extreme population density on starvation and ultimately death. A book detailing the dynamics of starvation was written by Jewish physicians, of whom all but one died at the hands of the Germans (Apfelbaum, 1946).

The polio immunization trials of the mid-1930s in the United States resulted from biomedical experiments in which Drs. Brodie and Park of New York grew polio virus in monkey tissue and then rendered the virus inactive with a drug. After about twenty monkey trials, together with another physician working independently with a different virus procedure, they inoculated several thousands of children. Several cases of polio, paralysis, and even death occurred as a result of these poorly designed experiments (Paul, 1971). Ultimately the successful polio vaccine was developed by Drs. Weller, Enders, and Robbins. Massive experimental trials occurred with many children receiving the vaccine and equally as many children in the control group given a placebo. The experimenters knew with certitude that all the control children would be unprotected and that polio, paralysis, and even death would strike some of these children for the simple reason that they fell into the control group by random selection.

The vagaries of randomness befell a group of black men who unwittingly found themselves in the control group of the following experiment: Tuskegee medical researchers designed a study of the long-term effects of untreated syphilis among men, and effective treatment was withheld from these men for twenty-five years to observe the outcomes (United States Department of

Health, Education, and Welfare, 1973). Similarly, cancer specialists at the famous Sloan-Kettering Cancer Foundation injected live cancer cells into the skins of unsuspecting patients (Katz, 1972). Public reaction to this news was so strong that the USPHS produced its 1966 policy on human experimentation, which requires biomedical researchers funded by USPHS to establish human experimentation review committees to review new projects and to monitor ongoing research. The main goal is to protect the rights and safety of research subjects by scrutinizing the methodology of the experiment and procedures for obtaining informed consent (United States Department of Health, Education, and Welfare, 1971).

Although this brief history covers only a few of the better known instances of human experimentation, nevertheless it offers some insight into the persistence, complexity, and high degree of ethical concerns associated with biomedical research and technology. These cases give the student a starting point for ideas about specific ethical concerns in medicine.

The norm of survival

The cultural conceptions of the primacy of life and the belief in the greatest good concept of morality form the basis for one societal norm that the profession of medicine adheres to: that the human species ought to do its best to work toward survival and the means to produce a decent life. Physicians and other biomedical researchers are faced with the uncertainities derived from the limited state of medical knowledge and the incomplete mastery of effective therapeutic procedures. What the physician ought to do, according to the norm of survival, is to act clinically in spite of the uncertainties for the good of the stricken patient. In a real sense, every clinical encounter is an experiment. Fox (1959) in her study of a metabolic group presents a picture of physicians attempting to cope with the great ethical concern about using dangerous drugs and surgical procedures in the light of limited knowledge. The physicians had to weigh the professional norm of advancing medical knowledge against the norm of helping the patient to survive. Leaning too hard in one direction could deprive the patient of a lifesaving or life-improving outcome, and the other direction could lead to great harm to the patient. The moral uncertainty and resultant stress among physicians were handled by establishing close unity within the professional group in which emotion was shared freely among colleagues, and patients were treated in privileged ways contrary to the aloof, logical-rational image of the scientist that is widely accepted in our society. In cases such as the one Fox studied, in which patients are critically ill but capable of interacting with others and performing their social roles, physicians evaluate the status of patients and tend to define them as "treatable." The risk-benefit ratio is low because the norm of advancing medical science is given lower priority than the norm of helping the patient to survive. Highly risky experimental procedures usually are forsaken for more conservative, albeit experimental, methods. The physician will battle to save the life of a "treatable" patient, and euthanasia in these cases is rare (Crane, 1975). However, as discussed in the next section, although this conservative approach is less experimental, it may conflict with the ethical question of the patient's right to life and death.

The norm of the integrity of the human body

Western social thought, particularly religious thought, has ascribed great value to rights concerning the viability and maintenance of the human body and all its organ systems. If one doubts the pervasiveness and strength of the norm of bodily integrity, imagine the reactions of members of a community where some individuals have commenced to capriciously mutilate their bodies. The community would react quickly and decisively to halt the self-mutilation because society has been vested with the authority to ensure that individuals treat their bodies according to the test of common sense and medical opinion. Less extreme examples of this proprietary interest has occurred with the advent of warning labels on cigarette packages and the proliferation of state-supported treatment programs for alcoholics.

This norm forms the basis for the concern in medicine about the ethics of the right to life and, conversely, the right to death. Ethical questions within medicine are raised whenever medicine intervenes and thereby somehow affects the complex relationships between human rights, life, and death. In this section, we shall examine one such intervention, namely fetal research, to draw out the ethical issues surrounding the norm of bodily integrity. We chose fetal research because it embodies one of the more common forms of medical intervention, that is, biomedical research. Furthermore, fetal research encompasses the difficult cases of children and the unconscious, condemned, or dying person, and thus the ethical questions emerge in clear contrast against these extreme or polar cases.

Fetal research: definitions. It is important for individuals who are analyzing ethical issues to be clear about what they are talking about. The simplest method for assuring some degree of common understanding is to define the major terms that will be used. In the present discussion, the term "research" is defined as those procedures which are not directly therapeutic or curative to the research subject. It seems reasonable to assume that all other medical research that is directly the most hopeful therapeutic regimen poses minimal ethical concerns. The term "fetus" is defined as nonviable or one that is incapable of surviving outside of the mother's uterus. All other fetuses could be considered in the same light as children for purposes of medical ethics.

Research on the nonviable fetus can be divided into the following types:

1. Research on fetuses in uteri
   a. No abortion planned
   b. Abortion planned
      (1) Dead
      (2) During abortion
2. Research on fetuses ex uteri
   a. Spontaneous abortion
      (1) Living
   b. Induced abortion
      (1) Living
      (2) Dead

The substance of research on live fetuses includes the following (McCormick, 1975; Walters, 1975):

1. Prenatal diagnosis
2. Intrauterine therapy
3. Fetal behavior
4. Nutrition
5. Placental transfer
6. Fetal physiology and metabolism
7. Abortion techniques
8. Tissue rejection
9. Oxygenation and life-prolongation
10. Delivery techniques

Fetal research: ethical issues. The position one takes concerning the norm of bodily integrity for fetuses is not dependent on what position one takes regarding the status of the fetus. Whether the fetus is considered to be like a fully developed adult human or whether it is defined as a lower animal such as a monkey or a dog does not appear to be particularly relevant to the major ethical concerns expressed by both medical and nonmedical persons. Experimentation on nonviable, living human fetuses outside of the uterus has led to two major ethical concerns that maintain their significance for society regardless of the position one takes concerning the status of the fetus.

The first of these concerns we call the "ethics of consequences." If experimentation is permitted on nonviable, live human fetuses, such practices over time will weaken the structure of the norm of bodily integrity. Of particular concern is that this weakening will manifest itself by members of society showing diminishing levels of concern for living entities that are incapable of looking out for their own bodies. Persons who are very old, comatose, very young, and severely retarded represent classes of humans that are highly vulnerable to this potential threat. Furthermore, if fetuses become valuable research commodities as a result of scarcity and the process of supply and demand, individuals and institutions may find it profitable to encourage the production of fetuses through abortion. This troublesome consequence is made more problematic by the real possibility that the powerless or poor members of society would be coerced to contribute more to the product than the more affluent and powerful members.

Informed consent

Fetal research poses ethical issues that relate to the first and last stages of life. In this sense, human fetuses share something important with many people who have reached the terminus of life either through fatal disease or the aging process. What people at the beginning and end of life have in common is nonviability and the problem of not having control over decisions that affect bodily integrity. Control over what happens to one's body in a medical setting presupposes that the person receiving the treatment or experiment be appraised of the procedures. The ethical concern is the extent to which the patient or experimental subject can decide whether to participate based on knowledge of the potential risks that the treatment or experimental condition holds for bodily integrity. For both fetuses and many patients at the end of their lives, informed consent becomes a serious ethical problem for medical researchers and clinicians. The inability to make decisions regarding one's body is particularly troublesome for society because it contradicts the norm of bodily integrity. Because of this, society has created a special category or role for those who cannot make decisions about their bodies for one reason or another. Their status is regarded as special and distinct from other classes of people and certainly superior to higher animals in the sense that the right to bodily integrity must be protected for them. This

special status rests on the scientific knowledge that human fetuses and individuals who are insane, senile, unconscious, and with other similar conditions have the potential or capacity to act autonomously, to experience reflection and consciousness of self, and to produce or create works of art, scientific investigations, and interpersonal relationships; in short, to become or return to the status of fully developed human being (Wasserstrom, 1975). Another dimension of this potential, one that the profession of medicine tends to deny, as discussed in Chapter 4, is the capacity for death as the natural end stage of life. Just as a human fetus has the potential to live, so the terminally ill or aged have the natural capacity to die. The issue of protecting bodily integrity through informed consent is the same for both ends of life's spectrum; however, that integrity for some is life and for others is death.

Specifically various positions have been formulated regarding that special class of persons unable to give informed consent. One perspective declares that those incapable of developing informed consent forfeit their rights directly to the next of kin or to the mother in the case of the human fetus (Bok, 1975). From this perspective, it is not necessary to obtain informed consent from the fetus or patient concerned. Another view says that consent must be obtained but may be done indirectly through proxy decisions by parents or next of kin. This position presupposes that the best interests of the bodily integrity of fetuses and others are taken to heart by the proxy. As Lappé (1975) points out, "while it is a noble thing to offer oneself to science it is somewhat less generous to sacrifice someone else." Neither of these positions, however, have demonstrated by their application to actual cases that bodily integrity has been preserved. This is due in part to the problem of someone making a life or death decision for someone else and partly due to the ambiguities associated with the concept of bodily integrity, particularly in cases in which the patient is near death but medical science sees hope for eventual recovery at some level of capacity. The first problem stems from research in sociology and social psychology, which consistently have demonstrated how difficult, if not impossible, it is to take on the perspective of someone other than ourselves. Although it may be possible to measure and understand the expressions of values and attitudes of others, it appears to be impossible to go through the process of internalizing those values and attitudes as others have done within their lives, and hence one cannot take the perspective of the other in any realistic empirical sense. For this reason, it is not possible to decide with any degree of confidence that a person's position regarding bodily integrity has been represented adequately.

Also one is constantly faced with medical cases in which the patient expresses a desire to die but a proxy has been established because the family or physicians treating the person have decided that the patient's ability to make rational decisions is suspect. Furthermore, the medical practitioner may have some grounds for hope that the patient will experience some degree of recovery. Of course, the more remote the grounds the greater the ethical problem of violating the patient's bodily integrity.

Finally, the third position, expressed extremely well by Ramsey (1975), negates the ethical concerns by insisting that fetal consent is absolutely necessary but unobtainable. For this reason, Ramsey rejects all experimentation on human fetuses as unethical.

Regardless of which of the two non-Ramsey positions one takes, informed consent is problematic under the best of circumstances, that is, when both the medical researcher and subject are fully capable of articulating and communicating their respective needs, the benefits of the research to society, and the potential risks involved. Studies of informed consent in which the subjects are fully cognizant and articulate about their needs have raised serious questions about how well the subject's bodily integrity is protected. For example, Gray's excellent study (1975) of a clinical research committee established to review proposed experiments to protect human subjects concluded that no prior review of research can assure the ethical participation of eventual subjects. He found that research proposals were rejected by the review committee primarily because the informed consent forms required of all research according to the current ruling of the Department of Health, Education, and Welfare contained omissions, inaccuracies, inconsistencies, or complex wording or because the design of the research posed risks to the subjects not outweighed by the value of the research. Nevertheless, some researchers evaded the committee recommendations, or even if they did comply, many subjects still did not know that they were participating in research, some did not know the risks, and others felt obligated to participate in spite of their concerns about their safety. Gray defined five types of medical research subjects based on their stated reasons for participating in a labor-induction study and a starvation-abortion study in which the women were starved for a few days prior to abortions to evaluate the effect of starvation on the fetus. Table 14-1 contains the types of subjects and the number in each category. The fact that 39% of the labor-induction subjects were totally unaware of the study is a rather dramatic example of the problem of informed consent.

In another study of organ transplantation, Fox and Swazey (1974) point out that even under ideal conditions in which the recipient of the organ and the donor are apprised of the risks involved, a great deal of coercion and constraint, both medical and social, is exerted on the patient, the organ donor, and the physician. Medical science has determined that a live, well-matched organ optimizes the chances of a favorable outcome to a transplant operation. Live organ donors theoretically should experience transcendental fulfillment and view the process as a moral act of the high-

Table 14-1. Distribution of subject types in two medical research projects*

Type	Labor-induction subjects		Starvation-abortion subjects	
	Number	*Percent*	*Number*	*Percent*
Unaware subjects	20	39	0	—
Unwilling subjects	4		0	—
Indifferent subjects	3		0	—
Benefiting subjects	22	43	5	71
Committed subjects	2		2	
Total	51	100%	7	100%

*From Gray, B. H. *Human subjects in medical experimentation: a sociological study of the conduct and regulation of clinical research.* New York: John Wiley & Sons, Inc., 1975, p. 128.

est, liberating order. Instead donors are often close relatives of the patient who will die without the donor organ. The evidence suggests that the donor experiences compelling social pressure to donate a kidney, for example, and once donated a new set of obligations may be created between donor and recipient. As Mauss (1954) describes the gift or exchange relationship, it contains the processes of giving, receiving, and repaying, which draw those who participate in the gift relationship into a closer relationship with emotional and moral bounds. This places the physician in a difficult position in which he must decide ethically about the motives of the donor (altruistic, self-mutilation, or desire to control the recipient), and these must be balanced against the probabilities of risk versus benefit to the patient.

The right to die

There are thousands of Karen Quinlans every year who are terminally ill in United States' hospitals, sustained by a respirator, and fed intravenously to stay death. Death control, an almost necessary consequence of high medical technology, is applied at the discretion of physicians who base their decisions to apply extraordinary means to keep the patient "alive" on two basic guidelines: (1) whether a treatment method is readily available, and (2) whether the patient is treatable, that is,

whether the patient has the potential to interact and communicate meaningfully with others. A technological force beyond the control of both physicians and patients has led to a condition in which death is viewed as something ultimately evil to be denied and defeated by medical science. In many cases the method of medical treatment takes precedence over concern with bodily integrity and the quality of life and death.

This technological force, consisting of machinery; scientific knowledge about human biochemistry, physiology, and microbiology; and the clinical application of this information, is in conflict with a movement among religious groups and other individuals who view the norm of bodily integrity as extending from the beginning of life to death. This movement represents the consumer's attempt to retrieve control over bodily integrity from technological and impersonal forces. Both direct and indirect euthanasia represent then a means or strategy designed to protect the right to die.[1] People place conditions on treatment with living wills in which they demand the right to die unencumbered by technological means of sustaining life beyond its "natural" terminus.

All this poses difficult ethical questions. First, there is the difficult practical problem of determining when in fact the death process sets in. Furthermore, given the death process, often one would have serious questions as to whether the patient is treatable, that is, can somehow recover, and if so, what the quality of the person's life will be. Many physicians maintain that ethical dilemmas regarding potential for survival and quality of life disappear when all the facts of the given case are established. Be this as it may, a recent study of physicians' behavior toward critically ill patients found that withdrawal of treatment was common in cases in which it was deemed that the patient no longer had the capacity to interact meaningfully with others (Crane, 1975). However, active euthanasia was described as a rare occurrence by the physicians surveyed. Even where this determination is made with a strong probability of accuracy based on the latest medical research, the possibility always exists that one is wrong in deciding that the patient will never function as viable human being again. Finally, the question of who makes this decision is of major ethical concern and importance. If the patient makes it, one can question if he is in a rational state of mind given the terminal condition. If the family, relatives, or friends make the decision, do they have the best interests of the patient at heart? If the physician makes it, is he able to temper the desire to preserve life with the facts of the case and the patient's desire to live the last days of his life according to natural processes? The great danger with this conflict between medicine, technology, and religion is that it is an easy step from passively allowing someone to die at his wish to actively taking the life of someone whose wish has been articulated by a proxy. At this juncture the fetus and the dying patient join to complete the cycle of life and its ethical paradoxes and dilemmas.

In concluding this discussion of medical ethical problems, it is worth noting that these problems are a direct result of the successes of medicine. By conquering infectious diseases such as polio, smallpox, tuberculosis, and others, medicine has upset the balance of nature and thereby allowed populations to explode beyond a society's capacity to provide for its members' basic needs. Medicine has made it possible for people to live longer, only to fall victims to the chronic diseases associated with the aging process. Medical technology makes it possible to maintain life well beyond its natural limits. Such limits are exceedingly difficult to define in light of modern scientific devices and techniques that extend life. The natural limit of life can be thought of as the point at which life would cease to exist in the absence of the application of high technology, which has been extraordinarily successful in thwarting natural death.

Faced with these horrific consequences of the successes of medicine, physicians have tended to adopt a utilitarian ethical stance in which each individual practitioner works out the solutions to ethical problems based in part on the facts of the case and in part on individual moral codes and notions of the greatest good. Formal ethics with its absolute first principles of goodness and evil is held up as something to strive for but not practically attainable in light of the struggle over control of the quality of life and death. As pointed out in earlier chapters, complex political, social, and economic processes are bound intimately with the growth of medical technology and scientific developments. Abortion as a means of population control or fetal experimentation as a means of death control cannot be separated analytically from the larger questions having to do with the control of scarce resources, access to opportunities within societies, and the priorities assigned to the distribution of goods and services based on structured inequalities and systems of human value.

The great danger in utilitarian medical ethics stems from the likelihood that the scales will be tipped in favor of benefits to science or the greatest good rather than recognition of the risks to the individual's bodily integrity. This could result in extensions of medical science in which acts considered reprehensible today are deemed justified tomorrow. Society hangs together in large measure because individuals assume responsibility for the rights of others, particularly of those weaker or less privileged than others. To create a utilitarian decision-making process in medicine is to run the risk of concentrating power in the hands of a few elite members of society, thereby disrupting the social balance created by many people assuming some degree of responsibility for others. Shared meanings based on shared responsibility and participation are a major force in developing understanding between health professionals and patients. To allow an infant with severe brain damage to die may be the greatest good for the family and for society. But what effect does the act have on the intensity of effort of the newborn nursery staff for the next infant with a less certain but problematic mental prognosis? Is it consistent with utilitarian ethics to have the greatest good for a few or less good for the masses? Similarly, is repression and killing such as in Vietnam justified if the majority of Americans will benefit from greater economic security? Formal ethics, which evaluates the methods, the principles behind actions, and the consequences, is a higher order of ethical development than utilitarian ethics because it posits absolute and essential principles of human behavior that are irreducible in any given medical situation.

Since scientific data cannot substantiate or decide ethical or moral questions, Firth (1952) has provided those who must make ethical judgments with a nonscientific-based model of the decision-making process. Firth's model can be used to assess the quality of moral or ethical decisions by presenting the qualities of an ideal ethical observer. Such an observer would be (1) omniscient (know all the facts), (2) omnipercipient (would imagine how all others would be affected by the decision), and (3) dispassionate (would not allow emotional bias to affect decision).

According to this model, Cooke (1975) has extrapolated the need for actively and formally involving three types of persons in the decision-making process when questions of medical ethics are concerned. First, the health professional must be involved to contribute all the facts that can be known about the case. Second, the consumer is involved to make known all points of view and perspectives concerning the impact that any given medical decision will have on others. This is an exchange process between provider and consumer, both the patient and significant others, which adds the dimension of omnipercipience (Hessler and New, 1972; Hessler and Walters, 1975). Finally, emotional biases and conflicts of interests can be mediated by group involvement in the decision process, whereby the group strives to maximize its own impartiality. This is extraordinarily difficult to achieve, and the process is subject to much error. However, as Cooke points out, this approach is far more desirable than what he identifies as a monolithic approach, and he cites the law as setting a precedent for medicine in this regard.

For both the new student and medical sociologist, the encounter with the interface of medicine and morality strikes hardest when the difficult case involves decisions affecting the bodily integrity of a loved one. It is then that the poverty of utilitarian ethics with its emphasis on consequences alone emerges to plague those who must make the decisions. Currently medicine is moving toward a more formal ethical structure with a broader base of societal participation in the decision processes. This development holds great fascination for most of us who someday may be the recipient of a difficult medical decision.

NOTES

1. Ethicists have taken the position recently that there is no difference between the two approaches in that they both seek the same end, that is, to contrive the death of a person in an act of mercy. We cannot fail to notice the difference inasmuch as in the direct method one brings about death by doing something directly, whereas with the indirect method, one allows death to occur by not doing something to forestall it.

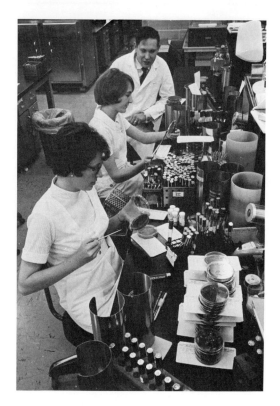

CHAPTER 15

American Medicine: a diagnostic workup

Centralization of the means of production and socialization of labor at last reached the point where they become incompatible with their capitalistic integument. This integument is burst asunder. The knell of capitalistic private property sounds, the expropriaters are expropriated.

Marx—Das Kapital

In early 1976 American Medicine entered Sociology Hospital complaining of high cost, impersonality, and a discrepancy between promise and performance. In the United States the cost of medical care had risen to nearly $100 billion per year. It was also suffering from a series of exposes in the press, several books complaining about poor quality and impersonality, and an acute episode of "Medical Story" on television. The implicit promise of medicine to cure all disease and eliminate death from all causes other than old age (some think, including old age) has been found insubstantial and has failed to keep pace with public expectations as reflected in both malpractice suits and the alienation of consumers on grounds of "breach of promise." The depth of the complaint can be seen by noticing that health providers have expressed growing concerns about impersonality and specialization and find themselves unable to cope with the rapid rise of technology and the ethical issues that have resulted from the discrepancy between technology and the ability to apply that technology to patient care.

HISTORY

Modern medicine was born in the late eighteenth and early nineteenth century as a child of capitalistic societies sired by the emergence of modern science. The right to practice medicine was assumed by individuals without licensing or examination and in most cases without adequate training. It suffered from expectable childhood diseases in the form of a number of divergent social movements, including homeopathy, thompsonianism, osteopathy, and chiropractic. In combatting these diseases, medicine organized its defenses, forming the national American Medical Association in 1849. Although accepting state control in the form of licensing and examinations and later in the form of regulation of the curriculum of medical schools, the main thrust of development has been toward increasing the power and autonomy of the individual practioner. Its adolescence was characterized by a need to cope with a burgeoning body of knowledge and heavy demand on the medical practitioner as the benefits of medicine became apparent to the public. The result has been a high degree of specialization that continues to the present and an acute crisis orientation with reference to disease. The major emphasis has been on saving lives and dealing with extremely severe conditions rather than with the care of sick people. It should be noted that the adoption of the fee-for-service free enterprise model has led to manpower shortages stemming primarily from unwillingness on the part of health practitioners to serve in rural areas and ghettos where financial remuneration would be a problem. The history of medicine in the United States has shown that the system has developed a pronounced caste structure and the physician has emerged as the most autonomous and powerful profession within the structure. Social mobility within the ranks of various health professionals is se-verely limited as a result, and American medicine appears to suffer from an ever-decreasing ability to adapt to a changing environment.

Medicine has been relatively inattentive to its own health. It has not reported for physical examination except on rare occasions. The last reported physical was conducted by Abraham Flexner in 1910. At that time it was found to be suffering from inability to absorb and utilize scientific protein. It was admitted to the metabolic research unit and provided with heavy doses of curriculum reform, which seemed to have resolved the problem of technical competence while aggravating the condition of specialism. It should be noted that solutions such as the Flexner treatment have tended to produce problems in their own rights, and this should be kept in mind as we proceed with this diagnostic workup. The emphasis on specialism and the acute crisis care orientation have resulted in other systems, such as those in education, religion, and the family, taking major responsibility for health maintenance. The medical care system in the United States both from within and in terms of the public is expressing great dissatisfaction with its current health.

PHYSICAL FINDINGS

On physical examination, medicine in the United States was found to have an infant mortality in excess of 20 per 1,000 which is higher than that of medical systems in other industrialized countries in the world. A palpably high level of specialization was found, with almost three out of four practitioners engaged in specialized practice. Metabolic findings include evidence of giantism as the health enterprise has grown to immense size. More than 2,000 occupational titles and over 2 million people are currently employed in the health enterprise. Further findings include extremely high costs of medical services, making them inaccessible to many who are intended recipients. This probably results from a high degree of bureaucratization as medicine has increasingly concentrated its practice in hospital settings. Since most people with diseases do not enter hospitals, this indicates a concentration of resources and effort in settings that are not only less accessible but also less useful to people in need of service. Medicine in the United States has begun to lose its sense of touch regarding its consumers, and the participation of consumers in the affairs of American medicine remains an extremely limited enterprise. The control of medicine is centered almost entirely with its practitioners, indicating a breakdown of normal homeostatic mechanisms and suggesting a loss of capacity for self-regulation. Accountability pressure has dropped to dangerously low levels, indicating a possible correlation with the low levels of consumer participation at this point. Serum analysis yielded evidence of infection with racism and sexism, and the inability of the system to successfully fight these is mysterious considering the high white count.

LABORATORY FINDINGS

Laboratory findings confirmed the physical observation of high mortality and point to the interrelationship of poverty, nutrition, and health status as causes of this high mortality rate. Furthermore, medicine was found to be suffering from shifting morbidity patterns because in its early years it was socialized to cope with acute illness and has not been able to handle the shift to an environment dominated by chronic and degenerative diseases. It is also unable to cope with increasing professionalism in its immediate work environment since these are a direct challenge to the autonomy of the medical practitioner. There is also some loss of efficiency in the support mechanisms because the occupations with which medicine most relates have become obsessed with professionalism and hence have focused more on the status of their respective occupations than on their work performance. Barriers have been erected across occupational boundaries, and the various health professions are less permeable than

required for teamwork and the kind of interaction needed to meet the challenges of the changing morbidity patterns. The high degree of stratification found suggests a structural rigidity, making the patient less flexible in dealing with external pressures. Furthermore, the high levels of status and income found among health professionals place the American medical system out of touch culturally and socially with the majority of consumers in the United States. Laboratory tests also confirm the presence of Freidson's disease (moral entrepreneurship), which is manifested in a process best described as the medicalization of deviance. Medicine is assuming responsibility for a larger range of behaviors that it regards as in need of changing and hence has emerged as a major force of social control in society. These added burdens are a major source of stress and are draining the vital energies of the patient. Rigidity is also confirmed by the bureausis test, which shows that medicine has generated a proliferation of red tape and organizational confusion, making use of the system next to impossible for many consumers. Not only is this difficult for the patient, but the system finds itself unable to use its own resources, resulting in high levels of metabolic waste. The social guiac is four plus. Relative to its giant intake of nutrients, its output is minimal.

PAST TREATMENT

The patient has had a long history of palliative and placebo treatments, resulting in repeated toxicities and interaction effects. The patient has engaged in a great deal of largely inappropriate self-treatment but recently has been seeing a local physician in Washington, D.C. by the name of Dr. H. E. Welfare. These self-treatments have included an acute symptom orientation in which the practitioners have expended their major energies on diseases that are largely under control, ignoring those that are uncontrolled. For the most of the diseases treated, the focus has been on symptomatic relief rather than cure.

The patient recently has attempted expansion of the number of physicians, thinking that this will cure the acute crisis of workloads; instead it contributed to its complaints of giantism and did nothing to resolve the problems of maldistribution. It then attempted the creation of new specialties such as family practice, falling prey to false advertising and the failure to recognize that new names for general practice do not a new specialty make. For several years it has been giving itself high doses of scientism, relying on new technology, new drugs, and new machineries to alleviate its problems. These have resulted in an increase in the labor intensiveness of the system and have aggravated the problem of cost. During the past several decades there has been a large increase in bureaucratization as more conditions are being managed in hospital settings. The problems raised by this treatment have already been indicated. In general, the patient seems to be one who is constantly tinkering with symptoms while denying its major complaints. It seems to have little awareness of the causes of its disorders as indicated in the following discussion on the differential diagnosis. Since the early 1960s the patient has been seen by Dr. Welfare, whose prescriptions include large doses of technology, most recently space technology in the form of communications satellites, to bring physicians to remote areas in spirit but not in body and a series of ever-increasingly complex institutional arrangements that have been identified as follows: neighborhood health centers, comprehensive mental health centers, emergency medical care systems, family health centers, experimental health centers, health maintenance organizations, and innumerable specialized treatment programs in maternal and child health, mental retardation, and alcoholism. Prescriptions have also taken the form of attempts to plan the organization of American medicine. These plans have included Comprehensive Health Planning, the Regional Medical Program, the Professional Standards Review Organization, and most recently, Regionalization and the Health Systems Agencies. As indicated in earlier chapters, each of these prescriptions has intensified the patient's problems while contributing little to their solution. All past treatments can be labeled as palliative, placebo, or quack. The patient has also indicated that he has had several other treatments but cannot remember what they were.

DIFFERENTIAL DIAGNOSIS

1. *Drug interaction.* This is the toxic combination of capitalism and socialism. As Marx pointed out in *Das Kapital,* the expropriators have been expropriated because the patient has fallen into a process which for want of a better term can be called the "medical industrial complex." We diagnose this complex as a process of medicine, government, and industry working together to patch up the holes and to stitch the lesions in the capitalistic integument. Thus we identify treatments that have conspired to socialize the losses in American medicine and to privatize the profits. Those aspects of medicine in the United States in which the resources have been totally exploited with no new investments of manpower or innovative thinking have been taken over by the government, and industry has continued to operate in those aspects of the system that are profitable. The health industry of the patient has become a mixed economy that is highly toxic to itself. In this mixed economy, practitioners can work under the auspices of the state, for example, receiving a salary as a state employee working under Medicaid and Medicare reimbursements, and still offer private services as well.

2. *Acute and chronic profit motive.* A particular symptom of the capitalist assumptions in the medical enterprise is the emphasis on profit as a motive in providing health services. As demonstrated by Waitzkin and Waterman (1974), the profits in medicine are enormous. Not only are medical practitioners in the United States the most highly paid in the world, but the

privatization of health resources yields enormous profits for industry. Most notorious are the drug and insurance industries.

3. *Consumer alienation.* The increasing centralization of the power and control in the hands of medicine has served to alienate consumers. The organization of services and the implementation of new technologies have driven up the cost of medical care making it inaccessible to many consumers. The increasing specialization of medical practice and the location of that practice in bureaucratic settings have yielded a higher level of impersonality at the point of delivery. Practitioners typically do not know their patients personally and have no interest in them beyond the disease process itself. Patients, on the other hand, have more trust in the physician who takes a personal interest in them and who knows enough about their life-styles to make reasonable inferences about the causes of their complaints and the effects of treatment alternatives.

4. *Cultural lag.* Much of the acute and chronic profit motive, particularly from the perspective of industry, results in a burgeoning technology of vast complexity. Physicians and other health practitioners have not developed the necessary defenses to integrate the technology with the norms of patient care. This has resulted in many problems, the most troublesome being a series of ethical concerns faced by both practitioners and patients. American medicine has responded with utilitarian solutions to ethical dilemmas, and patients have voiced the desire for a more formal set of ethical norms. This has exacerbated the confidence gap existing presently between patient and health professional.

5. *Psychogenic complaints.* It must be kept in mind that we are dealing with a highly knowledgeable and sophisticated patient who would be capable of feigning the full range of symptoms and signs discovered in this examination. We cannot rule out the possibility that the patient is malingering to continue the benefits of treatments under the auspices of Dr. Welfare.

TREATMENT PLAN

The definitive treatment plan is difficult to specify at the present time. Although we have some indications of what needs to be done, the question of how it is to be accomplished is illusive due to an inadequate research base. The sociology of health has the distinct disadvantage of having developed under the tutelage of the patient. Consequently the field has assumed or shared many of the patients' basic assumptions and finds itself in an embarrassing position when it comes to making a definitive diagnosis and specifying a treatment plan. Indeed, in this instance, one might say that the patient's problem is partly iatrogenic in that it has failed to receive adequate advice from practitioners in the past. The sociology of health is unable for the most part to differentially diagnose the problems of medicine in the United States because it has received a great deal of funding for research from Dr. H. E. Welfare. Although the field has developed to the point at which it can now recognize that past diagnoses and treatments were ineffective, work is just now beginning that would provide the adequate data base for definitive treatment. Recognizing that our recommendations are highly experimental and may run into difficulty with human subject committees, we would propose that the patient be admitted to the clinical research center and treated with the following protocol:

1. *Profitmotivectomy,* a surgical technique that removes the profit incentive from the practice of medicine, should be considered. We understand that it has been developed by practitioners in Cuba, the People's Republic of China, and Yugoslavia and requires major surgery on a systemic level. We are at present uncertain what effects this surgery would have on the patient in question, nor are we certain as to how the procedure should be carried out in the facilities available. A neurosurgical consult is needed to see if certain basic assumptions that are neurologically programmed can be altered.

2. High doses (in the neighborhood of

200 million units t.i.d.) of consumer participation are needed to make the system responsive to needs of the population. Greater emphasis should be placed on the prevention of disease and the provision of treatment, personnel, and facilities in a manner acceptable and accountable to the consumer. This requires considerable independence of decision making at the local level and the adaptation of resources to the specific needs of populations.

3. A radiological consult is required to set the dosage levels for high-voltage, public accountability irradiation. Basic policy decisions must be made and financing provided by public authorities. These, however, cannot rigidly specify the details of the patient's overall treatment program so as not to interfere with the consumer participation medications.

4. Physical therapy to change certain structural problems in American medicine is necessary. Specifically, we recommend that physicians be removed from the medical center for periods of their education and returned to the community for the majority of their medical education. Fur-

thermore, all members of the health care team should be educated together in this community context.

5. Public health is an important consideration, since little progress can be made in the management of this case without adequate attention to the environment that produced the disease. This requires attention not only to the economic and other incentives for the practice of medicine but also requires that consumers be trained to assume their role as overseers of the system. Quality control with external review must be initiated to make certain that the services provided are adequate and appropriate for consumer needs. Consumers need to take responsibility to see that the conditions under which services are delivered are acceptable, available, and accessible to the populations involved. Consumers must also assume greater responsibility for their own health maintenance, and toward this end, education must be provided to the consumers. In this regard the treatment plan includes informed consumers who assume greater responsibility for the maintenance of health within their community.

References

Abel-Smith, B. *The hospitals in England and Wales: 1800-1948.* London: William Heinemann, Ltd., 1964.

Abrams, H. K., and Snyder, R. A. Health center seeks to bridge the gap between hospital and neighborhood. *The Modern Hospital,* 1968, **110** (5), 96-100.

Abse, D. *Medicine on trial.* New York: Crown Publishers, Inc., 1969.

Ackerknecht, E. H. Problems of primitive medicine. *Bulletin of the History of Medicine,* 1942, **14,** 503-521.

Adams, S. Trends in occupational origins of physicians. *American Sociological Review,* 1953, **18,** 404-409.

Alchian, A. A., and Kessel, R. A. Competition, monopoly and the pursuit of pecuniary gain. In *Aspects of labor economics* (Bureau of Economic Research Special Conference Series, vol. 14). Princeton, N.J.: Princeton University Press, 1962.

Altshuler, A. A. *Community control: the black demand for participation in large American cities.* New York: Pegasus, 1970.

American Academy of Pediatrics. *Lengthening shadows: a report of the Council in Pediatric Practice of the American Academy of Pediatrics on the delivery of health care to children, 1970.* Evanston, Ill.: The Academy, 1971.

American Association of Medical Colleges. *Medical college application service: admission status.* Washington, D.C.: The Association, March 30, 1973.

American Hospital Association. *Classification of health care institutions.* Chicago: The Association, 1968.

American Hospital Association. *Hospital statistics.* Chicago: The Association, 1974.

American Medical Association. *Distribution of physicians, hospitals and hospital beds in the United States* (vols. for 1963, 1966, 1969, 1971). Chicago: The Association, 1971.

American Medical Association. *Recommendations of the Conference on the Guidelines for the Categorization of Hospitals Emergency Capabilities.* Chicago: The Association, 1971.

American Medical Association. *Survey of medical groups in the U.S. 1969.* Chicago: The Association, 1971.

American Nurses' Association. *Facts about nursing, 72-73.* Kansas City, Mo.: The Association, 1974.

American Nurses' Association. Guidelines on short term continuing education programs for pediatric nurse associates. *American Journal of Nursing,* 1971, **71,** 509-512.

American Nurses' Association and U.S. Department of Health, Education and Welfare. *Preparing registered nurses for expanded roles: a directory of programs* (DHEW Publication No. [NIH] 74-31). Washington, D.C., U.S. Government Printing Office, 1975.

American Osteopathic Association. *Directory of members.* Chicago: The Association, 1901.

Anderson, J. *Development of medical data information systems: final contract report under NASA* (Contract NAS9-11579). Nov. 1971.

Anderson, O. The utilization of health services. In Freeman, H., and Simmons, O. *The mental patient comes home.* New York: John Wiley & Sons, Inc., 1963.

Anderson, O. *Health care: can there be equity? The United States, Sweden and England.* New York: John Wiley & Sons, Inc., 1972.

Angrist, S., et al. Tolerance of deviant behavior: post hospital performance levels and rehospitalization. In *Proceedings of the Third World Congress of Psychiatry,* 1963.

Antonovsky, A. Breakdown: a needed fourth step in the conceptual armamentarium of modern medicine. *Social Science and Medicine,* 1972, **6,** 537-544.

Antonovsky, A. The utility of the breakdown concept. *Social Science and Medicine,* 1973, **7,** 605-612.

Apfelbaum, E. (ed.). *Choroba glodowa.* Warsaw: American Joint Distribution Committee,

Apple, D. How laymen define illness. *Journal of Health and Human Behavior,* Fall 1960, 219-225.

Atkinson, D. *Orthodox consensus and radical alternative.* New York: Basic Books, Inc., Publishers, 1971.

Aubert, V., and Messinger, S. The criminal and the sick. *Inquiry,* 1958, **1**(3), 137-160.

Bakst, H. J. The Roxbury Comprehensive Community Health Center. *Public Welfare,* 1969, **27,** 227-231.

Bakwin, H. Pseudodoxia pediatrics. *New England Journal of Medicine,* 1945, **232,** 691-697.

Balint, M. *The doctor, his patient and the illness.* London: Sir Isaac Pitman & Sons Ltd., 1957.

Bank, B., et al. *Readings in health care.* Columbia, Mo.: University of Missouri Medical Center, Section of Behavioral Sciences, 1973.

Banta, D., and Fox, R. Role strain of a health care team in a poverty community, *Social Science and Medicine,* 1972, **6,** 697-722.

Barker, R., et al. *Adjustment to physical handicap and illness* bulletin 55. New York: Social Science Research Council, 1953.

Barnard, C. I. *The functions of the executive.* Cambridge, Mass.: Harvard University Press, 1938.

Barnes, H. Herbert Spencer and the evolutionary defense of individualism. In Barnes, H. (ed.) *An introduction to the history of sociology.* Chicago: University of Chicago Press, 1948.

Basil, G. C., and Lewis, E. F. *Test tubes and dragon scales.* Chicago: University of Chicago Press, 1940.

Bauman, B. Diversities in conceptions of health and physical fitness. *Journal of Health and Human Behavior,* 1961, **2** (1), 39-46.

Beavert, C. S. *The hospital: a professional bureaucracy* (mimeograph). University of Missouri, 1972.

Beavert, C. S. *Caretakers of the intermittent dying: role strain of a hemodialysis team.* Masters thesis, University of Missouri, 1974.

Becker, H. *Outsiders: studies in the sociology of deviance.* New York: The Free Press, 1963.

Becker, H. S., Geer, B., Hughes, E., and Strauss, A. *Boys in white.* Chicago: University of Chicago Press, 1961.

Becker, H. S., Geer, B., and Miller, S. J. Medical education. In Freeman, H., Levine, S., and Reeder, L. (eds.) *Handbook of medical sociology.* Englewood Cliffs, N.J.: Prentice-Hall, Inc., 1972.

Bede, L., and Kriesberg, L. Career-relevant values in medical students: a research note. *Journal of the American Medical Association,* 1959, **171,** 1447-1448.

Beecher, H. K. *Research and the individual: human studies.* Boston: Little, Brown & Co., 1970.

Beecher, H., et al. A definition of irreversible coma. *Journal of the American Medical Association,* 1968, **205,** 85-88.

Behind the facade: too often a medical wasteland. *Medical World News,* 1971, **12** (4), 30.

Bellin, S., Geiger, J., and Gibson, C., Impact of ambulatory health care services on the demand for hospital beds. *New England Journal of Medicine,* 1969, **280,** 808-812.

Bendix, R., and Lipset, S. *Class, status and power.* New York: The Free Press, 1966.

Berg, R. (ed.) *Health status indices.* Chicago: Hospital Research and Educational Trust, 1973.

Berger, P. *Invitation to sociology: a humanistic perspective.* Garden City, N.Y.: Doubleday & Co., Inc., 1963.

Berry, R. E., Jr. On grouping hospitals for economic analysis. *Inquiry,* 1973 **10** (4), 5-12.

Bills, S. S. National health insurance—the battle

takes shape. *Journal of the American Hospital Association,* April 1971, **45,** 126-131.

Blau, P. *Dynamics of bureaucracy.* Chicago: University of Chicago Press, 1955.

Blau, P. *Bureaucracy in modern society.* New York: Random House, Inc., 1956.

Blau, P. *Exchange and power in social life.* New York: John Wiley & Sons, Inc., 1964.

Bloom, S. *The doctor and his patient.* New York: Russell Sage Foundation, 1963.

Bogardus, E. *The development of social thought.* New York: David McKay Co., Inc., 1960.

Bok, S. Research, casual or planned? *Hastings Center Report,* 1975, **5** (5), 25-26.

Borkenau, F. The concept of death. *The Twentieth Century,* 1955, **157,** 313-329.

Bott, E. *Family and social network.* London: Tavistock Publications Ltd., 1957.

Bourdillon, J. *Spinal manipulation.* New York: Appleton-Century-Crofts, 1973.

Bourgeois, C. *The situational perspectives of premedical students and their effect on academic career goals.* Unpublished doctoral dissertation, Brown University, 1975.

Boyd, D. R., Dunea, M., and Flashner, B. The Illinois plan for a statewide system of trauma centers, *Journal of Trauma,* 1973, **13** (1), 24-31.

Boylston, Z. *A historical account of the smallpox inoculated in New England.* London: S. Chandler, 1726.

Brecher, E. *Licit and illicit drugs.* Boston: Little, Brown & Co., 1972.

Breckinridge, M. *Wide neighborhoods, a story of the Frontier Nursing Service.* New York: Harper & Row, Publishers, 1952.

Breytspraak, L. M., and Pondy, L. R. Sociological evaluation of the physician's assistant's role. *Group Practice,* March 1969, 32-41.

Brightman, I. J., Notkin, H., Brumfield, W. A., Dorsey, S. A., and Solomon, H. S. Knowledge and utilization of health resources by public assistance recipients: public health and preventive medical resources. *American Journal of Public Health,* 1958, **48,** 188-199.

Brown, G. Post hospital adjustment of chronic mental patients. *Lancet,* 1958, **2,** 685-689.

Bucher, R., and Strauss, A. Professions in process. *American Journal of Sociology,* 1961, **46,** 325-344.

Buckley, W. *Sociology and modern systems theory.* Englewood Cliffs, N.J.: Prentice-Hall, Inc. 1967.

Bulletin of information: 1974-1975. Portland, Ore.: National College of Naturopathic Medicine, 1974.

Bullough, B., and Bullough, V. A brief history of medicine. In Freidson, E., and Lorber, J. *Medical men and their work.* Chicago: Aldine Publishing Co., 1972.

Bunker, J. P. Surgical manpower: a comparison of operations and surgeons in the United States and in England and Wales. *New England Journal of Medicine,* 1970, **282,** 135-144.

Buret, E. *La misere des classes. laborienses en angleterre et en France* (2 vols.). Paris, 1845-1846.

Burgess, A. M., Colton, T., and Peterson, O. L. Categorical programs for heart disease, cancer and stroke. *New England Journal of Medicine,* 1965, **273,** 533-537.

Bury, J. B. *The idea of progress.* New York: Dover Publications, Inc., 1955.

California reprise (editorial), *Journal of the American Osteopathic Association,* 1974, **73** (10), 140.

Callahan, D., Collette, P., and Hilmar, N. Career interests and expectations of U.S. medical students. *Journal of Medical Education,* 1957, **32,** 557-563.

Campbell, J. Working relationships between providers and consumers in a neighborhood health center. *American Journal of Public Health,* 1971, **61,** 97-103.

Caplow, T. *Ths sociology of work.* New York: The Free Press, 1954.

Carlton, C. O., and Hessler, R. M. *Space technology and medical care for Papago indians.* Unpublished manuscript, University of Missouri, 1973.

Carr-Saunders, A. M., and Wilson, P. A., *The professions.* Oxford: The Clarendon Press, 1933.

Carstairs, G. Medicine and faith in rural Rajasthan. In Paul, B. (ed.), *Health culture and community.* New York: Russell Sage Foundation, 1955.

Cartwright, A. *Patients and their doctors: a study of general practice.* London: Routledge & Kegan Paul Ltd., 1967.

Cartwright, N., and Marshall, R. General practice in 1963: its conditions, contents and satisfactions. *Medical Care,* 1965, **3,** 69-87.

Chadwick, E. *Report of the sanitary, condition of the labouring population of Great Britain.* London: W. Clowes & Sons, 1842.

Christie, R., and Merton, R. Procedures for the sociological study of the values climate of medical schools. *Journal of Medical Education,* 1958, **33** (Part II), 125-153.

Clark, M. *Health in the Mexican-American culture: a community study* (2nd ed.). Berkeley: University of California Press, 1970.

Cleland, V. *Nurse clinicians and nurse specialists: an overview.* Paper presented at the American Nurses' Association Convention, Detroit, Mich., May 1972.

Clements, F. E. Primitive concepts of disease. *Publications in American Archaeology and Ethnology,* 1939, **32,** 185-252.

Clendening, L. (ed.). *Source book of medical history.* New York: Dover Publications, Inc., 1942.

Cline, J. Report of the committee to study the relationships between osteopathy and medicine. *Journal of the American Medical Association,* 1953, **152** (8), 734-739.

Clute, K. *The general practitioner: a study of medical education and practice in Ontario and Nova Scotia.* Toronto: University of Toronto Press, 1963.

Cobb, B. Why do people detour to quacks? In Jaco, E. G. (ed.). *Patients, physicians, and illness.* Glencoe, Ill.: The Free Press, 1958.

Coe, R. *Sociology of medicine.* New York: McGraw-Hill Book Co., 1970.

Cohen, P. *Modern social theory.* New York: Basic Books, Inc., Publishers, 1968.

Cole, W. *An introduction to osteopathic medicine.* Marceline, Mo.: Wadsworth, 1957.

Coleman, F. C. Licensure problems of allied health personnel. *Federal Bulletin,* 1970, **57,** 204-213.

Coleman, J., Katz, E., and Mered, H. *Medical innovation: a diffusion study.* Indianapolis: The Bobbs-Merrill Co., Inc., 1966.

College of General Practitioners. *Report of a symposium on the art and the science of general practice.* Torquay, England: Devonshire Press, 1965.

Collins, R. *Conflict sociology: toward an explanatory science.* New York: Academic Press, Inc., 1975.

Commission on Chronic Illness. *Chronic illness in a large city,* Cambridge, Mass.: Harvard University Press, 1957.

Connelly, J. P., Stoeckle, J. D., Lepper, E. S., and Farrisey, R. M. The physician and nurse—their interprofessional work in office and ambulatory settings. *New England Journal of Medicine,* 1966, **275,** 765-769.

Cooke, R. E. The role of ethics in pediatrics. *The American Journal of Diseases of Children,* Oct. 1975, **129,** 1157-1161.

Corey, L., Saltman, S., and Epstein, M. *Medicine in a changing society.* St. Louis: The C. V. Mosby Co., 1972.

Cornaro, L. *Tratto della vita sobria.* Padva, 1558.

Corwin, R. G. Role conception and career aspirations: a study of identity in nursing. *Sociological Quarterly,* April 1961, **2,** 69-86.

Corwin, R. G., and Taves, M. J. Nursing and other health professions. In Freeman, H. F., Levine, S., and Reeder, L. G. (eds.). *Handbook of medical sociology.* Englewood Cliffs, N.J.: Prentice-Hall, Inc., 1963.

Coser, L. A. *The functions of social conflict.* New York: The Free Press, 1956.

Coser, R. Authority and decision-making in a hospital: a comparative analysis. *American Sociological Review,* 1958, **23,** 56-63.

Council on Dental Education. Dental auxiliary education, 1968-1969. *Journal of the American Dental Association,* 1969, **79,** 926-934.

Council on Interracial Books for Children. *Chronicles of American Indian protest.* Greenwich, Conn.: Fawcett Publishing, Inc., 1971.

Council on Pediatric Practice. *Lengthening shad-*

ows: a report of the Council on Pediatric Practice of the American Academy of Pediatrics on the delivery of health services to children, 1970. Evanston, Ill.: American Academy of Pediatrics, 1971.

Cox, C., and Mead, A. (eds.). *A sociology of medical practice.* London: Collier-Macmillan Ltd., 1975.

Crane, D. *The social potential of the patient: an alternative to the sick role.* Paper presented at the meeting of the International Sociological Association, Toronto, 1974.

Crane, D. *The sanctity of social life: physicians' treatment of critically ill patients.* New York: Russell Sage Foundation, 1975.

Croog, S., Levine, S., and Lurie, Z. The heart patient and the recovery process. *Social Science and Medicine,* 1969, **2,** 111-164.

Croog, S., and VerSteeg, D. The hospital as a social system. In Freeman, H., Levine, S., and Reeder, L. (eds.). *Handbook of medical sociology.* Englewood Cliffs, N.J.: Prentice-Hall, Inc., 1972.

Crowell, E. P. Osteopathic medicine. In *Encyclopedia Britannica* (Vol. 13). Chicago: Encyclopedia Britannica, Inc., 1974.

Crozier, M. *The bureaucratic phenomenon.* Chicago: University of Chicago Press, 1964.

Curran, W. Legal regulation and quality control of medical practice under the British health service. *New England Journal of Medicine,* 1966, **274,** 547-557.

Curran, W. J. New paramedical personnel. To license or not to license? *New England Journal of Medicine,* 1970, **282,** 1085-1086.

Danielson, R. *The Cuban health area and polyclinic: organizational focus in an emerging system.* Paper presented at the meeting of the International Sociological Association, Toronto, Aug. 1974.

Danielson, R. The Cuban health area and polyclinic, *Inquiry,* June 1975, **12** (supp.) 86-102.

Danielson, R. Personal communication, 1976.

Davis, F. *Passage through crisis.* Indianapolis: The Bobbs-Merrill Co., Inc., 1963.

Davis, F. *The nursing profession: five sociology essays.* New York: John Wiley & Sons, Inc., 1969.

Davis, J. Great books and small groups. In Hammond, P. (ed.). *Sociologists at work.* New York: Basic Books, Inc., Publishers, 1964.

Davis, K. *Production and cost function estimation for nonprofit hospitals,* unpublished manuscript.

Davis, M. The organization of medical service. *American Labor Legislation,* 1916, **6,** 18-20.

Davis, M., and Eichhorn, R. Compliance with medical regimens: a panel study. *Journal of Health and Human Behavior,* 1963, **4** (4), 240-250.

Davis, M. S., and Tranquada, R. E. Sociological evaluation of the Watts Neighborhood Health Centers. *Medical Care,* 1969, **7,** 105-117.

Davis, M., and von der Lippe, R. Discharge from hospital against medical advice: a study of reciprocity in the doctor-patient relationship. *Social Science and Medicine,* 1967, **1,** 336-344.

Dawson, G. G. *Healing: pagan and Christian.* London: Society for Promoting Christian Knowledge, 1935.

Dean, N. T. Personal communication, 1975.

Deloria, V. *Custer died for your sins.* New York: Avon Books, 1969.

Deloria, V. *We talk, you listen.* New York: Dell Publishing Co., Inc., 1970.

Deloria, V. *Forum for contemporary history* (letter). 1972.

Deloria, V. *God is red.* New York: Delta, 1973.

Department of Health, Education, and Welfare. *The institutional guide to DHEW policy on protection of human subjects.* Washington, D.C.: U.S. Government Printing Office, 1966.

Department of Health, Education, and Welfare. *Final report of the Tuskegee Syphilis Study Ad Hoc Advisory Panel.* Washington, D.C.: U.S. Government Printing Office, 1973.

Dinitz, S., Angrist, S., Lefton, M., and Pasamanick, B. Psychiatric and social attributes as predictors of case outcome in mental hospitalization. *Social Problems,* 1961a, **8,** 322-328.

Dinitz, S., Angrist, S., Lefton, M., and Pasamanick, B. The post-hospital psychological functioning of former mental hospital patients. *Mental Hygiene,* 1961b, **45,** 579-588.

Dinitz, S., Angrist, S., Lefton, M., and Pasamanick, B. Instrumental role expectations and post-hospital performance of female mental patients. *Social Forces,* 1962, **40,** 248-254.

Dohrenevend, B. S., and Dohrenevend, B. (eds.). *Stressful life events.* New York: John Wiley & Sons, Inc., 1974.

Donabedian, A. The quality of medical care. In Corey, L., and Saltman, S. (eds.). *Medicine in a changing society.* St. Louis: The C. V. Mosby Co., 1972.

Dorn, H. Mortality. In Hauser, P. and Duncan, O. (eds.). *The study of population.* Chicago: University of Chicago Press, 1959.

Dorozynski, A. *Doctors and healers.* Ottawa: International Development Research Center, 1975.

Douglas, J. The absurd and suicide. In Shneidman, E. (ed.). *On the nature of suicide.* San Francisco: Jossey-Bass, Inc., Publishers, 1969.

Downes, J., and Collins S. A study of illness among families in the Eastern Health District of Baltimore. *Milbank Memorial Fund Quarterly,* 1940, **18,** 5-26.

Drago, M. County osteopaths reject invitation to join medical society. *Arizona Daily Star,* Jan. 12, 1972.

Driscoll, V. Liberating nursing practice. *Nursing Outlook,* Jan. 1972, **20,** 24-28.

Dubbs, G. Tomorrow's chiropractic school. *The ACA Journal of Chiropractic*, 1970, **7**, 7-24.

Dube, W. F., Striller, F. T., and Nelson, B. C. Study of U.S. medical school applicants, 1970-1971. *Journal of Medical Education*, 1971, **46**, 845.

Dublin, L., Lotka, A. J., and Spiegelman, M. *Length of life: a study of the life table*. New York: Donald, 1949.

Dubos, R. *Mirage of health*. Garden City, N.Y.: Doubleday & Co., Inc., 1959.

Dubos, R. *Man adapting*. New Haven, Conn.: Yale University Press, 1965.

Dubos, R. *So human an animal*. New York: Charles Scribner's Sons, 1968.

Duesenberry, J. S. *Income, saving and the theory of consumer behavior*. Cambridge, Mass.: Harvard University Press, 1949.

Duff, R., and Hollingshead, A. *Sickness and society*. New York: Harper & Row, Publishers, 1968.

Dumont, R., and Foss, D. *The American view of death*. Cambridge, Mass.: Schenkman Publishing Co., Inc., 1972.

Durkheim, E. *The division of labor in society* (Simpson, G., trans.). New York: The Free Press, 1933.

Durkheim, E. *Suicide*. New York: The Free Press, 1951.

Duttera, M. J., and Harlan, N. R. *Evaluation of physicians extenders in the rural southeast: patterns of practice and patient care*. Paper presented at the meeting of the American College of Physicians, San Francisco, 1975.

Editors of the *Yale Law Review:* The American Medical Association: power, purpose and politics in organized medicine. *Yale Law Review*, 1954, **63**, 7.

Ehrenreich, B. and Ehrenreich, J. *The American health empire: a report from the Health Policy Advisory Center*. New York: Random House, Inc., 1971.

Ehrenreich, B., and English, D. *Witches, midwives and nurses: a history of women healers*. Old Westbury, N.Y.: The Feminist Press, 1973.

Eilers, R. D. National health insurance: what kind and how much (Part I). *New England Journal of Medicine*, 1971, **284**, 881-886.

Elling, R. H., and Halebsky, S. Organizational differentiation and support: a conceptual framework. *Administrative Science Quarterly*, 1961, **6** (2), 185-209.

Engel, G. A unified concept of health and disease. In Engel, G. (ed.). *Psychological development in health and disease*. Philadelphia: W. B. Saunders Co., 1962.

Erikson, E. Identity and the life cycle. In *Psychological issues*. New York: International Universities Press, 1959.

Eron, L. The effects of medical education on medical students. *Journal of Medical Education*, 1955, **10**, 559-566.

Estes, E. H., and Howard, D. R. Potential for newer classes of personnel: experiences of the Duke Physician's Assistant Program. *Journal of Medical Education*, 1970, **45**, 149-155.

Etzioni, A. *The semi professions and their organizations: teachers, nurses, social workers*. New York: The Free Press, 1969.

Evans, W. Is orthodox medicine adopting osteopathy? (reprint). *Physical Culture Magazine* 1941.

Farberow, N. (ed.) *Taboo topics*. New York: Atherton, 1963.

Fein, R. *The doctor shortage: an economic diagnosis*. Washington, D.C.: The Brookings Institute, 1967.

Feingold, E. A political scientist's view of the neighborhood health center as a new social institution. *Medical Care*, 1970, **8**, 108-115.

Feldman, J. *The dissemination of health information*. Chicago: Aldine Publishing Co., 1966.

Feldstein, M. S. The medical economy. In *Life, death and medicine* (Scientific American Book). San Francisco, W. H. Freeman & Co., Publishers, 1973.

Field, M. *Doctor and patient in Soviet Russia*. Cambridge, Mass.: Harvard University Press, 1957.

Field, M. The doctor-patient relationship in perspective: "fee-for-service" and "third party" medicine. *Journal of Health and Human Behavior*, 1961, **2**, 252-262.

Field, M. *Soviet socialized medicine*. New York: The Free Press, 1967.

The first hundred years (editorial). *Journal of the American Osteopathic Association*, 1974, **73** (10), 140.

Firth, R. Ethical absolution and the ideal observer, *Philosophy and Phenomenological Research*, 1952, **12**, 317-345.

Fischer, G. Socio economic factors and outcome of released mental patients. *Journal of Health and Human Behavior*, 1965, **6**, 105-110.

Fishman, D., and Zimel, C. Specialty choice and beliefs about specialties among freshman medical students. *Journal of Medical Education*, 1972, **17**, 524-533.

Fletcher, C. M. Diagnosis of pulmonary emphysema —an experimental study. *Proceedings of the Royal Society of Medicine*, 1952, **45**, 577-584.

Flexner, A. *Medical education in the United States and Canada*. (Bulletin No. 4). Carnegie Foundation for the Advancement of Teaching, 1910.

Fox, R. C. Training for uncertainty. In Merton, R., Reader, G., and Kendall, P. *The student physician*. Cambridge, Mass.: Harvard University Press, 1957.

Fox, R. C. *Experiment perilous: physicians and patients facing the unknown*. Glencoe, Ill. The Free Press, 1959.

Fox, R. C. Illness. In *International Encyclopedia of*

the Social Sciences. New York: The Free Press, 1968.

Fox, R. C., and Swazey, J. P. *The courage to fail: a social view of organ transplants and dialysis.* Chicago: The University of Chicago Press, 1974.

Frankel, M. S. *The Public Health Service guidelines governing research involving human subjects: an analysis of the policy-making process.* Washington, D.C.: George Washington University Program of Policy Studies in Science and Technology, 1972.

Franklin, B. *Some account of the Pennsylvania Hospital.* Baltimore: Johns Hopkins, 1754.

Freeman, H., Brim, O., and Williams, G. New dimensions of dying. In Brim, O., et al. (eds.) *The dying patient.* New York: Russell Sage Foundation, 1970.

Freeman, H., Levine, S., and Reeder, L. (eds.). *Handbook of medical sociology.* Englewood Cliffs, N.J.: Prentice-Hall, Inc., 1972.

Freeman, H., and Simmons, O. *The mental patient comes home.* New York: John Wiley & Sons, Inc., 1963.

Freidson, E. Client control and medical practice. *American Journal of Sociology,* 1960, **65**, 374-384.

Freidson, E. *Patients' views of medical practice.* New York: Russell Sage Foundation, 1961.

Freidson, E. Medical sociology. *Current Sociology,* 1962. 10/11.

Freidson, E. *The hospital in modern society.* Glencoe, Ill.: The Free Press, 1963.

Freidson, E. Disability as social deviance. In Sussman, M. (ed.). *Sociology and rehabilitation.* Washington, D.C.: American Sociological Association, 1966.

Freidson, E. *Profession of medicine.* New York: Dodd, Mead & Co., 1970.

Freidson, E. The organization of medical practice. In Freeman, H., Levine, S., and Reeder, L. (eds.). *Handbook of medical sociology.* Englewood Cliffs, N.J.: Prentice-Hall, Inc., 1972.

Freidson, E., and Lorber, J. *Medical men and their work.* Chicago: Aldine Publishing Co., 1972.

Freidson, E., and Rhea, B. Process of control in a company of equals. *Social Problems,* 1963, **2** (2), 119-131.

Freymann, J. G. *The American health care system: its genesis and trajectory.* New York: Medcom Press, 1974.

Friedl, E. Hospital care in provincial Greece, *Human Organization,* **16**, 24-27.

Friedrichs, R. *A sociology of sociology.* New York: The Free Press, 1970.

Frisch, E. *An historical survey of Jewish philanthropy.* New York: Macmillan, 1924.

Fromm, E. *The anatomy of human destructiveness.* New York: Holt, Rinehart & Winston, Inc., 1973.

Frontier Nursing Service. *Quarterly Bulletin,* Summer 1974, **50**.

Frost, E. *Christian healing.* London: Mowbray, 1940.

Garrett, A. E. *The Indian Health Service information system: summary description.* Washington, D.C.: U.S. Department of Health, Education, and Welfare, Office of Research and Development, Jan. 4, 1972.

Geertsma, R. H., and Grinoils, D. R. Specialty choices in medicine. *Journal of Medical Education,* 1972, **47**, 509-517.

Geiger, H. J. Of the poor, by the poor, or for the poor: the mental health implications of social control of poverty programs. *Psychiatric Research Report,* April 1967a, **21**, 55-65.

Geiger, H. J. The neighborhood health center: education of the faculty in preventive medicine. *Archives of Environmental Health,* 1967b, **14**, 912-916.

Geiger, H. J. Health center in Mississippi. *Hospital Practice,* Feb. 1969, 4, 68-81.

Geiger, H. J. The physician as reactionary, reformer, revolutionary. *Social Policy,* 1971, 1 (6), 24-33.

Geomet, Incorporated. *The impact on future health manpower requirements and supply of increasing productivity through use of technological advance,* Nov. 1972.

Gerth, H., and Mills, C. W. *From Max Weber.* New York: Oxford University Press, Inc., 1946.

Gibson, C. D. The neighborhood health center: the primary unit of health care. *American Journal of Public Health,* 1968, **58**, 1188-1191.

Gibson, G. Chinese medical practice and the thoughts of Chairman Mao. *Social Science and Medicine,* Feb. 1972, **6**, 67-93.

Gibson, G. Guidelines for research and education of emerging medical services. *Health Services Reports,* 1974, **89** (2), 99-111.

Giddings, F. *Sociology: a lecture.* New York, 1908.

Glaser, B., and Strauss, A. *Awareness of dying.* Chicago: Aldine Publishing Co., 1967.

Glaser, B., and Strauss, A. *Time for dying.* New York: Aldine Publishing Co., 1968.

Glaser, R. Innovations and heroic acts in prolonging life. In Brim, O., et al. (eds.). *The dying patient.* New York: Russell Sage Foundation, 1970.

Glaser, W. American and foreign hospitals. In Freidson, E. *The hospital in modern society.* Glencoe, Ill.: The Free Press, 1963.

Glaser, W. *Social settings and medical organization: a cross-national study of the hospital.* New York: Atherton Press, Inc., 1970.

Glasser, M. Consumer expectations of health services. In Corey, L., Saltmen, S., and Epstein, M. (eds.). *Medicine in a changing society.* St. Louis: The C. V. Mosby Co., 1972.

Goddard, J. L. The medical business. In *Life and death and medicine* (Scientific American Book). San Francisco: W. H. Freeman & Co., Publishers, 1973.

Godkins, T. R., Stanhope, W. D., and Lynn, T. N. Current status of the physician's assistant in Oklahoma. *Oklahoma State Medical Association Journal,* 1974, **67**, 102-107.

Goffman, E. *Presentation of self in everyday life.* Garden City, N.Y.: Doubleday-Anchor, 1959.

Goffman, E. *Stigma.* Englewood Cliffs, N.J.: Prentice-Hall, Inc., 1963.

Goldman, L. Factors related to physicians medical and political attitudes: a documentation of intra-professional variations. *Journal of Health and Social Behavior,* 1974, **15** (3), 177-187.

Goode, W. J. Community within a community: the professions. *American Sociological Review,* 1957, **22**, 194-199.

Goode, W. J. A theory of role strain. *American Sociological Review,* 1960a, **25**, 483-496.

Goode, W. J. Encroachment, charlatanism and the emerging profession: psychiatry, sociology and medicine. *American Sociological Review,* 1960b, **25**, 902-914.

Goode, W. J. The librarian: from occupation to profession? *The Library Quarterly,* 1961, **31**: (4), 306-318.

Goode, W. J. *Explorations in social theory.* New York: Oxford University Press, Inc., 1973.

Goodrich, C., Olendski, M., and Crocetti, A. Hospital based comprehensive care: is it a failure? *Medical Care,* 1972, **10**, 363-368.

Gordon, D. Health maintenance service: ambulatory patient care in the general medical clinic. *Medical Care,* 1974, **12**, 648-658.

Gordon, G. *Role theory and illness,* New Haven, Conn.: College & University Press, 1966.

Gordon, J. B. The politics of community medicine projects: a conflict analysis. *Medical Care,* 1969, **7**, 491-528.

Gordon, M. *Sick cities: psychology and pathology of American urban life.* Baltimore: Penguin Books, Inc., 1963.

Gouldner, A. Theoretical requirements of the applied social sciences. *American Sociological Review,* 1957, **22**, 92-102.

Graham, D., and Stevenson, I. Disease as a response to life stress. 1. The nature of the evidence. In Lief, H. I. et al. (eds.). *The psychological basis of medical practice.* New York: Harper & Row, Publishers, 1963.

Graham, F. Group versus solo practice: arguments and evidence. *Inquiry,* 1972, **9** (2), 49-60.

Graham, S. Socioeconomic status, illness and the use of medical services. In Jaco, E. G. (ed.). *Patients, physicians and illness.* Glencoe, Ill.: The Free Press, 1958.

Graham, S., and Reeder, L. Social factors in the chronic illnesses. In Freeman, H., Levine, S., and Reader, L. (eds.). *Handbook of medical sociology.* Englewood Cliffs, N. J.: Prentice-Hall, Inc., 1972.

Gray, B. H. *Human subjects in medical experimentation: a sociological study of the conduct and regulation of clinical research.* New York: John Wiley & Sons, Inc., 1975.

Gray, P. G., and Cartwright, A. Choosing and changing doctors. *Lancet,* 1953, **2**, 1308-1309.

Greenwood, E. Attributes of a profession. *Social Work,* 1957, **2** (3), 44-55.

Griffin, M. *Aged hospital patients: the process of occupying a new role.* Unpublished masters thesis, University of Missouri, 1975.

Grinker, R. *Psychosomatic research.* New York: W. W. Norton & Co., Inc., 1953.

Gross, Dan H. *The psychodynamics of religious healing.* Paper presented at the meeting of the Society for Applied Anthropology, Miami, Fla., April 18, 1971.

Gross, E. *Work and society.* New York: Thomas Y. Crowell Co., Inc., 1958.

Gurin, R., Veroff, J., and Feld, S. *Americans' view their mental health.* New York: Basic Books, Inc., Publishers, 1960.

Habenstein, R. W. and Christ, E. A. *Professionalizer, traditionalizer and utilizer.* Columbia: University of Missouri Press, 1955.

Habermas, J. *Technik und Wessenschaft als Ideologie.* Suhrkamp Verlag Kg., 1968.

Halberstam, M. J. Liberal thought, radical theory and medical practice. *New England Journal of Medicine,* 1971, **284**, 1180-1185.

Hall, O. The informal organization of the medical profession. *Canadian Journal of Economics and Political Science,* Feb. 1946, **12**, 30-44.

Hall, O. The stages of a medical career. *American Journal of Sociology,* 1947, **53**, 327-337.

Hall, O. Types of medical careers. *American Journal of Sociology,* 1949, **55**, 243-253.

Hall, O. Sociological research in the field of medicine. *American Sociological Review,* 1951, **16**, 639-649.

Hall, O. Some problems in the provision of medical services. *Canadian Journal of Economics and Political Science,* 1954, **20**, 456-466.

Harrington, M. *The other America.* Baltimore: Penguin Books, Inc., 1963.

Harris, D. The development of nurse midwifery in New York City. *Bulletin of the American College of Nurse-Midwives,* 1969, **14**, 1.

Harris, D., Daily, E. F., and Lang, D. M. Nurse-midwifery in New York City. *American Journal of Public Health,* 1971, **16** (1), 64-77.

Harris, R. *A sacred trust.* New York: The New American Library, Inc., 1966.

Hassinger, E. M. and Hobbs, D. J. Health service patterns in rural and urban areas: a test between availability and use. *University of Missouri Agricultural Experiment Station Bulletin,* April 1972, no. 987.

Hawley, A. *Human ecology: a theory of community structure.* New York: The Ronald Press Co., 1950.

Haynes, G. Educational standards for chiropractic colleges. *The ACA Journal of Chiropractic,* 1967, **4**, 60.

Haynes, G. Chiropractic education and curriculum

flexibility. *The ACA Journal of Chiropractic,* 1969, **8,** 13.

Henry, P. Pimps, prostitutes and policemen: education of consumers for participating in health planning. *American Journal of Public Health,* 1970, **60,** 2171-2174.

Hershey, N. The inhibiting effect upon innovation of the prevailing licensure system. *Annals of the New York Academy of Science,* 1969, **166,** 951-956.

Herzlich, C. Quelques aspects de la representation sociale de la sante et de la maladie. *Revue Psychologie Francaise,* 1964, **9,** 1-14.

Hessler, R. M., and Griffard, C. D. Community health paraprofessional: the occupation of not quite, *Inquiry,* March 1976, **13,** 90-96.

Hessler, R. M., and New, P. K.-M. Research as a process of exchange. *The American Sociologist,* Feb. 1972, **7,** 13-15.

Hessler, R. M., New, P. K.-M., Bellin, S., Schoepf, B., and Bagwell, P. *Neighborhood health centers: polarization of issues.* Paper presented at the meeting of the Society for Applied Anthropology, Boulder, Colo., April 1970.

Hessler, R., Nolan, M., Ogbru, B., and New, P. K.-M. Intraethnic diversity: health care of the Chinese-Americans. *Human Organization,* Fall 1975, **34,** 253; 262.

Hessler, R. M., and Walters, M. J. Consumer evaluation of health services: implications for methodology and health care policy. *Medical Care,* 1975, **13,** 683-693.

Hinkle, R. Durkheim in American sociology. In Wolff, K. (ed.). *Emile Durkheim, 1858-1917.* Columbus, Ohio: Ohio State University Press, 1960.

Hobbs, D. A comment on applied sociological research. *Rural Sociology,* June 1969, **34,** 241-245.

Hochbaum, G. M. Consumer participation in health planning: toward a conceptual clarification. *American Journal of Public Health,* 1969, **59,** 1968-1705.

Hofstadter, R. *Social darwinism in America.* Boston: Beacon Press, 1955.

Hollingshead, A., and Redlich, F., *Social class and mental illness.* New York: John Wiley & Sons, 1958.

Hollister, R. M. *From consumer participation to consumer control of neighborhood health centers.* Unpublished doctoral dissertation, Massachusetts Institute of Technology, 1970.

Hollister, R. M., Kramer, B. M., and Seymour S. B. *Neighborhood health centers.* Lexington, Mass., D. C. Heath & Co., 1974.

Holmes, O. *Homeopathy and its kindred delusion.* Boston, 1842.

Holton, W., New, P. K. and Hessler, R. M. *Citizen participation and inter agency relations.* Research report to the National Institute of Mental Health, Washington, D.C., 1972.

Homans, G. C. *The human group.* New York: Harcourt, Brace & Co., Inc., 1950.

Homans, G. C. *Social behavior: its elementary forms.* New York: Harcourt, Brace & World, 1961.

Hrdlicka, A. *Physiological and medical observations among the Indians of southwestern United States and northern Mexico* (Bureau of American Ethnology, Bulletin 34). Washington, D.C.: U.S. Government Printing Office, 1908.

Hsu, F. *Religion, science and human crises: a study of China in transition and its implications for the West.* London: Routledge & Kegan Paul Ltd., 1952.

Hsu, F. *China day by day.* New Haven, Conn.: Yale University Press, 1974.

Hudson, J. *Social policy and theoretical sociology.* Paper presented at the meeting of the Midwest Sociological Society, St. Louis, April 16, 1970.

Hughes, E. *Men and their work.* Minneapolis: University of Minnesota Press, 1958.

Hughes, E. C., Hughes, H. M., and Deutscher, I. *20,000 nurses tell their story.* Philadelphia: J. B. Lippincott Co., 1958.

Humbolt, A. *Personal narrative of travels to the equinoctial regions of America during the years 1799-1804* (3 vols.). London: G. Bell & Sons Ltd., 1877.

Humphreys, F. *Humphrey's manual for the administration of medicine and treatment of disease.* New York: Humphrey's Homeopathic Medical Co., 1927.

Huntington, M. J. The development of a professional self-image. In Merton, R., Reader G., and Kendall, P. (eds.). *The student physician.* Cambridge, Mass.: Harvard University Press, 1957.

Hyman, M. Medicine. In Lazarsfeld, P. F., Sewell, W., and Wilensky, H. (eds.). *The uses of sociology.* New York: Basic Books, Inc., Publishers, 1967.

Jaco, E. G. (ed.). *Patients, physicians and illness: a source book in behavioral science and health.* New York: The Free Press, 1972.

John, R., Kimmelman, D., Hoas, J., and Orris, P. Public health care in Cuba. *Social Policy,* Jan. 1971, **1,** 5; Feb. 1971, **1,** 41-46.

Johnson, W. Faces on a new China scroll. *Sports Illustrated,* 1973. **39,** Sept. 24, 82-100.

Johnson, W. G. To die as a man: disease, truth and christian ethics. *Journal of the Iowa Medical Society,* 1966, **56,** 813-816.

Johnson, W. L. *A study of family adjustment to the crisis of cardiac disease.* New York: American Nurses' Foundation, Inc., 1966.

Jungfer, C., and Last, M. Clinical performance in Australian general practice. *Medical Care,* 1964, **2,** 71-83.

Kadushin, C. Social class and the experience of ill health. *Sociological Inquiry,* 1964, **1,** 67-80.

Kane, R., and Kane, R. *Federal health care (with reservations).* New York: Springer Publishing Co., 1972.

Kant, E. On the supposed right to lie from altruistic motives. In Beck, L. W. (trans. and ed.). *Critique of practical reason.* Chicago: University of Chicago Press, 1949.

Kaplan, A. *The conduct of inquiry.* San Francisco: Chandler Publishing Co., 1964.

Katz, J. (ed.). *Experimentation with human beings.* New York: Russell Sage Foundation, 1972.

Katz, F. *Autonomy in organization: the limits of social control.* New York: Random House, Inc., 1968.

Kaufman, M. *Homeopathy in America.* Baltimore: The Johns Hopkins University Press, 1971.

Kemnitzer, L. *Yuwipi medicine: healing and the Indian response to the whiteman's culture.* Paper presented at the meeting of the Society for Applied Anthropology, Miami, Fla, April, 1971.

Kendall, P. The learning environment of hospitals. In Freidson, E. *The hospital in modern society.* Glencoe, Ill.: The Free Press, 1963.

Kendall, P. and Selvin, H. C. Tendencies toward specialization in medical training. In Merton, R. Reader, G. and Kendall, P. (eds.). *The student physician.* Cambridge, Mass.: Harvard University Press, 1957.

Kiev, A. *Curanderismo: Mexican-American folk psychiatry.* New York: The Free Press, 1968.

Kimmel, E. A critical evaluation of the chiropractic as profession. *The ACA Journal of Chiropractic,* 1964, **1,** 8.

King, S. Social psychological factors in illness. In Freeman, H., Levine, S., and Reeder, L. (eds.). *Handbook of medical sociology.* Englewood Cliffs, N.J.: Prentice-Hall, Inc., 1972.

Kittrie, N. *The right to be different.* Baltimore: The Johns Hopkins University Press, 1971.

Knowles, J. H. U.S. health: do we face a catastrophe? *Look Magazine,* June 1970, pp. 74-78.

Knutson, A. *The individual, society and health behavior.* New York: Russell Sage Foundation, 1965.

Koch, A. and Peden, W. (eds.). *The life and selected writings of Thomas Jefferson.* New York: Modern Library, 1944.

Kolb, J., and Sidel, V. Influence of utilization review on hospital length of stay. *Journal of the American Medical Association,* 1968, **203,** 117-119.

Koos, E. *The health of regionville.* New York: Columbia University Press, 1954.

Kosa, J., and Robertson, L. The social aspects of health and illness. In Kosa, J., Antonovsky, A., and Zola, I. (eds.). *Poverty and health.* Cambridge, Mass.: Harvard University Press, 1969.

Kramer, M. Comparative study of characteristics, attitudes and opinions of neophyte British and American nurses. *International Journal of Nursing Studies,* Dec. 1967, **4,** 281.

Kramer, M. Role conceptions of baccalaureate nurses and success in hospital nursing. *Nursing Research,* Sept.-Oct. 1970, **19,** 428-439.

Kramer, R. M. Participation of the poor: comparative community case studies in the war on poverty. Englewood Cliffs, N.J.: Prentice-Hall, Inc., 1969.

Kubler-Ross, E. *On death and dying.* New York: Macmillan, Inc., 1970.

Kuhn, T. *The structure of scientific revolutions.* Chicago: University of Chicago Press, 1970.

LaHargue, Z. Morbidity and marital status. *Journal of Chronic Diseases,* 1960, **12,** 476-498.

Lakatos, I., and Musgrave, P. *Criticism and the growth of knowledge.* Cambridge, Engl.: Cambridge University Press, 1970.

Lambert, W., Libman, E., and Posea, E. G. The effect of increased salience of a membership group on pain tolerance. *Journal of Personality,* 1960, **28,** 350-357.

Lame Deer, and Erdoes, R. *Lame Deer: seeker of visions.* New York: Simon & Schuster, Inc., 1972.

Langner, T., and Michael, S. *Life stress and mental health.* New York: The Free Press, 1963.

Lappé, M. Abortion and research. *Hastings Center Report,* June 21, 1975, **5.**

Lawson, J. *History of North Carolina 1714.* Richard, Garrett & Massie, 1937.

Lazarsfeld, P. F. The change of opinion during a political discussion. *Journal of Applied Psychology,* 1939, **23,** 131-147.

Lee, M. L. A conspicuous production theory of hospital behavior. *The Southern Economic Journal,* July 1971, **38,** 48-58.

Lee, M. L. *Adaptive utility function and the theory of economic behavior* (mimeographed). Columbia, Mo.: University of Missouri Medical Center, Section of Behavioral Sciences, 1975.

Lefton, M., Angrist, S., Dinitz, S., and Pasamanick, B. Social class, expectations and performance of mental patients. *American Journal of Sociology,* 1962, **68,** 79-87.

Lefton, M., Dinitz, S., Angrist, S. S., et al. Former mental patients and their neighbors: a comparison of performance levels. *Journal of Health and Human Behavior,* 1966, **7,** 106-113.

Lemert, E. Legal commitment and social control. *Sociology and Social Research,* 1946, **30,** 370-378.

Lemert, E. *Social pathology.* New York: McGraw-Hill Book Co., 1951.

Lennane, K. J., and Lennane, R. J. Alleged psychogenic disorders in women: a possible manifestation of sexual prejudice. *New England Journal of Medicine,* 1973, **288,** 288-292.

Leuret, F., and Bon, H. *Modern miraculous cures.* New York: Farrar, Straus & Cudahy, 1957.

Levine, S., and Scotch, N. *Social stress.* Chicago: Aldine Publishing Co., 1970.

Levinson, P., and Schiller, J. Role analysis of the indigenous nonprofessional. *Social Work,* 1966, **11,** 95-101.

Lewis, A. Health as a social concept. *British Journal of Sociology,* 1953, **11,** 109.

Lewis, C., and Resnick, B. The Norse Clinic—dynamics of ambulatory patient care. *Journal of the Kansas Medical Society*, 1967, **68** (3), 123-124.

Lewis, E. P. A role by any name (editorial). *Nursing Outlook*, Feb. 1974, **22**, 89.

Lewis, R. G. Osteopathic statements and definition. *Journal of Osteopathy*, 1902, p. 222.

Lin, P. *The chiropractic and process: a study of the sociology of an occupation*. Unpublished doctoral dissertation, University of Missouri, 1972.

Lindhardt, M. The Danish morbidity survey of 1950. In *Proceedings of the International Population Conference*, Wien, Austria, 1959.

Lindgren, H. *Psychology of personal and social adjustment*. New York: American Book Co., 1959.

Litman, T. J. Public perceptions of the physician's assistant—a survey of the attitudes and opinions of rural Iowa and Minnesota residents. *American Journal of Public Health*, 1972, **62**, 343-346.

Litwak, E. Models of bureaucracy that present conflict. *American Journal of Sociology*, 1961, **67**, 177-184.

Logan, W. P. D. National morbidity statistics in England and Wales. In *Proceedings of the International Population Conference*, Wien, Austria, 1959.

Lohrenz, F. N. The Marshfield Clinic physician-assistant concept: clinical evaluation of advanced ages, disadvantages and prospects. *New England Journal of Medicine*, 1971, **284**, 301-304.

Lorne, P. Doctors without patients! The anesthesiologist—a new specialist. Unpublished doctoral dissertation, University of Chicago, 1949.

Ludz, P. Alienation as a concept in the social sciences: a trend report and bibliography. *Current Sociology*, 1973, **21**, entire issue.

Lynd, R., and Lynd, H. *Middletown*. New York: Harcourt, Brace & Co., 1929.

Lynd, R., and Lynd, H. *Middletown in transition*. New York: Harcourt, Brace & Co., 1937.

MacGregor, F., Able, T. M., Byrt, A., Laver, E., and Weissmann, S. *Facial deformities and plastic surgery: a psychosocial study*. Springfield, Ill.: Charles C Thomas, Publisher, 1953.

MacLean, C. M. U. Traditional healers and their female clients: an aspect of Nigerian sickness behavior. *Journal of Health and Social Behavior*, Sept. 1969, **10**, 172-186.

Madigan, F. Are sex mortality differentials biologically caused? *Milbank Memorial Fund Quarterly*, 1957, **35** (2), 202-23.

Mahoney, A. Factors affecting physician's choice of group or independent practice. *Inquiry*, 1973, **10** (2), 9-18.

Mannheim, K. *Ideology and utopia* (Wirth, L., and Shils, E. trans.). New York: Harcourt, Brace & Co., 1936.

Marcuse, H. *One dimensional man*. Boston: Beacon Press, 1964.

Marriott, M. Western medicine in a village of northern India. In Paul, B. (ed.). *Health culture and community*. New York: Russell Sage Foundation, 1955.

Martel, M. Academentia praecox: the aims, merits and empirical scope of Parsons' multisystemic language rebellion. In Turk, H., and Simpson, R. *Institutions and exchange*. Indianapolis: The Bobbs-Merrill Co., Inc., 1971.

Martin, B. Physician manpower, 1972. In Vahovich, S. *'73 Profile of medical practice*. Chicago: American Medical Association, 1973.

Martin, W. Preferences for types of patients. In Merten, R., Reader, G., and Kendall, P. (eds.). *The student physician*. Cambridge, Mass.: Harvard University Press, 1957.

Martindale, D. *The nature and types of sociological theory*. Boston: Houghton-Mifflin Co., 1960.

Marx, K. *Das Kapital* (Engels, F., ed.). Chicago: Henry Regnery Co., 1961.

Marx, K., and Engels, F. *Manifesto of the communist party*. New York: International Publishers Co., Inc., 1932.

Maryon, E. E. *The new medical world*. Springfield, Mass.: Hampden Publishing Co., 1906.

Maslow, A. *Motivation and personality*, New York: Harper & Row Publishers, 1954.

Masterman, M. The nature of a paradigm. In Laktos, I., and Musgrave, P. *Criticism and the growth of knowledge*. Cambridge, Engl.: Cambridge University Press, 1970.

Mauksch, H. The organizational content of nursing practice. In Davis, F. *The nursing profession: five sociological essays*. New York: John Wiley & Sons, Inc., 1969.

Mauksch, H. Nursing: churning for change. In Freeman, H., Levine, S., and Reeder, L. (eds.). *Handbook of medical sociology*. Englewood Cliffs, N.J.: Prentice-Hall, Inc., 1972.

Mauksch, H. *A social science basis for conceptualizing family health*. Paper presented at Conference on Medical Sociology, Warsaw, Poland, 1973.

Mauksch, I. and David, M. Prescription for survival. *American Journal of Nursing*, 1972, **72**, 2189-2193.

Maus, H. *A short history of sociology*. London: Routledge & Kegan Paul Ltd., 1962.

Mauss, M. *The gift: forms and functions of exchange in archaic societies*. Cunnison, I. (trans.). Glencoe, Ill.: The Free Press, 1954.

Mayer, K. *Class and society*. New York: Random House, Inc., 1955.

McCallister, S. and Liccione, W. J. Medical student attitudes toward rural practice: before and after first year. In *Proceedings of the Fourteenth Annual Conference on Research in Medical Education*. Nov. 1975.

McCormick, R. A. Fetal research, morality, and public policy. *Hastings Center Report*, June 1975, **5**, 26-31.

McCorkle, T. Chiropractic: a deviant theory of disease and treatment in contemporary Western society. *Human Organization*, 1961, **20**, 20-23.

McDonald, B., Pugh, W., and Gunderson, E. Organizational factors and health status. *Journal of Health and Social Behavior*, 1973, **14** (4), 330-334.

McElrath, D. Physicians in prepaid group practice. *American Sociological Review*, **26**, 1961, 596-607.

McKinlay, J. The sick role—illness and pregnancy. *Social Science and Medicine*, 1972, **6**, 561-572.

McLuhan, T. *Touch the earth*. New York: Pocket Books, 1971.

McMahon, B., Pugh, T., and Ipsen, J. *Epidemiologic methods*. Boston: Little, Brown & Co., 1960.

Mechanic, D. The concept of illness behavior. *Journal of Chronic Diseases*, 1962a, **15**, 189-94.

Mechanic, D. Some factors in identifying and defining mental illness. *Mental Hygiene*, 1962b, **46**, 66-74.

Mechanic, D. Perceptions of parental responses to illness. *Journal of Health and Human Behavior*, 1965, **6** (4), 253-257.

Mechanic, D. General medical practice in England and Wales: its organization and future. *New England Journal of Medicine*, 1968a, **279**, 680.

Mechanic, D. *Medical sociology*. New York: The Free Press, 1968b.

Mechanic, D. Illness and cure. In Kosa, J., Antonovsky, and Zola, (eds.). *Poverty and health*. Cambridge, Mass.: Harvard University Press, 1969.

Mechanic, D. The organization of medical practice and practice orientation among physicians in pre-paid and non-paid primary care settings. *Medical Care*, 1975a, **13**, 189-204.

Mechanic, D. Practice orientations among general practitioners in England and Wales. In Cox, C. and Mead, A. (eds.) *A sociology of medical practice*. London: Collier-Macmillan Ltd., 1975b.

Mehorney, A. Factors affecting physicians' choice of group or independent practice. *Inquiry*, 1973, **10** (2), 9-18.

Merton, R., Reader, G., and Kendall, P. (eds.). *The student physician*. Cambridge, Mass.: Harvard University Press, 1957.

Meyer, H. J. Sociological comments. In Girosser, C., Henry, W. E., and Kelly, J. G. (eds.). *Nonprofessionals in the human services*. San Francisco: Jossey-Bass, Inc., Publishers, 1969.

Meyers, H. B. The medical industrial complex. *Fortune*, Jan. 1970, **81**, 90-91.

Millis, J. *The graduate education of physicians*. Chicago: American Medical Association, 1966.

Mills, C. *White collar*. New York: Oxford University Press, 1951.

Mills, D. *Study of chiropractors, osteopathic and naturopaths in Canada*. Ottawa: The Queen's Printer for Canada, 1966.

Mills, L. *The osteopathic profession and its colleges* (Booklet No. 20). Chicago: American Osteopathic Association, 1947.

Mitchell, D. *A hundred years of sociology*. Chicago: Aldine Publishing Co., 1968.

Montgomery, R. *Born to heal*. New York: Coward, McCann & Geoghegan, 1973.

Moore, H. H. *American medicine and the people's health*. New York: D. Appleton & Co., 1927.

Morris, J. N. Some current trends in public health. *Proceedings of the Royal Society*, 1963, **159B**, 66.

Moynihan, D. P. *Maximum feasible misunderstanding: community action in the War on Poverty*. New York: The Free Press, 1969.

Mullett, C. *The bubonic plague and England: as essay in the history of preventive medicine*. Lexington, Ky.: University of Kentucky Press, 1956.

Mumford, L. *The city in history*. New York: Harcourt, Brace & World, 1961.

Mussallem, H. K. The changing role of the nurse. *The American Journal of Nursing*, 1969, **69**, 514-517.

Nathanson, C., and Becker, M. Work satisfaction and performance of physicians in pediatric outpatient clinics. *Health Services Research*, 1973, **8** (1), 17-26.

National Academy of Sciences Board of Medicine Ad Hoc Panel for New Members of the Physicians' Health Team. *Physicians' assistants*. Washington, D.C.: National Academy of Sciences, 1970.

National Center for Health Statistics. *Origin, program and operation of the U.S. National Health Survey*. USPHS publication 1000, series 1, no. 1, 1963.

National Center for Health Statistics, Vital and Health Statistics. *Inpatient health facilities as reported from the 1969 MFI Survey*. Series 14. No. 6. Washington, D.C.: U.S. Government Printing Office, 1972.

National Center for Health Statistics, Vital and Health Statistics. *Average length of stay in short-stay hospitals: demographic factors, United States —1968*. Series 13. No. 13. Washington, D.C.: U.S. Government Printing Office, 1973.

National Center for Health Statistics. *Health resources statistics*. Washington, D.C.: U.S. Government Printing Office, 1974.

National Commission for the Study of Nursing and Nursing Education. Summary report and recommendations. *American Journal of Nursing*, 1970, **70**, 279-294.

The nation's hospitals: a statistical profile (Part 2: Hospital guide issue). *Hospitals*, 1970, **44**.

Navarro, V. Health, health services and health planning in Cuba. *International Journal of Health Services*, 1972, **2**, 409-410.

Navarro, V. A critique of the present and proposed strategies for redistributing resources in the health sector and a discussion of alternatives. *Medical Care*, 1974, **12**, 721-742.

New, P. K.-M. *The applications of reference group*

theory to shifts in values: the case of the osteopathic student. Unpublished doctoral dissertation, University of Missouri, 1960.

New, P. K.-M. The osteopathic students: a study of dilemma. In Jaco, E. G. (ed.). *Patients, physicians and illness: a source book in behavioral science and health* (2nd ed.). New York: The Free Press, 1972.

New, P. K.-M. Community health centers: five danger signals. In Browne, J. W. (ed.). *Community health center in Canada: background papers 4.* Ottawa: Information Canada, 1973.

New, P. K.-M. Barefoot doctors and health care in China. *Eastern Horizon,* 1974, **13** (3), 7-21.

New, P. K.-M., et al. *Hope and reality* (mimeograph). Boston: Tufts University School of Medicine, 1968.

New, P. K.-M., and Hessler, R. M. Neighborhood health centers: traditional medical care at an outpost? *Inquiry,* 1972, **9** (4), 45-58.

New, P. K.-M., Hessler, R. M., and Cater, P. B. Consumer control and public accountability. *Anthropological Quarterly,* July 1973, **46,** 196-213.

New, P. K.-M., and New, M. L. The links between health and the political structure in New China. *Human Organization,* Fall 1975, **34,** 237-251.

New, P. K.-M., Ricci, E. M., and Hessler, R. *The spirit is healed.* Paper presented at meeting of the Society for Applied Anthropology, Miami, Fla., April 18, 1971.

Newell, D. J. Problems in estimating demand for hospital beds. *Journal of Chronic Disease,* 1964, **17,** 749-759.

Nightingale, F. *Florence Nightingale to her nurses.* New York: The Macmillan Co., 1914.

Nisbet, R. *The sociological tradition.* New York: Basic Books, Inc., Publishers, 1966.

Normile, F. R. A formula for estimating bed needs. *Hospitals,* 1969, **43,** 57-58.

Northup, G. *Osteopathic medicine: an american reformation.* Chicago: American Osteopathic Association, 1966.

O'Dell, M. L. Physicians' perceptions of an extended role for the nurse. *Nursing Research,* July-Aug. 1974, **23,** 348-351.

Offer, D., and Sabshin, M. *Normality.* New York: Basic Books, Inc., Publishers, 1966.

Office of Economic Opportunity. *The comprehensive neighborhood health services program* (Guideline No. 6128-1). Washington, D.C.: U.S. Government Printing Office, 1968.

Ogburn, W. F. *Social change with respect to culture and original nature.* New York: B. W. Huebsch, 1922.

O'Neil, M. F. A study of baccalaureate nursing student values. *Nursing Research,* 1973, **22,** 437-441.

Ousler, W. *The healing power of faith.* New York: Hawthorne Books, Inc., 1957.

Parker, A. W. The consumer as policy maker—issues of training. *American Journal of Public Health,* 1970, **60,** 2139-2153.

Parsons, T. *The structure of social action.* New York: The Free Press, 1937.

Parsons, T. *The social system.* New York: The Free Press, 1951.

Parsons, T. Definitions of health and illness in the light of American values and social structure. In Jaco, E. G. (ed.). *Patients, physicians and illness.* Glencoe, Ill.: The Free Press, 1958.

Parsons, T. *Social structure and personality.* New York: The Free Press, 1964.

Parsons, T. Research with human subjects and the professional complex. *Daedalus,* Spring 1969, **98,** 325-360.

Parsons, T. The sick role and the role of the physician reconsidered. *Milbank Memorial Fund Quarterly,* 1975, **53** (3), 257-278.

Patient Care, **5** (3).

Paul, B. (ed.). *Health culture and community.* New York: Russell Sage Foundation, 1955.

Paul, J. R. *A history of poliomyelitis.* New Haven, Conn.: Yale University Press, 1971.

Pavalko, R. M. (ed.). *Sociological perspectives on occupations.* Itasca, Ill.: F. E. Peacock Publishers, Inc., 1972.

Pavia, R., and Haley, H. Intellectual, personality, and environmental factors in career specialty preferences. *Journal of Medical Education,* 1971, **46,** 281-289.

Pellette, E. Some differences between osteopathy and chiropractic (reprint). *Herald of Osteopathy.*

Penchansky, R., and Fox, D. Frequency of referral and patient characteristics in general practice. *Medical Care,* 1970, **8,** 368-385.

Pennell, M. Y., and Hoover, D. B. Allied health manpower supply and requirements: 1950-1980. *Health Manpower Source Book 21* (Public Health Service publication No. 263). Washington D.C.: U.S. Government Printing Office, 1970.

Perrott, G., Tibbitts, C., and Britten, R. The National Health Survey. *Public Health Reports,* 1939, **54,** 1663-1687.

Perrott, G. S. *The federal employees health benefits program, enrollment and utilization of health services 1961-68.* Rockville, M.: U.S. Department of Health, Education, and Welfare, 1971.

Perse, I., and Crocker, L. *The Peckham experiment.* London: George Allen & Unwin Ltd., 1944.

Peterson, B. Time capsule. *The Journal of the American Osteopathic Association,* 1973-1974.

Peterson, O., Andrews, L. P., Spain, R. S., and Greenberg, B. S. An analytical study of North Carolina general practice (Part 2). *Journal of Medical Education,* 1956, **31,** 12.

Peterson, P., and Pennell, M. *Health manpower science book: medical specialists.* Washington, D.C.: U.S. Government Printing Office, 1962.

Peterson, W. *Population*. New York: Macmillan, Inc., 1969.

Phillips, D. Self reliance and inclination to adopt the sick role. *Social Forces,* 1965, **43**, 555-563.

Piedmont, E. Referrals and reciprocity: psychiatrists, general practitioners and clergymen. *Journal of Health and Social Behavior,* 1968, **9** (1), 29-41.

Pierce, R. V. *The people's common sense medical advisor.* Buffalo, N.Y.: World's Dispensary Printing Office and Bindery, 1895.

Pitts, J. Social control. In *International encyclopedia of the social sciences.* New York: The Free Press, 1968.

Press, I. D. Urban illness: physicians curers and dual use in Bogota. *Journal of Health and Social Behavior,* 1969, **10** (3), 209-211.

Ramsey, P. *The patient as person.* New Haven, Conn.: Yale University Press, 1970.

Ramsey, P. *The ethics of fetal research.* New Haven, Conn.: *Yale Fastback,* 1975.

Record, J. C., and Cohen, H. R. The introduction of midwifery in a prepaid group practice. *American Journal of Public Health,* 1972, **62**, 3.

Redlich, F., Hollingshead, A. B., and Bellis, F. Social class differences in attitudes toward psychiatry. *American Journal of Orthopsychiatry,* 1955, **25**, 60-70.

Reeder, L. G. The patient-client as a consumer: some observations on the changing professional-client relationship. *Journal of Health and Social Behavior,* 1972, **13** (4), 406-412.

Reuther, W. The need for comprehensive national health insurance and the national service corps. In Corey, L., Saltman, S., and Epstein, M. *Medicine in a changing society.* St. Louis, The C. V. Mosby Co., 1972.

Ribicoff, A. *The American medical machine.* New York: Harper & Row, Publishers, 1972.

Rice, R. G. Analysis of the hospital as an economic organism. *Modern Hospital,* April 1966, 87-91.

Riessman, F. *Strategies against poverty.* New York: Random House, Inc., 1969.

Ritzer, G. *Sociology: a multiple paradigm science.* Boston: Allyn & Bacon, Inc., 1975.

Rivers, W. H. *Medicine, magic and religion.* New York: Harcourt, Brace & Co., Inc., 1924.

Ro, K. K. Patient characteristics, hospital characteristics and hospital use. *Medical Care,* 1969, **7**, 295-312.

Robinson, J. *The economics of imperfect competition.* London: Macmillan & Co. Ltd., 1933.

Roemer, M. I. On paying the doctor and the implications of different methods. *Journal of Health and Human Behavior,* Spring 1962, **3**, 4-14.

Roemer, M. I. Controlling hospital use through limiting hospital bed supply. In *Where is hospital use headed? Proceedings, Fifth Annual Symposium on Hospital Affairs.* Chicago: University of Chicago Health Information Foundation, 1963.

Roemer, M. I., and Elling, R. H. Sociological research on medical care. *Journal of Health and Human Behavior,* Spring 1963, **4**, 49-68.

Roemer, M., and Morris, R. Hospital regionalization in perspective. *Public Health Reports,* 1959, **74**, 916-922.

Rogers, E. *The philosophy and science of health.* Milwaukee: Lee Foundation for Nutrition Research, 1949.

Rogoff, N. The decision to study medicine. In Merton, R., Reader, G., and Kendall, P. (eds.). *The student physician,* Cambridge, Mass.: Harvard University Press, 1957.

Roll, W. G. The psi field. In Roll, W. G., and Pratt, J. G. (eds.). *Proceedings of the Para-Psychological Association: 1957-1964.* Durham, N.C.: Christian Printing Co., 1966.

Rose, A. *Sociology: the study of human relations.* New York: Alfred A. Knopf, Inc., 1965.

Rose, J. *Introduction to sociology.* Chicago: Rand-McNally & Co., 1971.

Rosen, G. An eighteenth century plan for a national health service. *Bulletin of the History of Medicine,* 1944, **16**, 429-463.

Rosen, G. Cameralism and concept of medical police. *Bulletin of the History of Medicine,* 1953, **27**, 21-42.

Rosen, G. The hospital: historical sociology of a community institution. In Freidson, E. (ed.). *The hospital in modern society.* Glencoe, Ill.: The Free Press, 1963.

Rosen, G. The evolution of social medicine. In Freeman, H., Levine, S., and Reeder, L. (eds.). *Handbook of medical sociology.* Englewood Cliffs, N.J.: Prentice-Hall, Inc., 1972.

Rosengren, W., and Lefton, M. *Hospitals and patients.* New York: Atherton Press, 1969.

Rosenstock, I. What research in motivation suggests for public health. *American Journal of Public Health,* 1960, **50**, 295-302.

Rosenthal, G. D. *The demand for general hospital facilities.* Hospital Monograph Series 14. Chicago: American Hospital Association, 1964.

Ross, J. Social class and medical care. *Journal of Health and Human Behavior,* Spring 1962, 35-40.

Roth, J. *Timetables.* Indianapolis: The Bobbs-Merrill Co., Inc., 1963.

Rothlisberger, F., and Dixon, W. *Management and the worker.* Cambridge, Mass.: Harvard University Press, 1939.

Royal Commission on Medical Education. *1965-68 Report* (Cmnd. 3569). London: HMSO, 1968.

Rozenfeld, I. I. *Curative and preventive aspects of public health services for rural populations* (trans. from Russian National Science Foundation, Washington, D.C.). Jerusalem: Israel Program for Scientific Translations, 1963.

Sadler, A. M., Sadler, B. L., and Bliss, A. *The physician's assistant: today and tomorrow.* New Haven, Conn.: Yale University Press, 1972.

Salloway, J., and Dillon, P. A comparison of family networks and friend networks in health care utilization. *Journal of Comparative Family Studies*, 1973, **4** (1), 131-142.

Samora, J., Saunders, L., and Larson, R. Medical vocabulary knowledge among hospital patients. *Journal of Health and Social Behavior*, 1961, **2**, 83-92.

Sanazaro, P. J. Physician support personnel in the 1970's. *Journal of the American Medical Association*, 1970, **214**, 98-100.

Saward, E. Personal communication, 1970.

Saward, E., Blank, J., and Greenlick, M. Documentation of twenty years of operation and growth of a prepaid group practice plan. *Medical Care*, 1968, **6**, 231-244.

Scherzer, C. J. *The church and healing*. Philadelphia: The Westminster Press, 1950.

Schneller, E. S. Perceptions of autonomy of prospective physicians' assistants. Paper presented at the Second National Conference on New Health Practitioners, 1974.

Schumacher, C. The 1960 medical school graduate: his biographical history. *Journal of Medical Education*, 1961, **36**, 398-406.

Schwartz, L. R. The hierarchy of resort in curative practices: the Admiralty Islands, Melanesia. *Journal of Health and Social Behavior*, Sept. 1969, **10**, 201-209.

Schwartz, J. L. *Medical plans and health care*. Springfield, Ill.: Charles C Thomas, Publisher, 1968.

Scott, W. R., and Volkart, E. H. *Medical care: readings in the sociology of medical institutes*. New York: John Wiley & Sons, Inc., 1966.

Sedlack, W. E. The study of applicants, 1965-1966. *Journal of Medical Education*, 1967, **42**, 28.

Sedlack, W. E. Applicants for the 1971-72 medical school entering class. *Journal of Medical Education*, 1973, **48**, 300-301.

Sellers, R. V. The black health workers and the black health consumer—new rules for both. *American Journal of Public Health*, 1970, **60**, 2154-2170.

Selye, H. *The stress of life*. New York: McGraw-Hill Book Co., 1956.

Shattuck, L. *Report of the sanitary commission of Massachusetts*, 1850. Cambridge, Mass.: Harvard University Press, 1948.

Shils, E. The sanctity of life. In Labby, D. H. (ed.). *Life or death: ethics and options*. Seattle: University of Washington Press, 1968.

Shortell, S. Patterns of referral among internists in private practice: a social exchange model. *Journal of Health and Social Behavior*, 1973, **14** (4), 335-347.

Shroyer, T. Toward a critical theory for advanced industrial society. In Dreitzel, H. P. (ed.). *Recent sociology No. 2*. New York: Macmillan, Inc., 1970.

Shryock, R. H. *Medicine in America*. Baltimore: The Johns Hopkins University Press, 1966.

Sidel, V. W. Feldshers and "feldsherism": the role and training of the feldsher in the USSR. *New England Journal of Medicine*, 1968, **278**, 934-939.

Sidel, V. *Serve the people: observations on medicine in the People's Republic of China*. New York: Josiah Macy, Jr., Foundation, 1973.

Sigerist, H. *A history of medicine: primitive and archaic medicine* (vol. 1). New York: Oxford, 1957.

Silver, H. K. New allied health professionals: implications of the Colorado Child Health Associate Law. *New England Journal of Medicine*, 1971, **284**, 304-307.

Silver, H. K., and Hecker, J. A. The pediatric nurse practitioner and the child health associate: new types of health professionals. *Journal of Medical Education*, 1970, **45**, 171-176.

Simon, H. A. *Models of man: social and rational*. New York: John Wiley & Sons, Inc., 1951.

Simon, H. A. *Administrative behavior*. New York: Macmillan, 1965.

Small, A. *The cameralists: pioneers of German Social Policy*. Chicago: University of Chicago Press, 1909.

Smith, H. Two lines of authority are one too many. *Modern Hospital*, 1955, **84**, 59-64.

Smith, R. T. Health and rehabilitation manpower strategy: new careers and the role of the indigenous paraprofessional. *Social Science and Medicine*, April 1973, **7**, 281-290.

Sokolowska, M. Personal communication, 1972.

Somers, A. *Health care in transition: directions for the future*. Chicago: Hospital Research and Educational Trust, 1971.

Somers, H., and Somers, A. *Doctors, patients and health insurance*. Garden City, N.Y.: Doubleday & Co., Inc., 1961.

Sorokin, P. *Contemporary sociological theories*. New York: Harper Torchbooks, 1928.

Sparer, G., Dines, G., and Smith, D. Consumer participation in OEO assisted neighborhood health centers. *American Journal of Public Health*, 1970, **60**, 1091-1102.

Spicer, E. H. *Pascua: a Yaqui village in Arizona*. Chicago: University of Chicago Press, 1940.

Spiegel, H. B. C. (ed.). *Citizen participation in urban development*. (Vols. 1 and 2). Washington, D.C.: Center for Community Affairs, National Training Laboratory Institute for Applied Behavioral Science.

Srole, L., et al. *Mental health in the metropolis*. New York: McGraw-Hill Book Co., 1962.

Stahl, S. *Illness among the aged: a study of the determinants of the perception of levels of health in an indigent urban population* (microfilm). Doctoral dissertation, Ann Arbor University, 1971.

Stanford Research Institute. *Chiropractic in Cali-*

fornia. Los Angeles: Haynes Foundation, 1960.

Stekert, E. J. Focus for conflict: southern mountain medical beliefs in Detroit. *Journal of American Folklore*, 1970, **83**, 115-147.

Stelling, J., and Bucher, R. Autonomy and monitoring on hospital wards. *Sociological Quarterly*, 1972, **13**, 431-446.

Stephen and the Farm. *Hey beatnick! This is the farm book*. Summertown, Tenn.: The Book Publishing Co., 1974.

Stevens, R. *Medical practice in modern England*. New Haven, Conn.: Yale University Press, 1966.

Stevens, R. *American medicine and the public interest*. New Haven, Conn.: Yale University Press, 1971.

Stewart, W., and Pennell, M. *Health manpower science book! Physician's age, type of practice and location*. Washington, D.C.: U.S.G.P.O. 1960.

Still, A. *Autobiography*. Kirksville, Mo. (no publisher indicated), 1908.

Stockwell, E. Socioeconomic status and mortality in the United States. *Public Health Reports*, 1961, **76**, 1081-1086.

Stockwell, E. *Population and people*. Chicago: Quadrangle, 1968.

Stoeckle, J. D., and Candib, L. M. The neighborhood health center: reform ideas of yesterday and today. *New England Journal of Medicine*, 1969, **280**, 1385-1391.

Stoeckle, J. D., and Zola, I. After everyone can pay for medical care: some perspectives on future treatment and practice. *Medical Care*, 1964, **2**, 36-41.

Stoeckle, J. D., Zola, I. K., and Davidson, G. G. The quantity and significance of psychological distress in medical patients: some preliminary observations about the decision to seek medical aid. *Journal of Chronic Disease*, 1964, **17**, 959-970.

Strauss, A., Schatzman, L., Earlich, D., Bucher, R., and Sabshin, M. The hospital and it's negotiated order. In Freidson, E. *The hospital in modern society*. Glencoe, Ill.: The Free Press, 1963.

Strauss, R. The nature and status of medical sociology. *American Sociological Review*, 1957, **22**, 200-204.

Suchman, E. *Sociology and the field of public health*. New York: Russell Sage Foundation, 1963.

Suchman, E. Social patterns of illness and medical care. *Journal of Health and Human Behavior*, 1965, **6**, 2-16.

Suchman, E. A model for research and evaluation on rehabilitation. In Sussman, M. (ed.). *Sociology and rehabilitation*. Washington, D.C.: American Sociological Association, 1966.

Sumner, W. *What social classes owe to each other*. Caldwell, Idaho: Caxton Printers, 1961.

Susser, M. *Community psychiatry*. New York: Random House, Inc., 1968.

Sussman, M. (ed.). *Sociology and rehabilitation*. Washington, D.C.: American Sociological Association, 1966.

Sussman, M. B., Kang, M. R. and Williams, G. K. *Paraprofessionalism and rehabilitation counseling: annotated bibliography*. Cleveland: Case Western Reserve University, Institute on the Family and the Bureaucratic Society, May, 1971.

Swanton, J. R. Social and religious beliefs and practices of the Chickasaw Indians. In *Forty-fourth Annual Report of the Bureau of American Ethnology, 1926-1927*. Washington, D.C.: U.S. Government Printing Office, 1928.

Sweet, R., and Twaddle, A. *Preventability Study: final report* (mimeograph). Boston: Massachusetts General Hospital, 1969a.

Sweet, R., and Twaddle, A. An exploration of delay in hospitalization. *Inquiry*, 4(2), 35-41, 1969b.

Sydenstricker, E. *Hagarstown morbidity studies*. Washington, D.C.: U.S. Government Printing Office, 1930.

Syme, L. The clinical bias in epidemiology. Paper presented at meeting of A.P.H.A., 1966.

Syme, L., and Reader, L. (eds.). Social stress and cardiovascular disease. *Milbank Memorial Fund Quarterly*, 1967, **45** (Part II), 2.

Syme, S. L., Hyman, M. M., and Enterline, P. E. Some social and cultural factors associated with the occurrence of coronary heart disease. *Journal of Chronic Disease*, 1964, **17**, 277-289.

Szasz, T. *The myth of mental illness*. New York: Harper & Row, Publishers, 1961.

Szasz, T., and Hollender, M. A contribution to the philosophy of medicine: the basic models of the doctor-patient relationship. *Archives of Internal Medicine*, 1956, **97**, 585-592.

Tagliacozzo, D., and Mauksch, H. The patient's view of the patient's role. In Jaco, E. G. (ed.). *Patients, physicians and illness: a source book in behavioral science and health*. New York: The Free Press, 1972.

Taylor, C. *In horizontal orbit*. New York: Holt, Rinehart & Winston, Inc., 1970.

Taylor, S. *Good general practice: a report of a survey*. London: Oxford Press, 1954.

Teich, A. H. (ed.). *Technology and man's future*. New York: St. Martin's Press, 1972.

Theodore, C. N., and Haig, J. N. *Selected characteristics of the physician population, 1963 and 1967*. Chicago: American Medical Association, 1968.

Theodore, C. N., Sutter, G., and Haig, J. *Medical school alumni, 1967*. Chicago: American Medical Association, 1968.

Thielens, W. Some comparisons of entrants to medical and law school. In Merton, R., Reader, G., and Kendall, P. (eds.). *The student physician*. Cambridge, Mass.: Harvard University Press, 1957.

Thompson, V. A. *Modern organization*. New York: Alfred A. Knopf, Inc., 1961.

Thompson, W. *Population problems*. New York: McGraw-Hill Book Co., 1953.

Timasheff, N. *Sociological theory: its nature and*

growth. New York: Random House, Publishers, 1957.

Titmuss, R. *The welfare state*. London: George Allen & Unwin, Ltd., 1958.

Todd, M. C., and Foy, D. F. Current status of the physician's assistant and related issues. *Journal of the American Medical Association*, 1972, **220**, 1714-1720.

Torrey, E. F. *The death of psychiatry*. New York: Penquin Books, Inc., 1974.

Tumin, M. *Social stratification*. Englewood Cliffs, N.J.: Prentice-Hall, Inc., 1967.

Tumin, M. *Patterns of society*. Boston: Little, Brown & Co., 1973.

Turk, H., and Simpson, R. *Institutions and exchange*. Indianapolis: The Bobbs-Merrill Co., Inc., 1971.

Twaddle, A. Aging, population growth and chronic disease. *Journal of Chronic Disease*, 1968a, **21**, 417-422.

Twaddle, A. *Influence and illness*. Unpublished doctoral dissertation, Brown University, 1968b.

Twaddle, A. Health decisions and sick role variations. *Journal of Health and Social Behavior*, 1969, **10**, 105-115.

Twaddle, A. Life values, life chances and life styles. *Journal of Operational Psychiatry*, Winter 1973a, 13-23.

Twaddle, A. Illness and deviance. *Social Science and Medicine*, 1973b, **7**, 751-762.

Twaddle, A. The concept of health status. *Social Science and Medicine*, 1974, **8**, 29-38.

Twaddle, A. *On crime and illness*. Paper presented at annual meeting of the American Sociological Association, 1976.

Twaddle, A. Utilization of medical services by a captive population: analysis of sick call in a state prison. *Journal of Health and Social Behavior*, 1976, **17** (3), 236-248.

Twaddle, A., and Stoeckle, J. *Pressures for change in medical care: a conceptual model*. Paper presented at the Third International Conference on Social Science and Medicine, Elsinore, Denmark, 1972.

Twaddle, A., and Sweet, R. Factors leading to preventable hospital admissions. *Medical Care*, 1970, **8**, 200-208.

United Nations. *Demographic Yearbook*. New York: United Nations, 1971.

United States Department of Health, Education, and Welfare. Independent practitioners under Medicare, Washington, D.C.: U.S. Government Printing Office, 1968.

United States Department of Labor. *Manpower report of the president*. Washington, D.C.: U.S. Government Printing Office, 1971.

Vahovich, S. *'73 Profile of medical practice*. Chicago: American Medical Association, 1973.

Veblen, T. *The theory of the leisure class*. New York: Macmillan, Inc., 1899.

Villermé, L. R. De la mortalite, dans les divers quartiers de la ville de Paris. *Annales d'hygiene publique*, 1830, **3**, 294-341.

Vincent, P. Factors influencing patient compliance: a theoretical approach. *Nursing Research*, 1971, **20**, 509-516.

Vogel, V. *American Indian medicine*. New York: Ballantine Books, Inc., 1970.

Vogel, V. *This country was ours*. New York: Harper Torchbook, 1972.

Volmer, H., and Mills, D. (eds.). *Professionalism*. Englewood Cliffs, N.J.: Prentice-Hall, Inc., 1966.

von der Lippe, R. Personal communication, 1968.

Waitzkin, H., and Waterman, B. *The exploitation of illness in capitalist societies*. Indianapolis: The Bobbs-Merrill Co., Inc., 1974.

Walker, V. *Nursing and ritualistic practice*. New York: The Macmillan Co., 1967.

Walters, L. Fetal research and the ethical issues. *Hastings Center Report*, June 1975, **5**, 13-18.

Ward, L. *Applied sociology: a treatise on the conscious improvement of society*. New York: Macmillan, Inc., 1906.

Wardwell, W. A marginal professional role: the chiropractor. *Social Forces*, 1952, **30**, 339-348.

Wardwell, W. Limited, marginal and quasi-practitioners. In Freeman, H., Levine, S., and Reeder, L. (eds.). *Handbook of medical sociology*. Englewood Cliffs, N.J.: Prentice-Hall, Inc., 1972.

Wasserstrom, R. The status of the fetus. *Hastings Center Report*, June 1975, **5**, 18-22.

Weber, M. *The theory of social and economic organization* (Henderson, A. M., and Parsons, T., trans.). New York: Oxford University Press, 1947.

Weber, M. *The Protestant ethic and the spirit of capitalism*. (Parsons, T., trans.). New York: Charles Scribner's Sons, 1958.

Weinerman, E. R. Research into the organization of medical practice. *Milbank Memorial Fund Quarterly*, 1966, **44** (4), 104-140.

Weinerman, E. R., Ratner, R. S., Robbins, A., et. al. Yale studies in ambulatory medical care. *American Journal of Public Health*, 1966, **56**, 1037-1056.

Weslager, C. A. *Magic medicine of the Indians*. Somerset, N.J.: Middle Atlantic Press, 1973.

Wheaton, E. *Long term hospitalization and the family: family adjustment to rehabilitation and reunion*. Unpublished manuscript, University of Pennsylvania, 1970.

Wheeler, C. E. *The case for homeopathy*. London: The British Homeopathic Association, 1914.

Wilensky, H. L. Sociological aspects of leisure. *The International Social Science Journal*, 1960, **12**, 555-558.

Wilensky, H. L. The professionalization of everyone? *American Journal of Sociology*, 1964, **70**, 137-158.

Willard, W. *Curanderismo and health care* (mimeograph). Division of Social Perspectives in Medicine, University of Arizona, College of Medicine, Tucson, Ariz., 1972.

Williams, R. Application of research to practice and intergroup relations. *American Sociological Review*, 1953, **18**, 78-83.

Williams, R. M., Jr., and Goldsen, R. K. *Selection or rejection of nursing as a career.* Ithaca, N.Y.: Cornell University Press, 1960.

Wilson, E. *Sociology: rules, roles and relationships.* Homewood, Ill.: Dorsey Press, 1971.

Wilson, R. *The sociology of health.* New York: Random House, Inc., 1970.

Winton, F. R., and Bayliss, L. E. *Human physiology.* Boston: Little, Brown & Co., 1955.

Wise, H. G. Montefiore Hospital neighborhood medical care demonstration. *Milbank Memorial Fund Quarterly*, 1968, **46** (3), 297-307.

Wolff, H. *Stress and disease.* Springfield, Ill.: Charles C Thomas, Publisher, 1953.

Wolff, H. Disease and the patterns of behavior. In McIver, R. M. (ed.). *The hour of insight.* New York: Institute for Religious and Social Studies, 1954.

Wolff, K. (ed.). *Emile Durkheim, 1858-1917.* Columbus: Ohio State University Press, 1960.

Wren, G. R. Some characteristics of freshmen students in baccalaureate, diploma and associate degree nursing programs. *Nursing Research,* March-April, 1971, **20**, 167-172.

Yankauer, A., Tripp, S., Andrews, P., and Connelly, J. P. The outcomes and service impact of a pediatric nurse practitioner traning program, nurse practitioner training outcomes. *American Journal of Public Health*, 1972, **62**, 347-353.

Yankelovitch, D., and Barrett, W. *Ego and instinct.* New York: Random House, Inc., 1970.

Zappel, G. Lecture at Harvard Medical School, 1967.

Zborowski, M. Cultural components in response to pain. *Journal of Social Issues*, 1952, **8**, 16-30.

Zborowski, M. *People in pain.* San Francisco: Jossey-Bass, Inc., Publishers, 1969.

Zinsser, H. *Rats, lice and history.* Boston: Little, Brown & Co., 1935.

Zola, I. Illness behavior of the working class. In Shostak, A. B., and Gomberg, W. (eds.). *Blue collar world.* Englewood Cliffs, N.J.: Prentice-Hall, Inc., 1964.

Zola, I. Culture and symptoms. *American Sociological Review*, 1966, **31**, 615-630.

Zola, I. Medicine as a system of social control. In Cox, C., and Mead, A. (eds.). *A sociology of medical practice.* London: Collier-MacMillan, Ltd., 1975.

Author index

Subject index

341